Nursing Assistant Textbook

Senior Care Principles for the CNA

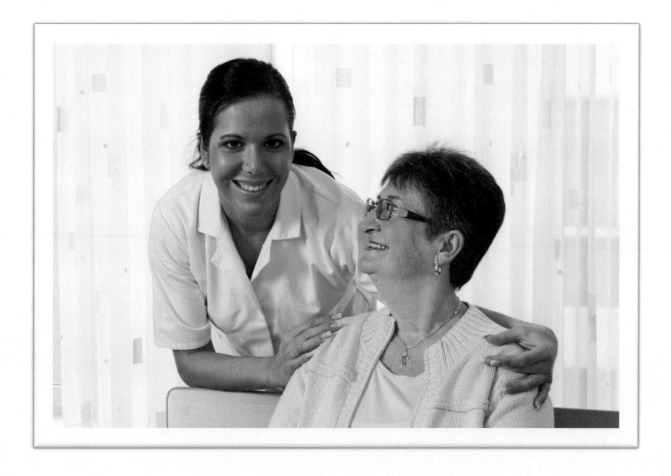

Jane John-Nwankwo   CPT, DSD, RN, MSN, Ph.D

Nursing Assistant Textbook

Senior Care Principles for the CNA

ISBN: 978-0-9889117-3-4

Printed in the United States of America.

Dedication

To my loving daughter, Jessica Chinyere John-Nwankwo

Table of Contents

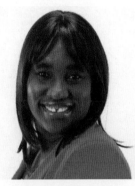

From the author

This book was written out of an inner passion to provide a quality, but concise textbook for Nursing Assistants as well as Caregivers.

- Jane John-Nwankwo RN, Ph.D

Author, Public speaker,

Educational consultant

support@janejohn-nwankwo.com

www.janejohn-nwankwo.com

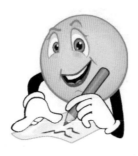

Chapter One

Introduction to Nursing Assistants

Outline

- What is the California Code of Regulations?
- Why Study this Legislation?
- Legal Implications of California Code of Regulations
- OBRA: Implications for Nursing Assistants
- Title 22, Division 5
- Nurse Assistant Requirements as set forth in Title 22 and OBRA
- Nurse Assistant Terminology
- What are the Legislated Nursing Assistant Duties?
- Nursing Units
- Patient Care Personnel
- Which duties are outside the scope of Nursing Assistants?
- Nursing Conditions
- Qualities of a Good Nursing Assistant
- Nursing Assistant Professionalism
- What is Professional Behavior?
- What is Unprofessional Behavior?
- Why Protect Patient Confidentiality?
- How to Maintain Patient Confidentiality
- The Nursing Assistant's Duty to the Employer

What is the California Code of Regulations?

The California Code of Regulations is a set of permanent rules and regulations.

These rules and regulations are reviewed, approved, and made available through the Office of Administrative Law. Any member of the public can access these regulations:

social services, welfare procedures, food and agriculture, business regulations, education, harbors and navigation, industrial law, rehabilitative and development services, investment, public health natural resources, motor vehicles, crime prevention and corrections, military and veterans.

It is sometimes referred to as administrative law. In the California Code of Regulations, there are twenty-eight titles.

Why do CNAs need to know?

Nursing assistant students need to know the content of California Code of Regulations, Division 5, Title 22. These rules regulate healthcare facilities. They contain vital legal information about the roles and responsibilities of the Nurse Assistant. The requirements for Nurse Assistant certification determine whether the nursing assistant will be part of medical profession or not.

The California Code of Regulations began in the early forties in an effort to codify state regulations. A free online version is provided online. Simply search for it.

Legal Implications of California Code of Regulations

These regulations are reviewed, approved, and published. Notices of proposed and about-to-be-repealed regulations are also announced.

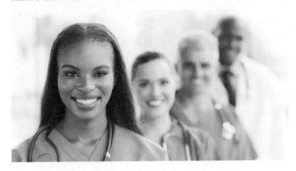

OBRA

The Omnibus Budget Reconciliation Act is more commonly known as the Nursing Home Reform Act of 1987. It has greatly improved nursing home facilities and patient care in those environments. OBRA set up federal standards for providing care to the residents of senior care facilities.

These improvements include limited and careful use of antipsychotic drugs, reducing both physical and medical restraints, reduction in and careful use of indwelling urinary catheters.

Nursing homes must have a written plan for provision of practical, enriching physical, social, mental, and psychosocial activities. Failure to provide items outlined in OBRA may result in fine, replacement of administration, civil and criminal lawsuits, or even closing of the facility.

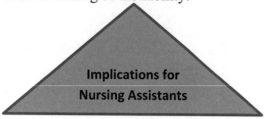

Implications for Nursing Assistants

As part of the nursing team, nursing assistants have a legal, professional, and moral obligation to ensure that the regulations under both Title 22 and OBRA are being met. If this is not the case, they need to document and report infractions to their immediate superiors. These regulations include:

- 42 CFR §483.15: Treating clients with dignity and respect.
- 42 CFR §483.15: Provision of measures to enhance patient's quality of life.
- 42 CFR §483.20: Reading and complying with the patient's comprehensive care plan.
- 42 CFR §483.20: Providing input into the assessment of each resident's overall health plan.
- 42 CFR §483.25: Working as part of the nursing team to ensure patients' daily living activities are met. These include assistance with eating, bathing, toileting, and mobility where required.
- 42 CFR §483.25: Prevention of pressure sores, and treatment to heal and prevent infection.
- 42 CFR §483.25: Providing appropriate care for urinary incontinence and bladder function if possible. Use of urinary catheters only temporarily and if necessary.

- 42 CFR §483.25: Working as part of the team to prevent accidents and injuries, falls.
- 42 CFR §483.25: Working as part of the medical team to avoid medication errors and overmedication.
- 42 CFR §483.25: Working as part of the nursing team to ensure residents are getting adequate nutrition and 42 CFR §483.25: sufficient fluid to prevent dehydration.
- 42 CFR §483.30: Noting and reporting when there is insufficient nursing staff.
- 42 CFR §483.40: Respecting and protecting resident's right to choose activities, schedules, and health care.
- 42 CFR §483.75: Working as part of the team to maintain accurate, complete, and accessible patient clinical records.

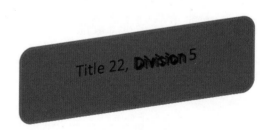

Title 22, Division 5

Title 22 chapter five concerns social security. More specifically, the Social Security California Code of Regulations outlines nurse-to-patient ratios. It deals with licensing and certification of structures including healthcare facilities, homecare agencies, and medical clinics.

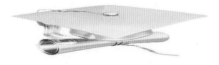

NURSE ASSISTANT REQUIREMENTS AS SET FORTH IN TITLE 22 AND OBRA

Becoming a Certified Nursing Assistant under California regulations does not require a high school diploma or GED. The next step is enrollment in a nursing assistant training program at a state-approved college, a trade school, or a healthcare facility.

The Certified Nursing Assistant program is currently 160 hours in duration. The CNA course includes a minimum of sixty hours of theory. There is time devoted to the study of Elder Abuse and Alzheimer's disease. Besides the sixty hours of in-class instruction and study, CNA students must also complete at least a hundred hours of clinical training in a facility that teaches skilled nursing.

All course content must comply with Title 22 and OBRA. While students are employed in a skilled nursing facility, they must receive an hourly wage even while they are in training.

Before being enrolled in the CNA program, all candidates have to pass a criminal background screening. They must also be tuberculosis negative taken as well as pass a physical exam.

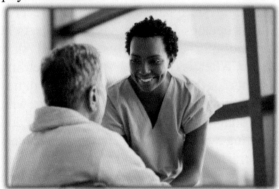

California Nursing Assistants can progress to Certified Nurse Assistants. To do this they need to complete state certification requirements. This is done under the supervision of a licensed nurse. Certified Nurse Assistants can provide basic nursing services to patients in an acute care, long-term, and intermediate healthcare facilities.

Becoming certified in California requires a graduate of the nursing assistant program to write a skills test. The candidate has three chances to pass the certification test.

Nurse Assistant Terminology

Under Title 22 and OBRA, Nursing Assistants are also called Certified Nurse Assistants, Geriatric Aides, Hospital Attendants, Nurse Aides, Nurse Assistants, and Patient Care Technicians, or orderlies.

No matter what the employer or facility calls them, nursing assistants have certain specific duties as outlined by Title 22 and OBRA.

What are the duties of a Nursing Assistant?

Nursing Assistants are expected to be trained for and ready to carry out general patient care. In performing these routine duties, they work under the supervision and direction of nursing and medical staff. Their duties depend on the nature of the facility and type of clients they are serving. It may also depend upon the training and additional qualifications they have received. Experienced nursing assistants may also have had on-the-job mentor training which ensured they could do additional procedures, and type of health care facility. Typically, the duties of nursing assistants would include things like responding to patients' call buttons, message delivery, stripping and making up beds, and assistance with patient activities like feeding, bathing, dressing, and safe mobility.

The job of a Certified Nursing Assistant puts them in direct contact with patients. As a CNA, patient care is the number one priority. Nursing assistants are key players in the every-day operations of the workplace in which they work. Their work

> *Certified Nursing Assistants are professionals who are expected to act with the skills they were taught as well as respect, caring, and compassion for their patients. Their expert care and empathy can ease the anxiety, suffering, and stress of those for whom they care*

environment might be a hospital or a long-term care facility, usually referred to as nursing homes.

Through knowledgeable measures and clinical experience, Certified Nursing Assistants assist those who through sickness or age are unable to care for themselves.

Certified Nursing Assistants work under the supervision of a designated healthcare professional who is usually a licensed Nurse. As part of a nursing team or unit, it is the job of the Certified Nursing Assistants to help their designated patients with specified activies of

daily living (ADL). These tasks may include help with eating, bathing, and dressing.

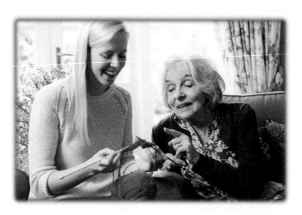

Because Certified Nursing Assistants spend long hours over long periods of time with the same patients, it is not unusual to develop close professional bonds with both the patients and their co-workers.

While there are common elements in the duties and patients, the job of a Certified Nursing Assistants demands flexibility and spontaneity. No two work days are the same. Change of shifts, staff changes, patients moving in and out of the facility, and the changing needs of those whom they serve make every day a new adventure.

The night shift Nursing Assistants receive patient updates from the day shift CNAs at the end of the shift. This is called shift report. After taking vital signs and settling patients for the night, there are always duties like answering call buttons, assisting with bathroom trips, emptying bedpans, and assisting with draining catheters. If patients are scheduled for morning surgery, they may need special care or support to comfort and reassure them.

During the day shift, the duties of Certified Nursing Assistants may include assistance with bathing, dressing and feeding. The morning rush often requires Certified Nursing Assistants to be efficient, organized, and calm in the middle of managing several patients at once. Breakfast tasks may be interrupted by the need to answer call lights.

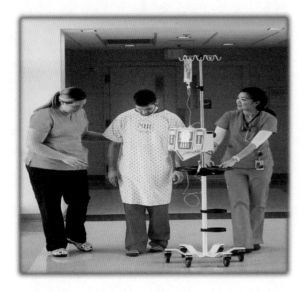

Certified Nursing Assistants are directly responsible to their supervisor. They will be expected to assist with updating chart information and furnishing the incoming shift with accurate, detailed patient information.

Certified Nursing Assistants may also be required to locate and collate medical supplies. They may be asked to assist the supervisor with a medical procedure, prepare a room for a new patient or help with patient admission or discharge.

Whether they are working in a hospital, a long-term patient facility, or a nursing home, the job expectations of a Certified Nursing Assistant are similar. Where hospital patients have meals brought to them, other facilities have dining rooms. In both environments, some patients may need feeding assistance. In all work environments, there will be call buttons to respond to and patient comfort and hygiene needs to be met.

Certified Nursing Assistants' assignments may be a specific hall, a department, or a designated nursing unit.

Nursing Units

Nursing assistants in hospitals, acute care settings, long-term care facilities, and intermediate care facilities work in nursing units. These units have areas and caseloads of designated patients. The nursing units and numbers of staff who provide this care are decided and assigned by facility administrators. Each unit shift has a supervisor who oversees the duties and nursing staff.

The safe organization, operation, and maintenance of the unit will include not only patient rooms but also liaison with support facilities, and services, outpatient services, and homecare providers.

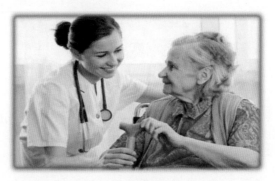

Patient Care Personnel

A Nursing Assistants is a vital part of the patient care personnel team. Included in this group may be both licensed and unlicensed caregivers. Together they assist in providing nursing care. CNAs do not always work in hospital settings. They may be hired to do work in various patient-care environments. They can be part of a nursing unit in acute care facilities, long-term and respite residential care. They also form part of healthcare teams in skilled nursing sections, outpatient departments, wellness clinics and special purpose hospitals. The conditions in which Certified Nursing Assistants are asked to work may be modern with high tech equipment. Many are heat and cooling controlled.

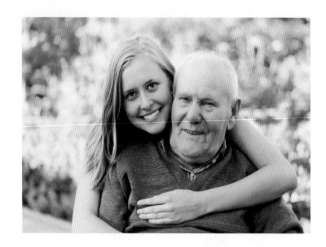

Which Duties are not for Nursing Assistants?

It is important to know what tasks are not within the scope of the training and legal obligations of Certified Nursing Assistants. Certified Nursing Assistants should not be asked to do any of these:

- *Supervise members of the nursing unit*

- *Give medication*

- *Change sterile dressings*

- *Give injections*

- *Change patient medications*

- *Give tube feedings*

- *Diagnose a patient illness*

- *Read and interpret X-ray or MRI results*

- *Interact with patient and/or support group regarding patient care*

- *Suggest alternative facilities or medical providers*

- *Prepare a resident care plan*

- *Make dietary suggestions*

- *Insert or remove tubes*

FLEXIBLE

A. Dependable

The ability to show up to work on time and perform required tasks is a quality of a good nurse assistant.

B. Considerate

An optimistic attitude will go a long way to preventing job burnout individually and within the nursing unit. Belief that patients benefit from the care of the nursing assistant should empower the considerate and empathetic care for the patients.

C. Pleasant

Mental stamina is important in a work environment where situations can get stressful. It is vital to the nursing assistants' wellbeing and that of their patients that they greet each day with a cheerful outlook and optimism. Even though clients and co-workers might not be so cheerful, a pleasant manner will go a long way in making the work environment more enjoyable for both patients, family and coworkers.

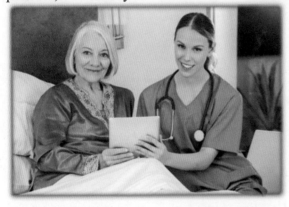

D. Empathetic

Empathy cannot be taught. It is the ability to put oneself in another's shoes. Good nursing assistants are compassionate to the suffering of their patients. They rejoice in small gains. They are cheerleaders for their patients when milestones are achieved. This attitude will lift the patients' spirits and encourage their perseverance.

E. Flexible

Assignments may change. Patient needs are always changing. Patients come and go. Nursing assignments may change from one shift to another to meet new patient needs. As part of a nursing team, a nursing assistant has to be flexible to meet these challenges with grace and the willingness to make the best of changes.

F. Honest

Legally, professionally, and morally, Nursing Assistants have an obligation to their patients, their colleagues, and their employer to follow the regulations and guidelines of their professional standards.

Certified Nursing Assistants are required by law and by the standards of their professional organization to adhere to the state laws and regulations as they pertain to their job and their work environment. One of the most valuable traits of a nursing assistant is honesty. Nursing units deal with sensitive patient information. They must be trustworthy to protect the confidentiality of those they serve. Honesty is required in all situations

G. Compassionate and caring

Caring for the needs of patients who cannot always care for themselves requires compassion. An important component of nursing assistants' ability to perform their job is physical stamina. An effective nursing assistant has to be physically strong to put in long hours standing and walking. He/she needs to be able to assist in safe patient transfers, moving heavy equipment, and bed making. Patients' safety is a major part of nursing assistants' responsibility. This includes tasks like lifting, transferring, and positioning.

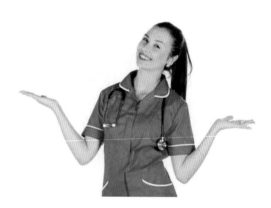

H. Sensitive to others

Certified Nursing Assistants must be sensitive to the needs of their patients, their patients' family, and their co-workers.

Effective, accurate communication skills are a critical part of the job. In both oral and written modes, Nursing Assistants must be able to provide precise patient information to the nursing team and receive information from other members of the team. Nursing Assistants must be able to share observations and document them on patient charts. They need to listen carefully to information patients provide and furnish patients with clear, concise instructions

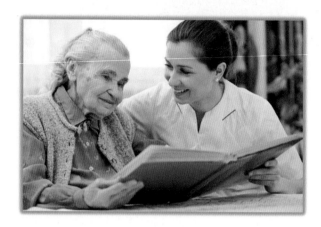

I. Respectful

Every person—no matter what their limitations or attitude—deserves to be treated with dignity. This includes the best care and respect for their privacy.

Besides a cheerful outlook, Nursing Assistants require the patience of Job. It takes time to assist a patient with ambulatory challenges to the bathroom. Helping a stroke victim dress may seem like an interminable task. Many daily assignments demand a calm, encouraging attitude.

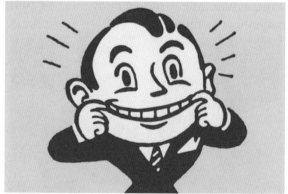

J. Cooperative

Emotional strength is a job requirement for CNAs. Caring for struggling patients can be stressful. Supporting them as they deal with their diagnosis and treatment calls for emotional stability of their nursing team.

Effective nursing units work well together to meet patient needs in a calm, cooperative spirit. The mark of a good team member is the willingness to help colleagues meet patient needs.

K. Team player

Nursing Assistants work as part of a nursing unit or healthcare team. That is why it is important to know how to work as an effective individual in a group. If team members help each other, more is accomplished, and patients receive a higher quality of care. Working as part of a team also improves staff morale and job satisfaction.

L. Observant

Hand in hand with good communication skills is the ability to be a keen observer. Certified Nursing Assistants should be on the lookout for visible changes in their patients. One of their responsibilities is noting any changes. These might include fluctuations in blood pressure, changes in appetite, a bruise, a scrape, swelling, or changes on mobility. Direct patient caregivers are in a position to observe even tiny changes that might be important.

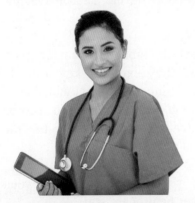

M. Well-groomed

Proper grooming reflects a Nursing Assistant's self-esteem and professionalism. Good grooming also instills a sense of confidence in residents. If Nursing Assistants don't make the effort to be well-groomed, it is natural for patients to feel that the staff isn't concerned about their care either.

As professionals, nursing assistants must come to work well-groomed and primly attired. Body jewelry, body art, dangling earrings and necklaces, and acrylic nails have no place in a clinical setting.

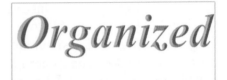

N. Organized

Nursing assistants are responsible for meeting the needs of several patients. It is important that they be organized in their attention to their patients, making keen observations, taking detailed notes for charts, and sharing patient changes both orally and in written form.

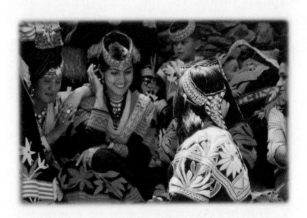

O. Respectful of cultural differences.

As healthcare professionals, Nursing Assistants need to understand and have compassion for their patients. This includes providing nonjudgmental care. Compassion includes respect for the patients' religious, ethnic, and cultural beliefs. It also includes being proactive in working to get them the services they require. Being able to put oneself in the patients' shoes is not something that can be taught in school.

Nursing Conditions

Besides the wide variety in work environment, other challenges face Certified Nursing Assistants. Other members of the nursing unit don't always hold Nursing Assistants in high regard. They are often given challenging or distasteful assignments that no one else wants to do. Patients are not always agreeable or diplomatic, or grateful when they are ill.

The work of Certified Nursing Assistants can be back-breaking. They are on their feet a good bit of their shift. Job demands can leave them caught between patients and supervisors. Many shifts are now twelve hours. Conditions can be emotionally stressful as well as physically demanding. Nursing Assistants must be careful not to expose themselves or their patients to contagious viruses, diseases, or bacteria.

> **Nursing Assistant Professionalism: What does Professionalism Mean?**

Being a healthcare professional obligates Nursing Assistants to provide competent caring and informed patient service in an ethical manner.

A Nursing Assistant should be committed to protecting patients' privacy, dignity, and health. As healthcare professionals Certified Nursing Assistants should fulfill their duties with the highest standards of professionalism in their manner and attitude.

It is understood that the professionalism of Nursing Assistants will include being responsible, honest, discrete, and trustworthy.

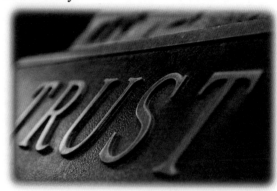

Professionalism includes keeping up to date in current patient services and availing themselves of opportunities for in-services, maintaining state certification, and being open to learning and professional development in the workplace. Professionalism also includes following the correct chain of command, knowing the scope of practice and being a team player. Most importantly, a professional Certified Nursing Assistant knows when to ask for assistance.

A Nursing Assistant is an important member of the medical profession. Part of becoming certified means adopting the standards of the profession.

Nurse aides have the most daily contact with patients. Thus, they have a key role in observation, listening to patients and family members, keeping accurate, detailed records and communicating information to the nursing team on a daily basis.

The CNA is a valuable liaison between patient and other healthcare staff.

In sharing this information, it is important to be professional in demeanor.

Professionalism also requires attention to personal grooming and good communication skills.

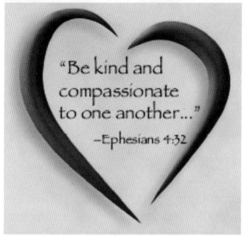

"Be kind and compassionate to one another..."
—Ephesians 4:32

It is a high priority to display compassion, enthusiasm, and the will to help others despite the fact that the job can be stressful, emotionally draining, and physically demanding. Keeping a calm, unruffled attitude in intense situations is the sign of a professional.

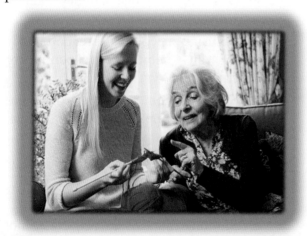

The code of ethics for Nursing Assistants acknowledges that, as healthcare professionals, their responsibility is to ease patient suffering and assist in restoring patient health. In doing so, part of their mandate is to acknowledge and address every part that makes up a patients' quality of life: physical, mental, emotional, social, and spiritual.

It is a part of the code of ethics to treat all patients with dignity and respect regardless of race, ethnicity, gender, or religion. It is also a professional obligation to be a good team player and to show loyalty to the employer.

Nursing Assistants also have an obligation to take care of themselves. This may seem selfish. But, consider this: If Nursing Assistants are not physically, mentally, and emotionally strong, they are not ready to look after the needs of their patients. The Nursing Assistant's employer and nursing unit team also needs them to be in good health. They do this by making sure they eat right, get eight hours of uninterrupted sleep, have hobbies and interests outside work, and stay home when they are ill.

Part of being a professional is appearing appropriately dressed and well groomed. Professional Nursing Assistants make a good impression in how they look, how they behave, and what they say. Patients respond with trust to their professionalism. The code of conduct reminds CNAs that they show respect for their patients by knocking before they enter the room, address the patient formally and introduce themselves, their title, and what they are going to do.

Nurse Assistants are expected to do everything they can to make the patient feel respected, informed, listened to, and confident that they are in good hands. There is no place in patient care for teasing, sarcasm, bullying, bossiness, or snide remarks. Patients already feel vulnerable and apprehensive. There is no need to add to their anxiety.

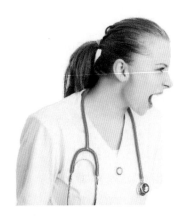

Applying the Code of Ethics in the workplace means doing the following:

- *Arriving on time in a mental, emotional, and physical condition to perform patient care duties.*

- *Taking time off work if the Nursing Assistant is unwell in order to recover and to avoid infecting others.*

- *Being absent only when it is unavoidable. Nursing Assistant teams and patients count on healthcare professionals. Certified Nursing Assistants have an obligation to their employer to fulfill their duties.*

- *Nursing Assistants have an obligation to notify the employer as far in advance as possible of a necessary absence.*

- *Certified Nursing Assistants have a duty to follow the instructions of their immediate superior within the scope of their professional duties.*

- *Being a team player, a good nursing assistant is loyal to the employer, colleagues, and patients.*

- *Being flexible and cooperative means accepting changes in assignments because of new patient demands and working with the nursing team to meet those demands.*

Work within your scope of practice

What is Unprofessional Behavior?

Unacceptable behavior may result in dismissal, reprimand, or a formal complaint on a Nursing Assistant's record. This could make it difficult to get a reference for another job.

Unprofessional behaviors may include:

- Abusing patients verbally, physically, or psychologically.

- Behaving is a discourteous manner with co-workers.

- Refusing a legitimate request made by an immediate superior or employer.

- Stealing from patient, colleagues and/or the employer.

- Deliberately damaging property of the facility.

- Insubordination.

- Neglecting responsibilities.

- Shirking duties—arriving late, not doing the assigned job, or leaving early.

- Altering patient records.

- Failing to report patient information in written and/or oral form.

- Appearing at the workplace under influence of drugs and/or alcohol

- Breeching patient confidentiality.

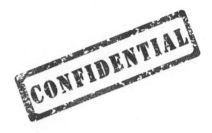

Why Protect Patient Confidentiality?

It is the nurse assistant's ethical, legal, professional, and moral duty to protect patient confidentiality.

Patient confidentiality is essential to patient trust.

Medical treatment is based on trust. Patients disclose sensitive, personal information to healthcare professionals, confident that this information will be shared only for treatment purposes and used only to help them. Without the assurance of confidentiality, those seeking medical assistance are likely to divert to an institution or professional in which they have greater trust or refuse to seek medical aid. This can create the potential for increased illness in the family or community.

Today, almost all patient information is stored digitally. While more convenient for accessing and sharing among the medical team, this increases the risk of digital hacking of sensitive patient data. In fact, Ponemon Institute's Fifth Annual Study on Medical Identity Theft notes that reported attacks on healthcare information increased by 125% over 2010 numbers. The stolen data can lead to identity theft, damaging patients' finances and careers.

Failing to protect patient confidentiality can result in dismissal, removal of certification, fines, civil lawsuits, and even prison. A Nursing Assistant's best professional action is to fulfill his/her ethical responsibility to protect patient confidentiality.

Increasing digital storage requires even more effort to protect patient information.

Is there ever a time when patient confidentiality may be breached? Perhaps. But these situations rest with family, attorneys, and facility administrators. In short, these decisions are made in dire circumstances and never at the nursing team level. The Nursing Assistant's job and ethical responsibility is to protect patient information at all costs.

How to Maintain Patient Confidentiality

Here are some ways the Nursing Assistant and the facility can maintain patient confidentiality in a digital world that has increased the need for heightened security measures.

Have clearly laid out wide-ranging confidentiality policies which staff has been in-serviced in and follows consistently and exactly. Confidentiality agreements are legal document between patients and the medical facility. They specify exactly the information that can and cannot be shared both inside the facility and outside with other medical personnel. It is the professional responsibility of Nursing Assistants to know this policy and to uphold its contents and confidentiality procedures.

Policies are best adhered to when ongoing regular retraining opportunities are provided not only for new staff but also for staff members who have already had in-service in confidentiality policies. Holding regular training for all facility staff including doctors, nursing unit members, clerical staff, and administrators helps build understanding of the policies and practices and why they exist. Refreshing the duties of all staff members reinforces the importance of confidentiality requirements.

If refresher training sessions have a social component, staff would be encouraged to attend with interest and commitment. It is also a great opportunity to build team morale and professionalism. Every effort should be made by all members of the facility to make in-service a positive experience.

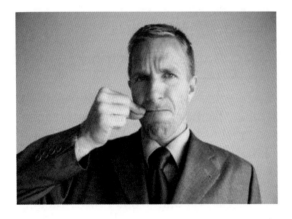

It is the duty of the medical facility to ensure that all patient files are stored on secure systems. Data increase astronomically with every year. This has created a challenge for hospitals, seniors' facilities, doctors' offices, and medical clinics. Saving and storing information and making it accessible to medical facilities is increasingly challenging.

It is vital that every medical facility and every person who handles these files do so within the highest level of security and digital protection. To that end, it is vital that the only personnel who have access to patient data are those who need this information as part of their patient contact and care. As a Nursing Assistant, it is crucial to patient confidentiality. Using only their password to access the needed information and protecting that password against use by any others' use is a wise policy.

An obvious threat to patient confidentiality is patient and staff cell phones. By eliminating their use within the facility possible threats to patient confidentiality are curtailed. With no cell phones available, the threat that patient data could be deliberately or accidentally recorded or photographed is avoided. When the use of cell phones is strictly prohibited, it helps to reduce the possibility of a breach of patient confidentiality.

The manner in which patient information is legitimately shared among professionals is a growing concern. In Imperial College research, it was revealed that nearly three in four medical professionals communicated with their colleagues about patients using SMS and other methods of dubious confidentiality. When sharing patient data, only secure systems approved by the facility should be used.

It is easy to overlook printed patient information as a source of information theft. Printed materials may look innocent but things like forms, notes, and labels can contain a wealth of information that can be easily misplaced, lost, or stolen in busy facilities. As professionals, Nursing Assistants have a duty to adhere to the rules for printing, safeguarding, and disseminating printed information put in place by their employers and for bringing to the attention of the immediate superior potential breaches in patient confidentiality posed by printed materials.

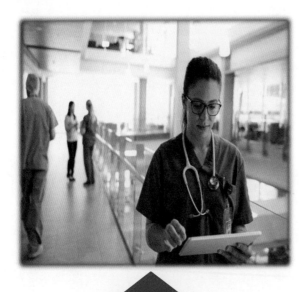

**Nursing Assistants'
Duty to Employer**

Nursing Assistants have an ethical and legal responsibility to their employer. These obligations include:

- Treating clients and staff in a courteous, respectful manner at all times.
- Reporting to work on time, ready to fulfill specified duties.
- Working as a team member to attend to patient needs reliably.
- Fulfilling the assignments outlined by the supervisor competently and cheerfully.

- Notifying the supervisor and the nursing team of patient observations in written and oral form.
- Keeping accurate patient records within the confidentiality guidelines as set out by the facility.
- Notifying the supervisor when the Nursing Assistant is unable to work as soon as possible.
- Assisting the nursing team in meeting patient needs, actively looking for areas where assistance is required.
- Performing prescribed duties as competently as possible, at all times.
- Asking for help or information in situations where instructions are unclear or the Nursing Assistant does not feel competent to complete a task.
- Taking the initiative to volunteer for assignments where something needs to be done.
- Building a good rapport with colleagues, patients, clerical staff, administrators, and others who enter the facility.
- Communicating accurately and succinctly, information about patient's status and recent changes with other members of the medical staff as needed.
- Establishing open and honest communication with facility personnel.
- Treating changes and modifications in patient assignments with co-operation and flexibility.
- Keeping patient needs and comfort always at the forefront of what is said and done.
- Reporting patient difficulties immediately to the nursing team and immediate supervisor.

- Seeking information from the previous shift staff before reporting to work.

- Communicating clearly in oral and written form information about patients to incoming staff at the end of the shift.

Helpful Resources

California Department of Health. "Licensing and Certification Program"
https://www.cdph.ca.gov/Programs/CHCQ/LCP/Pages/CNA.aspx.

CNA Plus Academy. "Sweet Sixteen: Top Qualities of a Great CNA" https://cna.plus/certified-nurse-assistant-top-qualities/

Hegner, Barbara. *Nursing Assistant: A Nursing Process Approach.*
https://www.amazon.ca/Nursing-Assistant-Process-Approach/dp/1418066079

National Library of Medicine. "The OBRA-87 nursing home regulations and implementation of the Resident Assessment Instrument: effects on process quality"
https://pubmed.ncbi.nlm.nih.gov/9256852/

NurseAlliance.org. "Title 22 Code of Regulations"
http://www.nursellianceca.org/files/2012/06/Title-22-Chapter-5.pdf

NurseJournal.org. "How to become a Certified Nursing Assistant"
https://nursejournal.org/certified-nursing-assistant/certified-nursing-assistant-responsibilities/

NursingLicensure.org. "Certified Nursing Assistant Requirements in California"
https://www.nursinglicensure.org/cna/california-nursing-assistant.html.

Pulliam, JoLynn. *Nursing Assistant, The: Acute, Subacute, and Long-Term Care.*
https://www.amazon.ca/Nursing-Assistant-Acute-Subacute-Long-Term/dp/0132622556.

RN.Com. "I Said what? Professionalism for the CNA" https://www.rn.com/featured-stories/professionalism-cna/

We Care Online. "Nursing Assistants: Tips on Improving Your Professionalism"
https://wecareonlineclasses.com/nursing-assistants-tips-on-improving-your-professionalism/

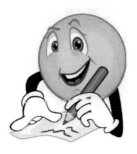

Chapter Two

Patient or Resident Rights

Outline

- The purpose of a long-term care facility

- The role of the Nurse Assistant in maintaining patient/resident rights, as stated in federal and state regulation

- California Code of Regulations Title 22, Division 5, Chapter 3, 72527 and Title 42 Code of Federal Regulations 483.10: A Comparison regarding patient/resident rights

- The Nurse Assistant role in preventing negligent acts and violation of patient/resident rights

- The Nurse Assistant role in reporting patient/resident rights violations

- The role of an ombudsman

- Examples of patient/resident rights, which support a patient's/resident's need for security, belonging and self-esteem

The purpose of a long-term care facility is to provide a variety of services. These services are designed to meet the residents' health and personal care needs. The services also assist residents to live as independently, safely, and happily as possible. Patients are encouraged to perform everyday activities on their own wherever feasible. Nursing Assistants have a key role to play in achieving these long-term facility goals.

A. Provide physical care

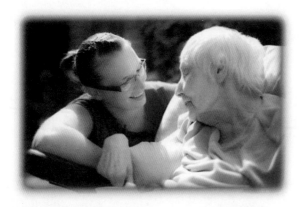

Residents often require long-term care because of serious, ongoing health issue or disability. The need for long-term physical care might come suddenly as a result of surgery, a broken bone, a heart attack, or stroke. Many physical needs develop gradually as residents age. They may become frailer or develop an illness or a disability that worsens.

Nursing Assistants provide skilled care, assisting residents to do daily living activities like eating, bathing, dressing, grooming, and mobility where help is required. These physical care activities are collectively called Activities of Daily Living (ADLs)

B. Provide focused care for patients/residents with special needs

American Senior Communities (https://www.asccare.com/types-long-term-care-services/) note that some residents have special challenges. These residents may have a developmental disability that may affect their physical, behavioral, intellectual, or cognitive functioning. Examples include cerebral palsy, muscular dystrophy, Parkinson's, neural muscular conditions, or autism. Nursing Assistants are trained to meet the special needs of these residents.

C. Provide a team approach to care and services

Nursing Assistants work in teams or units to care for an assigned group of residents. They share patient conditions, observe and report changes both orally and in written form in patient charts. Both physical tasks and sharing patient information are enhanced by this team approach. Nursing Assistants need to be cooperative, enthusiastic, energetic team workers. They also need good communication skills. Nursing Assistants should be willing to volunteer assistance and ask for help.

D. Prevent illness/injury and loss of function

In long-term care facilities, falls are the number one cause of death. An estimated 11,000 patients die from falls in American care facilities each year (https://www.myamericannurse.com/preventing-injuries-patient-falls/). Prevention is key. When residents are admitted, the nursing team does a review of patients' medications and drug interactions that could impair mobility and balance.

The nursing team offers patient-centered care that assesses and intervenes for fall risks. Environmental hazards like mats or slippery floors or steps or uneven terrain are eliminated.

Toileting, shower, and bed program are devised for each resident to minimize the risk of falls. Assistive aids are put in place where needed. The nursing team teaches balance techniques.

American Nurse (https://www.myamericannurse.com/prevent ing-injuries-patient-falls/) suggests these strategies for prevention of injuries from falls.

Implement fall prevention measures like bed rails and chair alarms, lap belts, gait belts, Bed and chair alarms, lap belts, gait belts, chair wedges, and nonslip footwear and chair wedges. These are designed to prevent falls.

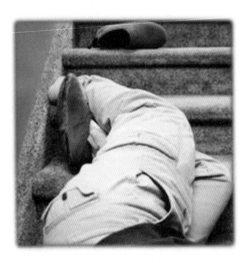

Injury-prevention interventions are an important part of the Nursing Assistant's critical components of quality care. Examples include floor matting/, hip protectors, low-low beds, raised toilet seats and safety bars in the shower, around the toilet, and in hallways.

It is important that nursing assistants know what fall prevention equipment is available. Nursing assistants also need to know fall prevention strategies. The final step is to decide which residents need which equipment and to teach them safe mobility strategies using this adaptive equipment.

E. Promote recovery and health in a setting that serves as both care facility and residence

Some residents may be short-term as the rehab after a fall, surgery, or an injury. It is the nursing team's role to aid in their recovery with a goal to resident independent living and return to their home.

F. Assist patient/resident in reaching their maximum potential both physically and mentally

Nursing Assistants have a vital role to play in helping residents reach their full potential physically and mentally or intellectually. These strategies improve Nursing Assistant-patient engagement.

1. When talking to the patient, the nursing assistant should strive to keep the information simple. Medical terms are neither understood nor helpful. Professionals should avoid medical jargon and acronyms. Communicating as clearly and specifically as possible is the goal.

2. The nursing unit should aim to get their patients involved goal setting and charting progress toward their goals.

3. It is important to ensure that all caregivers, the patient, and family members are on the same page. Nursing Assistant's oral and written communication must be clear enough for sharing among the nursing unit, with other medical professionals who interact with the patient, and with the patient and the patient's family, if the medical team decides this is important.

4. Nursing Assistants must be accountable for all patient interactions.
5. Nursing Assistants can ensure patient engagement by asking and answering patients.

The role of the Nurse Assistant in maintaining patient/resident rights, as stated in federal and state regulation

State and federal regulations require long-term resident facilities to have written policies. These must outline the rights of residents. Moreover, the facility must explain these policies to the resident and his/her family. The policies must be implemented. Individuals requiring nursing home care have a right to expect appropriate care. Residents have a legal right be treated with courtesy and respect regardless of race, ethnicity, gender, physical, or mental challenges.

A. The Nurse Assistant is responsible for being familiar with regulations that provide for patient/resident rights and for assisting patients/residents to exercise their rights

While Nursing Assistants play little part in creating the facility's policies, they are responsible for knowing and fulfilling these patient rights. As professionals, Nursing Assistants also need to know state and federal regulations regarding patient rights.

B. Patient/resident rights are protected by federal regulations for long-term care facilities

Residents' Rights are protected by the federal Nursing Home Reform Law of 1987. Under this law long-term care facilities must "promote and protect the rights of each resident." The law puts strong emphasis on individual dignity and the right of patients to make decisions concerning their care. Nursing homes funding under Medicare and Medicaid must meet these requirements in order to receive the government funding. Some states also have residents' rights regulations for facilities including nursing homes, licensed assisted living centers, adult care homes, and other care facilities. Residents" rights legislation is in place to ensure that those living in a long-term care facility have the same rights as others in the surrounding community.

C. Title 42, Code of Federal Regulations Resident Rights (483.10): Residents living in a health care facility should have the same rights as those held by all U.S. Citizens.

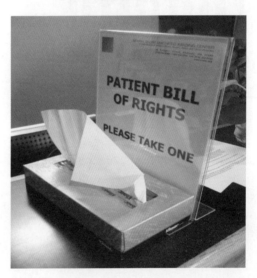

Resident rights are also protected by Title 42, regulation 483.10. This regulation outlines resident rights in any healthcare facility. Many of them mirror those in the Nursing Home Reform Law of 1987. The scope of the facility is wider under these regulations.

1. Residents have the right to be free of interference, coercion, discrimination, or reprisal from the facility in exercising their rights. They include: a. Quality of life

1) Residents have the right to the best care available

It is the duty of Nursing Assistants to ensure that residents do not feel pressured or coerced in exercising their rights to the highest quality of life and care the facility has within their power to offer. All residents have the right to expect the same quality care regardless of physical, mental, cultural differences, or socioeconomic difference.

2) Dignity, choice, and independence are important

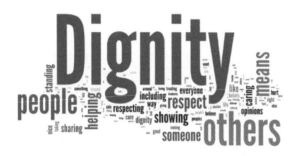

Regulation 483.10 emphasizes that residents must be treated with dignity. Nursing Assistants' care need to focus on empowering residents to be independent and offering them realistic choices.

3) Services and activities to maintain high level of wellness

The residential facility must offer residents programs, activities, and services which nurture residents' physical, mental, and social health. Residents should be informed of these activities and encouraged to participate.

4) Residents must have the correct care that should keep them as healthy as possible every day

A well-planned, long-range resident care plan considers the resident's medical, intellectual, social, and spiritual health. Nursing Assistants should strive in their resident care to address these facets of daily resident care.

5) Health should not decline as a direct result of the facility's care

Residents and their families have the right to quality care that will maintain the residents' health. The quality of care received from the facility should not lead to the detriment of the health of the residents.

6) The right to be fully informed about rights and services

Residents should not be kept in the dark about the services they are receiving and why they are receiving them. While it is not the job of a Nursing Assistant to discuss a resident's diagnosis, it is the resident's right to know what procedures Nursing Assistants are performing.

7) Residents must be told what care and services are available

Residents and their families have the right to know what services and patient care options are available to them. They have the right to make informed choices about the care they wish to receive.

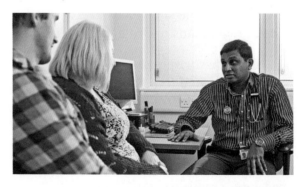

8) They must be told the charges for each service

When care options and available, services are explained to residents by medical staff, residents have the right to be fully informed about the costs of these services. Residents have the right to know a detailed cost breakdown.

9)Legal rights must be explained in a language they understand, a written copy is given to them

Legal rights can be complicated by technical language. Residents have the right to have this explained in language they can understand by medical and/or law personnel. They also have the right to receive a written explanation of these rights in simple, understandable, jargon-free form.

10) Right to be notified in advance of any room change or roommate

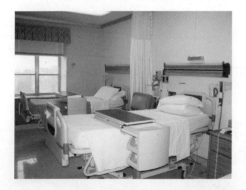

If there are proposed changes to a resident's room location or rooming arrangement, the resident has the right to be informed in advance of these proposed changes by the designated staff member.

11) Right to communicate with someone who speaks their language

If a resident does not speak and understand English, he has the right to receive and give his communication through an interpreter, a family member, or staff member who speaks his mother tongue. Nursing Assistants should be aware of and sensitive to any language barrier.

12) Right to obtain assistance for any sensory impairment, e.g., blindness

If a resident has a communication challenge like a visual or hearing deficit, he had the right to assistance in dealing with this sensory impairment. Every avenue for accommodation should be explored through community and medical organizations and caregivers. Residents should be fully informed about available accommodations.

13) Informed consent is a concept that goes along with this. A person has the right to direct what happens to his or her body: The right to make independent choices

No resident should be denied the right to informed consent regarding any medical treatment and care. Residents have the right to make informed choices with or without input from staff or family members. In every situation, resident rights come first.

14) Residents have the right to make choices about their doctors, care and treatments

If residents wish to change their doctor, the medical treatment they are receiving, or patient care options, they have the right to make these decisions. It is the Nursing Assistant's responsibility to listen to resident concerns and to share these with the nursing unit. The nursing supervisor will pass these on to medical staff where this is indicated. Patient concerns should also be documented in the resident's chart.

15) Rights to make personal decisions. These include what to wear and how to spend their time. They can join in community activities, both inside, and

It is a resident's right to make decisions regarding what to wear, what to do, and which groups/activities to associate with. Moreover, residents have the right to decide what amenities both inside the facility and in the community, they wish to access. The facility personnel should make residents aware of what is available. They can make helpful suggestions. But, ultimately, the decision rests with the resident. He/she should feel free to choose and encouraged to do so.

d) Resident Behavior and Facility Practices (483.13)

This requirement is aimed at having every resident maintaining the highest possible well-being. It protects the resident from the use of restraints for the purpose of control, punishment, or containment. The regulation limits restraint only in situations where it is medically necessary to protect the resident.

> *1. The resident has the right to be free from any physical restraints imposed, or from psychoactive drugs that are administered for the purpose of discipline or convenience and are not required for treatment of the resident's medical symptoms*

Whether restraints are physical or in the form of drugs, residents have the right to be free of these restraints unless these restraints are prescribed by the resident's doctor in treating his/her medical condition. Nursing Assistants should never use restraints of any kind unless the resident's doctor has advised the use of these restraints and stipulated how and when restraints may be used. Immediate supervisors should be consulted regarding any restraint decision.

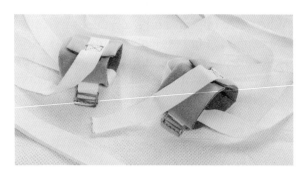

2. Restraint

Restrain involves any device or medication, or verbal threat which restricts the resident's right to freely access the grounds and equipment of the long-term facility. Restraint is a violation of resident rights.

a. *Physical (i.e., soft belt, bed rails, geri-chair, mittens, soft ties, locked wheelchair, lap buddy-if cannot be removed by patient)*

"Physical Restraints" are physical or mechanical devices or equipment. These may be attached or adjacent to the resident. Physical restraints may include leg or arm restraints, hand mitts, soft ties or vests, lap cushions, or lap trays.

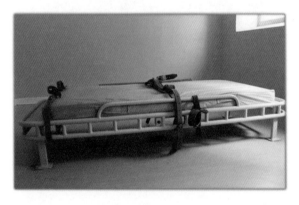

In order to prevent the resident from getting out of bed physical restraints may include side rails, tucking in sheets or using Velcro to hold clothing or bedding tight.

Physical restraint may involve restriction of movement using devices like chairs, trays, tables, gates, bars, or belts that prevent the resident from rising and/or moving to an area where he/she wants to go.

Physical restraints are deemed restraints if the resident cannot remove them easily. They restrict the resident's access to areas and/or freedom of movement.

b. Chemical (i.e., psychotropic drugs)

"Chemical Restraints" are drugs used for restrict the movement of the resident for the purposes of protecting his/her safety, disciplining him/her or providing convenience for the facility staff.

Chemical restraints are not used in the treatment of the resident's medical symptoms.

3. Freedom from abuse

The intent of this regulation is to ensure residents' right to be free from abuse, corporal punishment, and involuntary seclusion. Residents have the right not to be subjected to abuse by facility staff, other residents, consultants or volunteers, medical staff, service agency personnel, family members, friends, or other individuals visiting the facility.

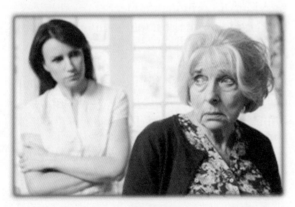

a. Financial; stealing or borrowing items or accepting gifts

Nursing Assistants should never steal, borrow, or accept items as gifts from residents. They should also be alert to residents' stealing or borrowing items that

don't belong to them. While residents are encouraged to mark possessions clearly and not to keep valuable items and cash on hand, they have the right to expect that their living space it private. Signs of this should be reported to the nursing unit supervisor.

b. Verbal; teasing, profanity, racial slanders, threats

Verbal abuse includes oral, written language or gestures that are disparaging or derogatory. These might be directed at the residents, their friends, or their families. The remarks might make reference to their age, their appearance, their inability to comprehend, or their physical or mental disability. Verbal abuse take the form of threats or ridicule. As professionals who have the most daily contact with residents, Nursing Assistants need to be aware of verbal abuse and report it to their supervisor.

c. Sexual; overtures, innuendo, gestures, inappropriate touching

"Sexual abuse" includes, but is not limited to, sexual harassment, sexual coercion, or sexual assault. Nursing Assistants have significant daily contact with patients. They need to be alert to signs of sexual abuse or resident comments alluding to sexual abuse.

d. Physical; battery, kicking, biting, hitting, shoving, pulling hair, rough handling

As professionals who have daily contact with residents, Nursing Assistants should be alert to signs of physical abuse. This includes hitting, spitting, slapping, hair pulling, pinching, and kicking of residents by staff, visitors, family members, or other residents. Physical abuse also includes controlling behavior through physical punishment.

e. **Psychological; ridiculing, ignoring, manipulating**

Also defined as "mental abuse" this is a form of verbal abuse. It includes humiliation, harassment, ignoring, threatening punishment, verbal manipulation, or deprivation. As professionals who see residents every day, Nursing Assistants need to be alert to mental abuse of residents by staff, other residents, visitors, and family members. Such conduct should be documented and reported to the nursing supervisor.

f. **Involuntary seclusion; isolation**

"Involuntary seclusion" involves the separation of a resident from other residents. He/she may be confined to her/his room against the resident's will. At times, for the safety of that resident or other residents it may be necessary for physical health reasons to do an emergency, short-term isolation or monitored separation. Involuntary seclusion and may be permitted only if it is used for a limited period of time as a therapeutic intervention. Its intent is to reduce agitation, ensure resident safety, and/or de-escalate a situation until professional staff can create an alternative to ameliorate the situation and address the resident's needs. As a professional, it is import that Nursing Assistants take this measure only in extreme circumstances and only if immediate supervisors and/or medical staff order it.

g. **Abandonment; leaving someone unattended**

It is a physical and emotional mistake to leave a resident unattended in bed, on the toilet, in the shower, outdoors, in the hallway, or in the dining room if this resident cannot safely transfer or move about freely. Falls can occur when residents who require assistance for daily living activities are left alone. Nursing Assistants often have to juggle working with multiple residents. They have to be master organizers not to abandon residents.

h. **Neglect; failure to provide care that a reasonable person would provide. (i.e., not answering call light, smells of urine and not being cleaned/changed)**

Neglect can take many forms. In many cases, it is simply the result of nursing staff with too many high-needs residents. Sometimes, neglect comes from not checking on residents often enough or closely enough. Deliberately ignoring obvious resident needs is abuse.

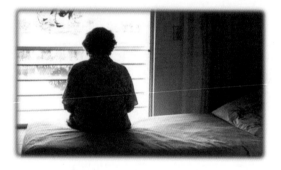

Neglect involves the failure of the nursing staff, the facility, and/or outside service providers to provide the necessary services and goods for the resident's physical health. Neglect can result in pain, mental anguish, and/or emotional distress. Neglect may be untreated bedsores, failure to provide clean sheets, being unresponsive to resident requests for assistance, failure to provide food and/or liquids such that residents experience dehydration, weight loss, and/or poor hygiene. Neglect might also involve failure to contact medical personnel. Neglect can also include residents wandering away from the facility, unexplained falls or injuries, and unsanitary facility conditions.

Nursing Assistants have a significant role to

Role of Nurse Assistants

play in protecting residents from neglect and abuse. As professionals who have the most daily contact with residents, Nursing Assistants are in a position to observe resident behavior. They are also the first to receive resident complaints and concerns. Nursing Assistants need to have a clear idea of the signs of abuse and neglect.

1. Self-care

As professionals, Nursing Assistant must take care of themselves. They cannot care effectively for others if they not in good physical and mental health. This means eating well, getting sufficient exercise. It means getting eight hours of uninterrupted sleep every night. Personal care also requires personal stress management strategies taking breaks, having a nutritious lunch, spending time with family and friends, and seeking professional intervention when needed

2. *Communication with supervisors*

In communicating observations of abuse or neglect, Nursing Assistants must be explicit in their written and oral communication.

3. *Identify resident abuse; signs and symptoms, suspected, verbal account, witnessed or known*

In reporting signs of abuse or neglect, Nursing Assistants need to note the time of the observation, who was present, the suspected incident, and whether it was witnessed, or reported by someone else. Both oral and written reports need to be made.

4. *Mandated reporter; SOC341 (reporting form), aiding and abetting, ombudsman, California Department of Public Health (CDPH)*

This form was adopted by the California Department of Social Services. It is required under Welfare and Institutions Code Sections 15630 and 15658(a)(1)

SOC341 documents information given by the reporting party of suspected incident of abuse or neglect of a long-term care elder or dependent adult.

As the professional who witnessed or was told of an incident of abuse or neglect it is the Nursing Assistant's responsibility to report this incident to her/his immediate supervisor. It is also the Nursing Assistant's legal responsibility under the California Department of Social Services to fill out the elder abuse report form, sign and date it.

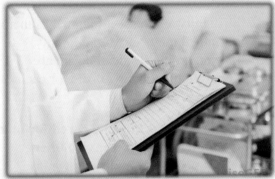

5. Documentation

Those who live in residential settings with long-term supportive services are at risk for abuse and neglect. Most suffer from several chronic diseases that have affected physical and cognitive functioning. Many are dependent on others for their daily living needs. Some cannot report abuse or neglect. Others are afraid to do so.

Residents in skilled nursing facilities are highly needy and thus highly vulnerable. Many cannot speak for their own rights. As front-line caregivers, Nursing Assistants are in a position to observe abuse and neglect. They have a legal, moral, and professional duty to document abuse and neglect. Often their reports implicate the employer, a co-worker, a medical professional, or a resident's family member. Reporting the incident may have career backlash. It is important for Nursing Assistants to know the signs of abuse and neglect. It is vital to know the laws regarding reporting these incidents and to follow documentation procedures exactly.

G. Quality of Life (483.15)

The intent of this clause is to specify the long-term care facility's responsibilities toward creating and sustaining an environment where residents are treated with the dignity and respect that makes them feel like valued members of the facility. Decisions regarding residential care are based on providing quality of life for each resident.

1. **The resident must be cared for in a manner and in an environment that promotes maintenance or enhancement of each resident's quality of life**

The resident's long-term care plan outlines care and maintenance of the resident's physical, mental, social, and spiritual wellbeing. Nursing staff works with other facility providers to achieve this quality of life for their clients.

2. **Care and environment includes:**

a. Dignity

Dignity involves resident/staff interactions that assist the resident to maintain and enhance his/her self-esteem and confidence. Residents are assisted as required to be dressed in well fitting, clean clothes, hair combed and styled, shaved, nails clean and clipped.

Residents are encouraged to dress themselves and assisted where necessary.

Resident independence and dignity is nurtured in the dining room. Staff assist wherever necessary, interacting and conversing with residents while assisting them.

b. Self-determination and participation

Residents are encouraged to choose and participate in activities.

c. Participation in resident and family groups

Residents are encouraged to take an active role in family group meetings with facility staff and to be pro-active in decision making about their resident care plan.

d. Participation in other activities

Residents should be informed both verbally and in writing of the day's activities both within the facility and in the community. Nursing Assistants can play a key role in encouraging participation and getting residents to the right location at the appointed time.

e. Accommodation of needs

Accommodation of needs must be done in a way that addresses physical and/or mental disabilities while respecting the resident's dignity. As primary care professionals, Nursing Assistants have an important role in seeing that accommodations encompass individual self-respect and self-worth.

f. Activities

To promote resident mental and physical health, the facility should provide a variety of activities to appeal to residents of various interests, ages and mobility.

g. Social Services

Quality of life sometimes requires that social service agencies to become involved to ensure residents are accessing all the resources they need to live an enriched life.

h. Personal living environment

Our quality of life is affected by our surroundings.
Environmental conditions affect physical health, mental health, and emotional well-being directly and indirectly. Pollution may affect our health. It may also darken our emotional outlook. A clean, bright, cheerful setting will brighten our days and actually lengthen a life span.

3. Identify environmental and personal living area hazards to prevent incidents and/or accidents

Part of respecting the dignity of residents is ensuring that their environment is barrier free and does not contain hazardous terrain that could cause accidents. This includes floor surfaces, chairs, and other furniture.

California Code of Regulations Title 22, Division 5, Chapter 3, 72527 and Title 42 Code of Federal Regulations 483.10: A Comparison regarding patient/resident rights

A: Residents shall be encouraged/assisted to exercise their rights as a patient and as a citizen, 72527(a). Written policies regarding patient rights must be established and available

1. Patient must be informed of rights, rules and regulations regarding patient conduct

2. Patient must be informed of services and charges

3. Patient must be informed of medical condition by doctor and have opportunity to participate in planning of medical treatment

4. Patient can refuse treatment and be informed of consequences (informed consent)

5. Patient can be transferred or discharged only for medical reasons, welfare, other patients' welfare, or for nonpayment

6. Patient shall be assisted to exercise rights, voice grievances, recommend changes in policy and services, have outside representation, and freedom from restraint, interference, coercion, discrimination and reprisal

7. Patient allowed to manage their personal finances

8. Patient has right to be free from mental and physical abuse and chemical and physical restraints

9. Confidential treatment of records

a. Health Insurance Portability and Accountability Act (HIPAA)

b. Standards and safeguards for documentation and transmission of health records to assure privacy and security of this data

10. Patient has right to be treated with consideration, respect, dignity, and individuality, including privacy

11. Patient has right to not be required to perform work

12. Patient has right to be able to communicate privately and send/receive mail

13. Patient has right to participate in social or religious activities

14. Patient has right to be allowed to retain and use personal clothing and possessions

15. If married, to be provided privacy and share a room if both are patients in the facility

16. Patient has right to have daily visiting hours

17. Patient has right to have visit by clergy at any time

18. Patient has right to have relatives, or person responsible to visit critically ill patient at any time

B. Patient rights may only be denied or limited for good cause evidenced by doctor's order and may be denied or limited only if allowed by law

C. California Health and Safety Code (Skilled Nursing and Intermediate Care Facility Patient's Bill of Rights)

1. [1599.1] Written policies regarding the rights of patients shall be established and made available to patient, guardian, next of kin, sponsor, and public a. In addition to patient rights and obligations defined in the regulations

1) The facility shall employ adequate, qualified staff

2) Assure personal hygiene of patients, including prevention of pressure ulcers and incontinence

3) Provide diet to meet patient needs

4) Activities and promotion of self-care

b. The facility shall be clean, sanitary and in good repair including the nurses call system

2. [1599.2] Written information informing patients of their rights include facility requirements in the Health and Safety Code and Title 22. a. Violations of either code may be grounds for civil or criminal proceedings against the facility or its personnel b. Patients have the right to voice grievances free of reprisal and to submit complaints to the Department of Public Health Services (CDPH)

3. [1599.3] Rights of patients who are determined to be incompetent, incapable of understanding, exhibits a communication barrier are to be carried out/protected by guardian, next of kin, conservator, sponsoring agency or representative unless it is the facility

The Nurse Assistant role in preventing negligent acts and violation of patient/resident rights:

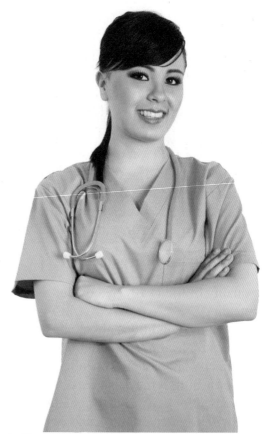

A. Explain the difference between negligence and abuse

B. Recognize the evidence of negligent acts and violations of patient/resident rights

C. Explain how to prevent violations of patient/resident rights

D. Define facility, state, and federal policies and procedures related to violation of patient/resident rights

The Nurse Assistant role in reporting patient/resident rights violations

A. Identify patient/resident rights violations

Through daily interaction with residents, Nursing Assistants see and hear resident information. As professionals, it is their duty to know the legislation regarding patient rights, to recognize and report incidents of violation of resident rights.

B. Discuss your observations with a licensed nurse/appropriate personnel

Nursing Assistants have a duty to report their observations regarding the residents they serve clearly and in detail to their immediate superior.

D. Report observations as a mandated reporter, following federal mandate for reporting suspected or actual patient/resident rights violations

Nursing Assistants have a legal obligation to make a written report of violation of patient rights.

E. Follow up on reported incident with licensed personnel

Nursing Assistants also have a professional and legal responsibility to follow up on their report. Nursing Assistants should check with their immediate supervisors to ensure that the injury reports they submitted was acted upon appropriately.

The supervisor should take immediate steps to prevent recurrence of a hazardous condition. Reports generated from an incident must be forwarded to the Safety Officer who will fill out the appropriate section of the report

---

The role of an ombudsman

An Ombudsman is a government agency employee. People can seek the assistance of an Ombudsman for help in navigating programs and/or policies related to residents' rights in a long-term care facility.

A. Patient advocate and member of the health care team
Sitting on the healthcare team, the ombudsman advocates for patient rights within federal and state legislation concerning long-term care facilities.

B. Impartial person who investigates complaints and acts as an advocate for patients/residents and/or families to resolve conflicts

Ombudsmen help resolve problems. They provide a neutral party standpoint between the resident and the long-term care facility. The ombudsman's role while impartial is to investigate resident complaints and advocate for the resident.

C. Legal responsibility of an ombudsman to follow facility protocol

While the ombudsman advocate for the resident, he/she does so with the federal, state regulations, and the written statements of the care facility.

F. Gives information to the public

Part of the ombudsman's role is to educate the public on issue which have been resolved. This may prevent future issues arising.

Maslow's Hierarchy of needs simplified in patient needs

A. Physiological
1. Food
2. Water
3. Oxygen
4. Sleep
5. Sex
6. Temperature extremes

B. Safety & Security: asepsis, knowledge of patient's/resident's individual needs
1. Freedom from fear and anxiety
2. Stability
3. Consistency in routine
4. Freedom from pain

C. Belonging: love and affection
1. This is the patient's/resident's home
2. Sense of belonging (psychosocial needs)
3. Acceptance and love
4. Receive family, friends, and visitors in home-like environment

D. Self-esteem
1. Ask opinion and really listen
2. Feeling competent
3. Gaining respect, approval and recognition

E. Self-actualization
1. Pride in accomplishment; opportunity to do their best
2. Attain full learning, creative, and spiritual potential

Helpful Resources

AARP. "The 1987 Nursing Home Reform Act" https://www.aarp.org/home-garden/livable-communities/info-2001/the_1987_nursing_home_reform_act.html.

Acello, B. & Hegner, B. (2016). *Nursing Assistant: A Nursing Process Approach.* (11th ed.) Boston, MA. Cengage Learning.

American Nurse. "Preventing Injuries from Falls" https://www.myamericannurse.com/preventing-injuries-patient-falls/.

American Senior Communities. "Types of Long Term Services" https://www.asccare.com/types-long-term-care-services.

ANE. Abuse, Neglect, Exploitation, and Misappropriation of Property in Nursing Homes: What You Need to Know" *The Consumer Voice.* https://theconsumervoice.org/uploads/files/issues/ANE_Prezi_Script-_FINAL_-_2018.pdf

Clinipace.com. "They're Talking. Are You Listening?" Nursing Assistant webinar https://www.clinipace.com/knowledge-hub/theyre-talking-are-you-listening-improve-your-clinical-trial-with-patient-insights/?gclid=CjwKCAjwwab7BRBAEiwAapqpTJnYfg_cncSX_3hfOnR1GBTLZNkOW0BPnN9iF0y7AxWA8MLsgQ62iBoCAo4QAvD_BwE

CMS. "Patient's Bill of Rights from Center for Medicare & Medicaid Services" https://www.cms.gov/CCIIO/Programs-and-Initiatives/Health-Insurance-Market-Reforms/Patients-Bill-of-Rights

Cornell Law School. "42 CFR 483.10 Resident Rights" https://www.law.cornell.edu/cfr/text/42/483.10

DHCS. "The Role of an Ombudsman" https://www.dhcs.ca.gov/services/MH/Pages/mh-ombudsman.aspx.

Elsevier. *Mosby's Textbook for Long-Term Care Nursing Assistants* (8th ed.)
https://www.elsevier.com/books/mosbys-textbook-for-long-term-care-nursing-
assistants/kostelnick/978-0-323-53073-6

Foundation for Assisting in Home Care. "Working with People with Developmental Disabilities"
https://courses.lumenlearning.com/suny-home-health-aide/chapter/working-with-people-with-
developmental-disabilities/.

Hawes, C. "Elder Abuse in Residential Care Settings: What is Known and what Information is
Needed" https://www.ncbi.nlm.nih.gov/books/NBK98786/

HealthDirect.com. "What You Need to Know about Fall Risk Interventions"
https://www.hdrxservices.com/blog/what-you-need-to-know-about-fall-risk-interventions/.

Lt.com. Ombudsman. "Nursing Home Residents' Rights"
https://ltcombudsman.org/uploads/files/support/Module-2.pdf

National Institute on Aging. "What is Long-Term Care?" https://www.nia.nih.gov/health/what-
long-term-care.

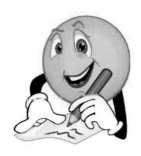

Chapter Three:

Effective Communication

Outline

I: Maslow's Hierarchy of Needs

II: Behaviors of patient/resident that reflect unmet human needs.

III: Forms of communication.

IV: Major steps in the communication process

V: Communication breakdown

VI: Effective Communication/Interpersonal Skills

VII: Conflict and conflict resolution.

VIII: Touch as a form of communication

IX: Common psychological defense mechanisms.

X: Nursing Assistant's role in family communication/interaction patterns

XI: Social and cultural factors influencing communication and emotional reactions to illness and disability

XIII: Communication within the healthcare team

Created by Abraham Maslow, a psychologist, in the forties, Maslow's hierarchy of needs is a five-tier model of human needs from basic to complex:

- Biological and Physiological basic life needs: air, food, drink, shelter, warmth, sex, sleep.
- Safety needs. protection, security, order, law, limits, stability,
- Belongingness, love, a sense of community needs. ...
- Esteem needs
- Self-actualization.

Widely accepted even though there is little research supporting it, Maslow's hierarchy of needs is still very popular.

The purpose of this unit is to introduce concepts and skills required for the Nurse Assistant to communicate effectively and interact appropriately with residents, the nursing team, residents' families and friends, and outside service providers who are members of the health care team.

Basic human needs

Nursing Assistants have a professional and legal duty to ensure residents' basic human needs are met. The seven basic needs are further subdivided into subcategories. In each need, the Nursing Assistant has a key role to play. If these needs are not met, Maslow contended that the outcome would be physical illness, mental health issues, and/or psychiatric illness. Maslow warned

that if physiological needs are not met, those under a Nursing Assistant's care could become very ill or even die, If a resident's safety needs are not met, posttraumatic stress could occur.

Typically, humans arrive at different stages of the hierarchy along life's path. At different times they might have a deficit in a certain stage. If this happens, that person may abandon the pursuit of a higher stage. He/she regresses to a lower stage to have more fundamental needs met. Not everyone reaches the top of the hierarchy. Things like poverty, injury, financial setbacks or illness may interfere with development in Maslow's hierarchy.

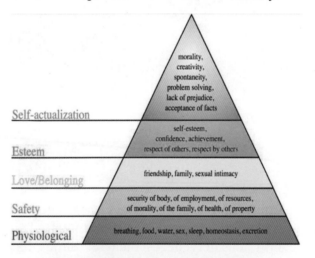

1. Physiological

Physiological needs are necessary to maintain life. These basic needs are required by all animals—including humans. They are the primary focus of infants.

Every human being has some basic physiological needs including food, oxygen, water, shelter, elimination, sleep, and sex.

It is important that Nursing Assistants recognize the importance of meeting residents' physiological needs. As front-line resident care providers, Nursing Assistants are in a position to note whether residents' basic needs are being met.

Example

When Nursing Assistants deliver meal trays, assists patient/resident with set-up, assist with feeding where needed, they are fulfilling Maslow's physiological needs.

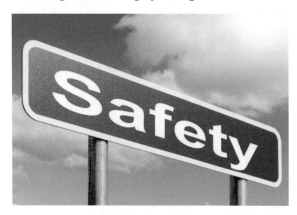

2. Safety and security needs

Safety and security issues gain attention after physiological needs are met. This shift to safety needs includes things like physical and mental health concerns, freedom from war, physical and financial security. Safety and security needs may include clothing, protection from a danger or harm, freedom from illness, injury, harm, fear, stability and order, family, economics

Example

When Nursing Assistants responds promptly to the resident's call light, he/she feels secure. Aiding residents with dressing, and helping resident's with showering, toileting, and mobility challenges are all part of Maslow's safety and security.

3. Sense of belongingness

Once physiological, safety, and security needs are met, residents will seek a sense of belonging. The resident will begin to focus on the need to have a feeling of community and being loved. These needs are usually met by friends, family, and romantic partners. In residential long-term care facilities this need to belong is often met by residents, staff, caregivers, and/or outside service providers.

Often residents in a long-term care facility lose contact with friends and family. Other residents, facility staff, and service providers become a community for these residents. As primary caregivers, Nursing Assistants are in a position to nurture resident interaction and encourage involvement.

Example

Nursing Assistants can help meet this need by encouraging family and friends to visit and making them feel welcome. They can encourage residents to reach out to family and friends. They can familiarize themselves with activities which might interest specific residents and encourage residents to become involved in activities offered at the facility and in the community. They can act as a link, getting residents to group activities.

4. Esteem

Esteem is feeling good about oneself. It is a sense of self-worth. Esteem is necessary for self-actualization. When a sense of community is met a resident may work toward esteem. Before esteem can be achieved, a resident needs love and a sense of belonging. Self-confidence and acceptance from others are important components of esteem.

The Nursing Assistant has a vital role to play in building resident esteem. Caring is at the heart of the Nursing Assistant–resident relationship. Through verbal and nonverbal interaction, the Nursing Assistant can develop resident self-esteem and confidence.

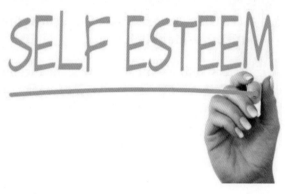

Example

When Nursing Assistants introduce themselves, address each resident by the name they prefer, and tell them in plain language what they are going to do, it increases the resident's confidence.

By listening to residents, and asking follow-up questions, the Nursing Assistant demonstrates caring, concern, and a willingness to help.

5. Self-actualization

Self-actualization involves the ability to be self-sufficient. It is the ability to achieve one's potential. Self-actualization varies from person to person. Engineers have self-actualized when they can complete a project satisfactorily. When architects complete a drawing that excites their clients, they have achieved self-actualization.

When a resident can complete his daily activities unassisted and is happily involved in the activities of the facility, he is self-actualized.

Example

Nursing Assistants can help residents achieve self-actualization by having a good understanding of what residents can do and assisting them to be as independent as they can. Sincerely acknowledgement and praise of a resident's sincere accomplishments is excellent motivation.

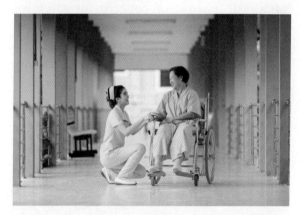

Importance of using Maslow's Hierarchy of needs

Maslow's hierarchy describes simply the structural truth of human existence. With deftness and precision, Maslow addressed deep questions about what humanity was really after. It looks at what humans long for. It speaks to how humans arrange their priorities. It explores competing claims on people's attention. Reaching the self-actualization stage is the mark of a life well lived.

The hierarchy notes that humans cannot look after our higher needs—social-emotional and spiritual—until more basic needs are met.

The hierarchy also serves as a reminder that there is more to serving residents than addressing their basic physiological needs. Understanding Maslow's hierarchy helps

Nursing Assistants understand how they can assist their residents in all five levels.

1. Basis of satisfactory achievement of each level

Before anyone can proceed to the next level, his needs at the previous level must be met. Those who are scraping to feed themselves have little interest or concern for safety or financial security for example. As professionals, Nursing Assistants need to know at what level of Maslow's hierarchy each of their residents is operating to help them address those needs.

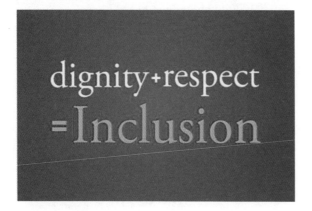

2. Meeting basic physiological needs

If physiological needs are not met, individuals will become ill or die. Meeting these basic needs is a Nursing Assistant's first priority.

3. A way for setting priorities and organizing activities

Assessing resident health and establishing a long-range plan for residents is facilitated by examining where the resident is functioning on Maslow's hierarchy. Resident care also needs to acknowledge that in times of stress, trauma, loss, or ill health residents may revert to a lower level on the hierarchy temporarily or permanently.

4. Promoting a holistic approach to patient/resident care planning

Using Maslow's hierarchy of needs the skilled nursing staff at a residential care facility can design an individual resident long-term care plan that addresses physical, mental, social, and spiritual needs of the resident.

5. Increasing awareness of reasons for patient/resident behaviors

An understanding of Maslow's hierarchy helps hone Nursing Assistants' awareness of resident behaviors and motivation. A study of Maslow reminds healthcare professionals that each unique resident's needs must be met so that they feel satisfied, listened to, cared for and valued.

The hierarchy helps the nursing team identify the level of care each resident requires. Nursing Assistants need to note whether residents in a long-term care setting have their need for food and water met. Are they eating and drinking enough? Do they need assistance and encouragement with basic physiological needs? Are residents' need for safety and privacy being met? What resident behaviors, comments, body language are red flags of unmet needs?

6. Consequence of Unmet basic needs

When residents' basic needs are unmet, it may result in illness, injury, or even death. Nursing Assistants, as primary caregivers, have a professional responsibility to know Maslow's physiological needs, to recognize when these are not being met, and to report their finding to the nursing unit.

Recognition and reporting of patient/resident behaviors that reflect unmet needs

In meeting recognized it is a matter of noting resident behaviors that reflect unmet needs.

Nursing Assistants need to adjust their behavior to show residents that they are attuned to their needs. This includes things like treating even grumpy residents with good humor and expressing concern for their wellbeing.

Nursing professionals must be transparent about what they are doing and why. This calms the anxiety of insecure residents and makes them feel safe.

Addressing residents courteously and respectfully shows residents their opinions and concerns matter. Nursing Assistants need to form a bond with residents. Residents in long-term care facilities benefit from bonding with their caregivers. Conversation, laughter, jokes, and sharing family anecdotes make residents feel a sense of belonging.

Behaviors that depict unmet human needs

When needs are unmet, tensions and anxiety arise. These feelings manifest themselves in verbal and nonverbal indicators. As trained professionals in daily contact with residents, Nursing Assistants need to listen for and watch for these indicators of unmet needs. These observations should be noted in residents' charts and shared with the nursing team.

1. Unmet physiological needs

Unmet physiological needs may cause illness or even death. Lack of appetite or inability to feed themselves can result in residents not getting sufficient nourishing food or hydration.

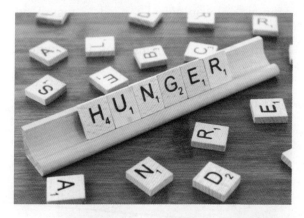

a. Complaints of hunger, irritability, weakness, and complaints of being cold or too warm

The most logical way for Nursing Assistants to discover residents' unmet physiological needs is through resident self-report of feeling hungry or thirsty. However, Nursing Assistants may have to discover these unmet needs through observation of resident lethargy, weakness, complaints of feeling achy or tired or too cold or too hot. If residents seem irritable, distracted, anxious, or tired, this may indicate unmet needs.

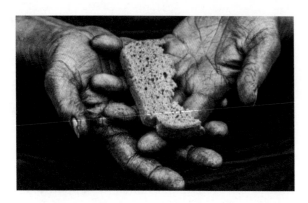

b. Alterations in vital signs and mental status

Unmet physiological needs may be indicated in residents' changes in vital signs. Nursing Assistants should look for a pattern in daily charting of vital signs. Residents may also present as not being as aware of their surroundings, slow of speech, lethargic, or disoriented.

2. Unmet psychological needs

Psychosocial needs of residents involve a sense of belonging and being loved. These needs may be met by the resident's family, friends, other residents, and caregivers. Psychosocial needs include mental, social, cultural, spiritual, and developmental needs.

a. Depression, anger, anxiety, and isolation

When psychosocial needs are unmet, residents may express anger, depression, irritation, or anxiety. They may withdraw from others, isolate themselves, and refuse to interact. Nursing Assistants who have daily contact with residents can aid in interaction by talking with residents, making them aware of activities in the long-term care facility and the community. They can aid is residents' accessing these social opportunities.

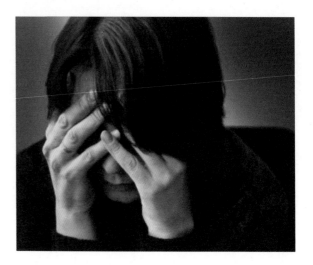

b. Physical ailments without an apparent cause

When social needs are unmet, residents may develop real or psychosomatic physical ailments. Nursing Assistants who have daily contact with residents should be sensitive to these physical ailments that have no apparent cause and report these symptoms to the nursing unit. Spending time with residents and getting them involved in facility activities is a good way to deal with these symptoms.

c. Expressions of feelings of worthlessness and loneliness

When residents are not actively involved in the facility, with their family or friends they can become despondent. They can feel lonely or worthless. Nursing Assistants who have daily contact with residents can help combat these feelings by listening to residents, conversing with them, and getting them involved in activities.

When their needs are not being met, residents can become uncooperative, stubborn, irritable, cantankerous, and physically and/or verbally abusive. Nursing Assistants who have daily contact with residents need to look beyond what residents are doing or saying to the root causes.

1. Looking beyond uncooperative along with having demanding and rude behavior

Some residents display consistent or occasional behavior that is rude and demanding. If their needs are not immediately met then they can become physically and/or verbally abusive. Nursing Assistants who have daily contact with residents need to look beyond what residents are doing or saying to what motivates this behavior .Perhaps, the resident is reacting to frustration over unmet needs. Maybe the resident has dementia symptoms or a reaction to medication.

2. Recognizing that a patient/resident has underlying needs for understanding and comfort

Nursing Assistants who have daily contact with residents need to look beyond what residents are doing or saying. Their behavior may be a cry for attention or comfort.

3. Responding with patience, kindness, and empathy

Regardless of how inappropriate residents' behavior is, as professionals, Nursing Assistants need to greet all residents with empathy and respect. Patience, kindness,

and caring concern for each resident are the sign of an introspective caregiver.

4. Consulting licensed nurse for assistance

If a resident continues to exhibit behavior that is physically or mentally hurtful to nursing staff and/or other residents, the Nursing Assistant should document this behavior and inform his/her immediate superior. Nursing Assistants are not expected to deal with continuing problems. It is their duty to report the situation to their supervisor.

In every instance of giving and receiving messages or information, there is a giver, a receiver, and a medium by which the information is conveyed. As part of the communication process, Nursing Assistants give and receive information with residents, with nursing supervisors and with other medical personnel.

When nursing staff receives information from others in the nursing unit or from residents it is the act of communicating. Communication also involves giving out information to the nursing team, to residents, or to outside care providers. Communication may be one-on –one or in a group.

Why is good communication so important? Good communication can help Nursing Assistants share accurate information necessary to deliver effective nursing care.

Poor communication skills can result in errors, omissions, and mistakes. These could endanger resident care.

Verbal or non-verbal communication

Communication may be spoken or written. It may be sent electronically or in the form of gestures. As a Nursing Assistant, it is very important that communication be accurate and understood. Where residents are nonverbal, message boards, written notes, and/or signing may need to be used. Where there is a language barrier, an interpreter may be needed.

Communication may take any or all of the following forms:

- **Establishing an eye contact**
  In an era when far too many residents and medical caregivers are staring at mobile devices, eye contact has become a lost nonverbal communication skill. When Nursing Assistants look residents and other medical staff in the eyes, it shows the resident or co-worker they are being listened to. It establishes attention and understanding what the information giver is saying. Eye contact when Nursing Assistants are communicating important information to residents and co-workers.

- **Addressing the resident by name**
  In a long-term care facility, residents don't always think their point of view is listened to or heeded. By using the resident's preferred name, Nursing Assistants create a link. Residents need to feel they are respected people—not just numbers. By taking the time to address residents by their names, it sends a message of empathy and concern.

- **Using appropriate oral and written language for each listener**
  When speaking with residents, Nursing Assistants will use different language than when they are talking to a healthcare professional. Nursing Assistants need to avoid medical terms and jargon when addressing residents.

- **Asking open-ended questions**
  When Nursing Assistants are trying to get an accurate picture of residents' health, a good strategy is to ask open-ended questions and wait for answer. So instead of asking a yes/no question, like: "Are you feeling okay today?" ask a more open-ended question, like: "How are you feeling today?" Open-ended questions seek resident input.

- **Making listening an art**
  Nursing Assistants are busy. They are responsible for several residents. However, listening carefully to what the resident is saying is an important part of skilled nursing care. Nursing Assistants need to listen to residents' complaints, concerns, and symptoms.

  It is also vital for Nursing Assistants to listen carefully to reports from other caregivers. If there is a request or data the Nursing Assistant does not understand, it is important to ask clarifying questions.

  A good strategy for making sure resident or healthcare professional information is understood is to repeat that information.

- **Using Positive Body Language**
  Body language is a powerful nonverbal communicator. A smile, a pat on the hand, a hug, a laugh, and an eye roll can communicate volumes to residents and staff. It is important for Nursing

Assistants to avoid negative body languages. These gestures: a frown, a sigh, a foot tap, arms crossed, glancing at the clock can send the wrong message to people.

Nursing Assistants are part of a helping profession. Positive body language is important in staff/resident communication but also in communicating with the nursing team.

- **Exuding respect and trust**
  Every resident has unique needs. Nursing Assistants, as primary caregivers, need to be respectful and compassionate to every resident. Every resident's concerns, needs, or fears are important and need to be taken seriously.

  If resident requests cannot be met, the Nursing Assistant needs to calmly explain why. Nursing Assistants should never make promise s for things they cannot provide. Residents appreciate honesty. It builds trust between the resident and the nursing team.

- **Sharing information in an accurate, timely manner**
  Sharing resident information with other members of the nursing team is extremely important. Whether this information is communicated orally or in written resident charts, it is vital that it be shared in accurate, professional language and that it be shared quickly. Charts and reports need to be provided for the next healthcare worker to see.

  Residents with hearing and/or vision challenges may require adaptive communication strategies.

Therapeutic communication: Use of therapeutic communication to promote optimum wellness

Therapeutic communication makes use of various techniques. These are aimed at preserving and enhancing the resident's physical, mental, and emotional well-being. Nursing Assistants provide patients with empathy, information, support and caring. It is also important that they maintain professional distance and objectivity with residents.

1. **Patient/resident-centered and goal oriented**

Therapeutic communication involves face-to-face interaction between the residents and their caregivers. The goal is to inform residents and involve them in decision making about their care. Therapeutic communication focuses on maintaining and advancing the physical and emotional well-being of each resident. The nursing team uses therapeutic communication techniques to provide information, engage, and support residents.

2. **Verbal or non-verbal communication**

While many therapeutic communication techniques involve getting and giving information from residents, Nursing Assistants also use non-verbal techniques.

Routes of communication

Routes of communication are often referred to as communication flow. Information flows from a source to a receiver. This flow can be lateral or horizontal. Horizontal communication is the flow of messages across an organization. Thus, information would be shared among colleagues in the nursing team. Horizontal communication goes directly without going through several levels of the facility. Reports during shift changes are an example of lateral communication.

The other route is downward, vertical, or top-down communication. This occurs in a facility when communication between those at different levels of authority within the facility. The communication flows from higher level to lower level. For example, if the employer issues a memo regarding Nursing Assistant procedures or attire, this would be vertical information flow. Downward communication is most often one-way communication. It gives Nursing Assistants directives or feedback about their job. It explains facility policies. Decisions are made and Nursing Assistants are expected to follow these directives.

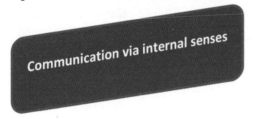

Nonverbal communication is unspoken or unwritten. It is information received by hearing, touching, smelling, and tasting. Nursing Assistants are keen observers of resident appearance, gestures, complaints, and concerns. Using their senses, they amass important information about residents' medical and psychosocial needs.

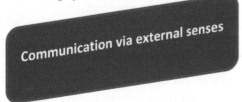

Verbal communication includes written information, oral report, body languages such as nods and gestures. Language shared by external senses gives clues to resident

health. This information is shared in written form in resident charts and orally at nursing team shift meetings.

Key steps and methods used in the communication process

Communicating involves series of actions or steps. There are several components. Understanding the communication process helps Nursing Assistants communicate effectively.

Important steps in communication

Nursing Assistants communicate several times in a given day in their long-term care facility. To communicate effectively with residents, nursing staff, and others, it's important to understand how the communication process works.

1. **Message**

This is the information that the sender is sharing with the receiver. This might be resident data.

2. **Sender**

The sender is the person providing the information. The sender might be the Nursing Assistant, the supervisor, an outside healthcare provider, the employer, or a resident.

3. **Receiver**

The receiver is the person for whom the written, oral, or nonverbal message is intended. The receiver might be the Nursing

Assistant, the supervisor, an outside healthcare provider, the employer, or a resident.

4. Interpretation

Often referred to as decoding, interpretation is done by the receiver. This is the meaning he/she takes from the message. Not all information is interpreted the way the sender intended. Several things might interfere: the complexity of the language, the resident's hearing or vision, the receiver's ability to comprehend, even a language barrier may interfere. Nursing Assistants need to be sensitive to a resident's ability to get meaning from the message.

Ensuring accurate interpretation can be accomplished by asking the sender clarifying questions. It can also be ensured by repeating or paraphrasing the information the sender gave.

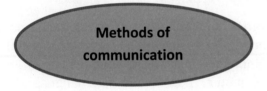

Methods of communication

Messages can be sent and received in a variety of ways. The chosen method of sharing may depend on the nature, complexity, or length of the message, the sender's preferred communication, or the age, mental acuity, or challenges of the receiver.

1. Verbal

Verbal messages are quicker and easier to send. They could be misinterpreted by the receiver. Sometimes, for legal reasons verbal messages is not the best medium.

2. Non-verbal

Consciously or unconsciously, Nursing Assistants can send positive or negative messages through a smile, a hug, a pat on the shoulder, a nod, a frown, or a sigh. These messages can be very powerful.

Types of non-verbal communication

a) Body language

Body language is nonverbal communicate of feelings or intentions. Body language includes posture, facial expressions, and hand gestures. Folded arms, toe tapping, and frowns are negative body language. Smiles, hand pats, high-fives, and thumbs up are positive body language.

b) Touch

Human touch is a powerful message of love and belonging. Most residents crave human touch. Nursing Assistants are primary caregivers. The power of touch can be a healing gesture.

c) Eye contact at patient's eye level

Establishing eye contact with the resident so he/she can look directly at the Nursing Assistant lets the resident know he/she is listened to and his/her comment, request, or complaint is acknowledged. Before Nursing Assistants ask for or deliver information, establishing eye contact is a good way to be sure the resident is focused on the communication.

Written

In a long-term care facility, residents and staff are surrounded by written information.

a) Labels; stickers or armbands for patient/resident precautions, room numbers, unit signs

These communication methods organize the facility. They provide vital information to staff and residents. They offer safety precautions to keep those who live and work there safe.

b) Visual labels; name tag, picture, uniform, picture board

For those who cannot read, do not read English, or have visual challenges room labels, photographs, illustrated name tags and bulletin boards, and picture displays provide important directional and social information.

3. Electronic

Because of improved technology, an aging population and those with special needs are finding new devices to extend their independence and make them more comfortable in their residential setting. As primary caregivers, Nursing Assistants have a role to play in helping residents access and use these assistive electronic devices.

Devices to develop sounds of words (verbal)

Called augmentative and alternative communication devices these electronic inventions help residents with communication disorders express themselves. These devices include everything from simple picture boards to computer programs that synthesize speech from text.

4. Computers/touch pads to type words or phrases onto screen (non-verbal)

For those who are physically incapable of speaking because of an illness, and injury, or mental or physical deterioration, electronic devices allow them to communicate. Picture boards or touch screens use pictures or symbols of items or activities used in daily life. A resident might touch the image of a glass to signal he/she wants a drink. Picture boards can be customized and expanded to fit the resident's education, age, and interests.

Keyboards, touch screens, and the resident's limited speech may be used in text displays. Both the sender and the receiver can exchange information while facing each other.

Speech-generating devices can now translate words or pictures into speech. Software programs convert personal computers into speaking devices.

5. Special communication skills

In order to assist special needs residents, Nursing Assistants need special communication skills. These range from using picture boards and sign language to employing electronic hardware and software programs.

a) Dementia-related communication skills

Over time, dementia will affect the ability to remember and understand such as names, dates and places. It also affects communication. Nursing Assistants working with residents who have dementia need special communication techniques. These include:

- Speaking slowly, clearly and in short sentences.
- Establishing eye contact before asking questions.

- Giving the resident time to respond, waiting calmly.
- Encouraging joining in conversations.
- Allowing the residents to speak for themselves.
- Maintaining a pleasant, respectful manner.
- Acknowledging what the resident has said.
- Offering the resident simple uncomplicated choices.
- Using alternative or augmented speech devices.

b) Use of a continuum of verbal and non-physical techniques

Combative residents can be physically dangerous to themselves, to other residents, and to staff. As first-line caregivers, Nursing Assistants need to know and use techniques to diffuse situations.

- Keeping the resident at arm's length.
- Being always on the alert to self-protection.
- Making sure the resident feels heard and listening to acknowledge what the resident has said by repeating the request.
- Addressing resident's demands calmly even if they are unreasonable.
- Explaining the situation simply an clearly.
- Telling the resident what you need him/her to do.
- Always working in teams when attending to combative residents.

Reasons for communication breakdown

Sometimes messages are not received or not understood. There may be a lot of reasons for a communication breakdown.

Verbal factors

The sender's message may not have reached the receiver. The receiver may have misunderstood the message or had an adverse reaction to it.

1. Criticism

Criticism is fault-finding. Nursing Assistants don't like to receive criticism from residents, co-workers, superiors, or their employer. Good Nursing Assistants consider the criticism, acknowledge it, and consider its merits, and act accordingly.

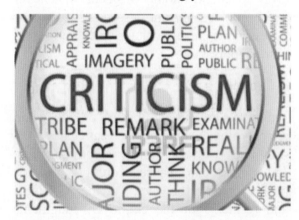

2. Value statements

Value statements are declarations about how the long-term care facility plans to value its residents, staff, and outside service providers. Value statements define how the residents, administration, and employees behave toward each other. A facility's priorities and actions are based on its stated values.

The purpose of a facility's value statement is to encourage behaviors from its staff, the residents, and administration. Value statements define the behavior of those who live and work at the facility. They also set the tone for visitors and outside service providers. Communication can break down when individuals don't know, don't understand, or refuse to follow stipulated value statements.

3. Interruptions

When interruptions in conversation occur, meaning can be lost. These interruptions may be electronic. They could be deliberate interruptions by the sender or the receiver. Nursing Assistants may encounter interruptions because of resident inability to hear or comprehend, or attend to what is being said. Outside noise may interrupt the message. Nursing Assistants may be called away to attend another resident. Whenever and however interruptions occur, it may be necessary to resume the conversation at a more opportune time.

4. Judgment

Judgments are based of biases, prejudice and stereotyping. Judgments can have a profound effect on communication. Judgments can cause conflict between professionals or between Nursing Assistants and residents or the employer. Judgments can create misunderstandings. Judgments may result in a communication breakdown.

Nursing Assistants should avoid making stereotypical judgments based on their prejudices towards the aged or those from a different religious or cultural background.

Stereotypical judgments often develop from ignorance, being misinformed, or making assumptions. If healthcare professionals are working with, or attending to the need of an individual, that person needs to be treated with respect and dignity. Conscious and unconscious beliefs should not enter into interactions. Judgments will unknowingly influence the communication of health professionals with potentially unpleasant results.

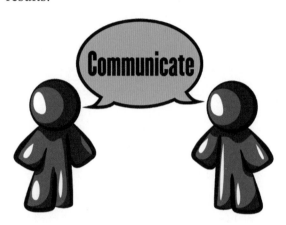

5. Language differences

Language barriers include linguistic barriers to communication. This might include difficulties in communication experienced by people or groups who speak a different language, or dialect. It might be that legal or medical jargon causes a lack of communication or comprehension.

Language barriers cause misunderstandings and misinterpretations. It is important that Nursing Assistants speak in simple, clear language when communicating with residents. Interpreters may be required.

Language barriers are the most common reason for ineffective communication that prevents the message from being conveyed or received.

6. Changing subjects

When conveying a message, it is important not to change the topic. It can be easy for this to occur if the receiver introduces extraneous information or deliberately steers the conversation away from the intent of the communication. Nursing Assistants can avoid digression by thinking through what they want to say or even rehearsing beforehand.

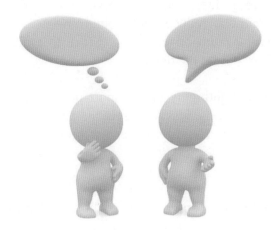

7. Excessive talking

When conveying a message it is always wise to keep it short and simple. Nursing Assistants should say what they have to say succinctly and stop talking. Repetition and needless explanations obscure communication.

8. Cliché and automatic answers

Residents and colleagues do not need or want to hear clichés. These often irritate or anger them. Nursing Assistants need to consider a heartfelt, "I'm sorry for your troubles." Sometimes, a sympathetic ear and silence are the best communicators of empathy.

Non-verbal factors

1. Body language

Negative body language can block communication or send the wrong message. Nursing Assistants need to be aware of their body language and avoid close positions like arms crossed or fist clenched.

2. Eye contact

To ensure the receiver is getting the message, it is important for the Nursing Assistant to establish eye contact with the message receiver. This establishes attention, focus, and trust.

3. Cultural beliefs, customs, and practices

The culture in which the sender of the message and the receiver of the information have been socialized influences the way they communicate. Traditions and beliefs affect the way both senders and receivers view communication. Culture, tradition, and beliefs of people are maintained through communication between individuals and groups.

Nursing Assistants need to be aware of and sensitive to the culture, custom, and beliefs of those with whom they interact. Differences may become communication barriers.

4. Environmental

Environment can have positive or negative effects on communication. Time, space, extraneous noise, distracting activities can produce barriers that inhibit effective communication. Nursing Assistants need to be sensitive to how things like the time of day, location, temperature, or competing groups can become barriers for effective communication

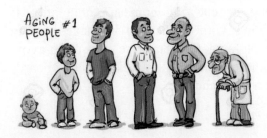

As residents' age or their medical conditions change, physiological communication barriers may develop. As primary caregivers, Nursing Assistants need to be aware of these barriers and compensate for them.

1. Hearing impairment

Besides noting to the nursing supervisor that a resident is having trouble communicating because of a hearing loss, there are several things Nursing Assistants can do to accommodate a hearing loss.

The Nursing Assistant can make sure he/she has the listener's attention before speaking. Touching a shoulder or hand is effective but simple.

Face-to-face contact and establishing eye contact are also important.

Nursing Assistants should try to support their message with facial expressions and body language.

Nursing Assistants should be careful to keep their hands away from their face. Speech will be clearer and the listener can use speech reading and other visual cues to get the message.

Speaking loudly or very slowly or exaggerating speech are not helpful to the person with a hearing loss. Talking while eating or chewing gum are unhelpful. If working with residents who have hearing loss Nursing Assistants are advised to avoid lip and tongue rings as well as heavy beards and moustaches.

If the listener has difficulty understanding Nursing Assistants should repeat it once. If there is still a difficulty, they should find a different way of giving the information.

When conversing with those who have a hearing loss, Nursing Assistants should attempt to reduce background noises. Turn off the radio or television. Move to a quiet space. Close the door.

Good lighting is also important. Residents with hearing loss can speechread. Nursing Assistants should ensure the lighting on in their face.

Thanks to today's technology, there are numerous apps that allow Nursing Assistants to speak into a smart phone and have the words show up on the screen. The person with hearing loss can then read the message. A good example is Dragon. The use of texting is also an efficient use to supplement communication.

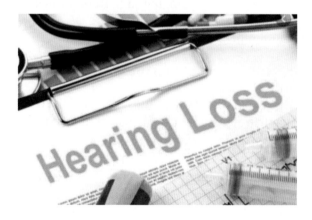

2. Loss of vision

It is important to report diminishing vision to the nursing supervisor. This may be corrected or improved by surgery or corrective lenses. There are several things Nursing Assistants can do to accommodate a vision loss.

- Nursing Assistants should identify themselves.
- Speaking naturally and clearly assists communication.
- Continuing to use facial expressions and body language can provide clues for visually challenged. Even when they cannot see these, body language and facial expressions are picked up in tone.
- Avoiding stilted language is a good communication strategy.
- Nursing Assistants should address the resident by name and speak directly to the person. He/she should strive for a dialogue.

3. Slowing of response time

Aging, medication, or medical condition may affect response time. The Nursing Assistant should wait patiently for a response, avoiding filling the space with talking or negative body language like toe tapping, sighing, frowning, finger tapping or glancing at the clock.

4. Drugs and Medication

Certain medications or dosages may make it difficult for residents to talk or to understand information. Nursing Assistants need to be aware that response time or comprehension may be affected by medication. If there are changes in communication, slurred words, lack of response, lethargy, or inattention, these should be reported to the nursing supervisor.

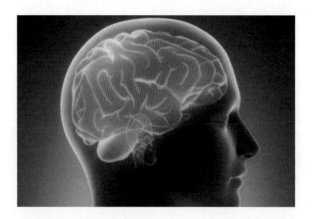

5. Cognitive changes

Cognitive functions like memory, concentration, attention, response, language, and focus may be affected by aging or deteriorated by disease, medication, or illness.

6. Loss of speech

Residents who have Dementia, Parkinson's, brain injury, or stroke may suffer from aphasia. Loss of the ability to communicate their needs, wants, fears, and concerns can be isolating for resident. It can leave them feeling angry, frustrated, terrified, and lonely.

Clearly, loss of speech can be a major communication barrier. If the loss is temporary, speech therapy may be effective. Augmented speech devices and software can help.

There are things Nursing Assistants can do to help bridge the communication gap.

When relying on touch to communicate with a senior, you resident, Nursing Assistants must be attentive to resident's nonverbal cues, such as body language.

Nursing Assistants provide hands-on care. They can express physical affection with a pat, a hug, or other gesture. Rubbing lotion on their arms or face, brushing or styling hair, and aiding with daily life functions show caring and respect. Touch therapy can be a simple gesture like holding hands. It goes a long way to show that someone is physically there for them.

When talking to a resident who has no speech, encourage the use of a picture board and yes/no signals. Signing is also a good way to bridge the gap.

Music and art therapy are also ways to aid in communication.

Not listening

Communication barriers may be caused by the receiver's not listening to the message. There may be several reasons for this.

1. Lack of concentration

The receiver may not be concentrating. This may be deliberated or unintentional.

a. Preoccupied

Perhaps the receiver is preoccupied with other issues or events in his/her life. Maybe the listener has little interest or doesn't understand the content.

b. Distracting noises

Background noises can obscure the messaged and can make hearing difficult.

c. Monotone voice

When the sender speaks in a monotone, it is easy for the listener to lose interest.

d. Negative behavior

If the listener has negative feelings about the topic or the speaker, his attention and/or response will be affected.

2. Selective hearing

Many people have selective hearing. They are emotionally deaf to the sender and/or the message. They simply tune out the speaker.

Use of effective communication/interpersonal skills

When communicating with resident, their family members, or guests, there are a few professional and legal things Nursing Assistants should keep in mind.

1. Communicating isn't just about talking. It is also about active listening
2. Nursing Assistants should watch the message their nonverbal communication is sending. They should also pay close attentions to the clues the nonverbal communication of others is giving.
3. Nursing Assistants should be very they are acting within the bounds of patient confidentiality under Health Insurance Portability and Accountability Act that protects patient privacy and personal information.

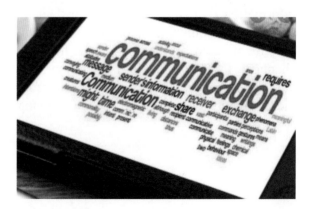

1. Introducing self

When communicating with residents, their family, or friends, Nursing Assistants should introduce themselves, giving their full name and title.

2. Using the patient's/resident's formal name initially

When first addressing residents, their family, or friends, Nursing Assistants should use their full name.

3. After initial introductions, asking patient/resident how he or she would like to be addressed

If invited to use a first name or a nickname, Nursing Assistants should note this on the resident's chart for future reference by the nursing team.

4. Explaining all tasks to the patient/resident before doing them

Before beginning a task, Nursing Assistants should explain in clear, simple language what is going to be done and why.

5. Patience

Nursing Assistants should listen actively and patiently to what a resident has to say, noting concerns, conditions, and symptoms on the resident's chart. These data should also be shared with the nursing team at shift change.

6. Using short sentences and asking for feedback

When communicating with residents, Nursing Assistants should use plain, jargon-free language and simple sentences. Seeking feedback involves residents in the decision-making process about their care.

7. Using eye contact

When communicating with residents, Nursing Assistants should establish eye contact to ensure resident engagement, focus, and understanding.

8. Speaking clearly, avoiding criticism, and avoiding interruption

When communicating with residents, Nursing Assistants should use positive verbal and nonverbal language. Interrupting the resident sends the message that what they have to say in unimportant. Speak clearly. Avoid contentious topics like religion or politics. Communication should not be critical, demeaning, off color, or disrespectful.

9. Clarifying information or conversation as needed

When communicating with residents, Nursing Assistants should use be sure the resident has received and understood the message by asking questions or having the resident repeat the information. A written reminder of key facts is also a good idea.

10. Knowing of body language of self and others

When communicating with residents, Nursing Assistants should remember how powerful body language is. It shows the receiver important information about emotions, attitudes, and relationships. Body language works in conjunction with the verbal clues. If there is a conflict between body language and words, the speaker may seem untrustworthy or deceptive.

11. Verbal and non-verbal messages

If there is a conflict between body language and words, the speaker may seem untrustworthy or deceptive. This sends the receiver a mixed message.

12. Using words that are easily understood

When communicating with residents, Nursing Assistants should avoid medical terms and complicated language. However, it is demeaning if the speaker is being condescending or patronizing.

13. Showing interest and respect

When communicating with residents, Nursing Assistants should attend to what the resident is saying and respond in a respectful tone.

14. Using a friendly tone of voice

When communicating with residents, Nursing Assistants should respond in a cheerful, professional manner.

15. Being positive while each interaction

When communicating with residents, Nursing Assistants should respond with positive affirmations to residents' questions, queries, comments, and complaints.

16. Ensuring confidentiality

When communicating medical information about residents in written and oral mode, Nursing Assistants should remember federal and state laws as well as facility policy regarding patient confidentiality. Nursing Assistants should share medical information only with the nursing team. The supervisor will decide what information should be shared and with whom.

Additional skills when communicating with patients/residents with special needs

When communicating with residents, Nursing Assistants should remember that those with special needs often require additional special equipment, technique, or personnel.

1. Cultural/language differences

When communicating with special needs residents whose mother tongue is not English, Nursing Assistants should seek the assistance of an interpreter or family member to ensure the message is understood.

Because of cultural differences, residents may receive verbal and nonverbal information through a different filter. When communicating with residents, Nursing Assistants should be aware of these differences.

2. Visual impairment

Visual impairment might require communicating with special needs residents using different techniques, hardware, and software.

a) Demonstrating surroundings to a visually impaired patient/resident

Modifications can be made to make residents' environment easier to navigate if they have visual challenges. Describe the room for them so they have a mental picture. Increase lighting—especially where rooms are dimly lit. When communicating with residents with visual challenges, Nursing

Assistants should approach them from their better vision side. Fall proof the room to avoid shiny surfaces that reflect glare and things like mats which could pose a threat.

b) Encouraging use of other senses

When communicating with residents, Nursing Assistants should encourage those with vision challenges to use other senses like hearing, smell, and touch to augment what residual vision they have.

c) Identifying self when entering patient's/resident's room

When communicating with residents, Nursing Assistants should identify themselves, their title, and why they are there.

d) Speaking aloud before touching patient/resident

When communicating with residents, Nursing Assistants should speak to the visually impaired resident before touching him/her.

e) Exploring the room with patient/resident

When orienting visually challenged residents to new rooms, Nursing Assistants should first provide a description of the room so the resident has a good mental picture. Then they should go on a physical tour of the room.

f) No rearrangement of the room

When interacting with residents, Nursing Assistants should never move objects or furniture. This sets up an obstacle course that could be dangerous.

g) Providing patient/resident with explanations about what will be and is being done

When working with residents, regardless of their special needs, Nursing Assistants should describe what they are doing. This dispels anxiety.

h) Letting patient/resident know when the nurse assistant is entering and leaving the room

When working with residents with special vision needs, Nursing Assistants should announce when they are leaving.

i) Keeping doors open

When working with residents with special vision needs, Nursing Assistants should leave the door open

j) Assisting as needed with meal set-up and eating

By assisting with table setting or tray set up, Nursing Assistants promoted independent feeding for visually impaired residents.

k) Speaking in a normal tone of voice

When working with residents with special vision needs, Nursing Assistants should speak directly to the resident in a normal conversational tone. Avoid words like blind, visually impaired, seeing, looking, and watching.

3. Hearing impairment

a) Gaining the attention of the patient/resident, using touch as appropriate

When working with residents with special hearing needs, Nursing Assistants should use touch or visual clues to get their attention.

b) Determining which ear has hearing loss

When working with residents with special hearing needs, Nursing Assistants should address them on the side of their better hearing.

c) **Checking to see if hearing aids are in, turned on and working**

When working with residents with special hearing needs, Nursing Assistants should ascertain that resident's hearing aids in place, turned on, cleaned, and have active batteries.

d) **Facing the patient/resident directly**

When working with residents with special hearing needs, Nursing Assistants should face the resident directly and at his/her eye level.

e) **Not blocking/covering your mouth or chewing gum**

When working with residents with special hearing needs, Nursing Assistants should not block their lips with hands, facial hair, body jewelry, gum, food, or other obstruction to speech reading.

f) **Reducing/eliminating background noise and other distractions**

When working with residents with special hearing needs, Nursing Assistants should turn off TV or radio, block competing noises by going to a quiet area, another room, or by closing the door.

g) **Speaking slowly, directly, and clearly when addressing a hearing-impaired patient/resident**

When communicating with residents with special hearing needs, Nursing Assistants should speak slowly, naturally, in a normal tone an in an appropriate tone. Nursing Assistants should address the resident directly by name.

h) **Using short sentences and simple words**

When communicating with residents with special hearing needs, Nursing Assistants should use short sentences and language the resident will understand.

i) **Repeating and rephrasing statements as needed**

When communicating with residents with special hearing needs, Nursing Assistants should repeat the message once. If the resident does not understand, the Nursing Assistant should then rephrase the message.

j) **Asking the patient/resident to repeat instructions to ensure understanding**

When communicating with residents with special hearing needs, a good way to ascertain whether the resident understood is to have him/her repeat the message to the Nursing Assistant.

k) **Knowing of messages sent by facial expressions and body language**

When communicating with residents with special hearing needs, Nursing Assistants should be hyperaware of the power of nonverbal communication.

4. Speech impairment

Dysphasia is partial loss of speech. Aphasia is total loss of speech. The two are often referred to as aphasia. When communicating with residents with speech impairment, Nursing Assistants should be aware of special equipment to help those residents.

a) **Providing writing materials and assistance as needed**

When communicating with residents with speech impairment, Nursing Assistants should provide written materials, tablets, computer programs, and software assistive speech materials and techniques.

b) Letting patient/resident use own words

Where residents have some speaking ability, when communicating with residents with speech impairment, Nursing Assistants should encourage them to use their own words. Residents should be allowed time to send or respond to messages.

c) Using picture boards or point boards

When communicating with residents with speech impairment, Nursing Assistants should be a use language augmentative devices such as pictured boards, video and audio/video hardware and software.

d) Standing in front of patient/resident

When communicating with residents with speech impairment, Nursing Assistants should stand directly in front of the resident so he/she can see the Nursing Assistant's face and mouth.

e) Avoiding finishing words and sentences for the patient/resident

When communicating with residents with speech impairment, Nursing Assistants should be patient and wait for the resident to finish a thought. Professionals should never fill in words for the resident or appear impatient.

5. Mental impairment (confusion, dementia)

When communicating with residents with a mental impairment, Nursing Assistants should know the symptoms and special techniques required.

a) Keeping directions simple

When communicating with residents with a mental impairment, it is important for Nursing Assistants to keep directions simple and one-step.

b) Repeating information as needed

When communicating with residents with a mental impairment, it is important for Nursing Assistants to repeat directions slowly and simply as often as needed.

c) Offering frequent general reassurance

Those with mental impairments can become confused and agitated. When communicating with residents with a mental impairment, it is important for Nursing Assistants to remain calm and offer verbal and nonverbal assurance to the resident.

d) Always having patient's/resident's attention before speaking

When communicating with residents with a mental impairment, it is important for Nursing Assistants to make sure they have the resident's attention before sharing information.

Conflicts and measures for conflict resolution

Conflict resolution offers a way for residents and nursing staff, nursing staff and administration, or residents' families and administration to reach a peaceful solution to a disagreement or issue. This dispute may concern personal, financial, political, or emotional concerns.

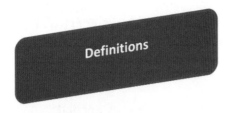

Definitions

Conflict

Conflict occurs when two sides cannot agree. There are four basic types: Inner conflict is within oneself. Conflict with others might be a dispute or disagreement. Conflict with the environment might include people fighting a storm, a flood, a drought, or a hurricane. Conflict with the supernatural might be between an individual and a higher power.

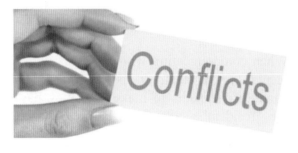

A controversy or disagreement

A disagreement ensues when two sides have opposing opinions about an issue. They can't agree.

When what a person has and what a person wants is different

A controversial issue results in a dispute or disagreement when there is a difference of opinion or values held by two opposing sides.

A pattern of energy

The way in which the disputants feel about a conflict is referred to as emotional resolution or emotional energy

Nature's primary motivation for change

Basically, humans' drive for change can come from within or it can be external. Seeking improvement, happiness, greater comfort, security, or well-being motivates people to seek change.

Conflict resolution

Conflict resolution is a way for opposing parties to attempt a peaceful solution to a disagreement. When a dispute arises, conflict resolution is often the best course of action to negotiate an agreement.

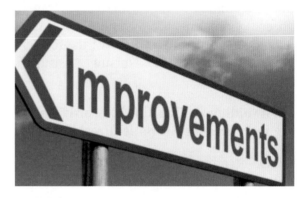

The aim of conflict resolution is to eliminate acrimony that could devolve into physical conflict.

Conflict myths

There are several myths regarding conflict.

1. Conflict is a negative

There is a belief that harmony is positive and conflict is negative. Conflict is inevitable. It is part of the cycle of human relationships.

2. Conflict is a contest

Some people use the words competition and conflict interchangeably. C ompetition is a rivalry between two groups or two individuals over an outcome. They both want to win. In conflict resolution, sides want to reach an agreement pleasing to both sides.

3. The presence of conflict is a sign of poor management

The presence of conflict means two sides have differing opinions. It is no reflection of poor or good management.

4. Conflict, if left alone, will take care of itself

It is rare that conflict can be resolved without opposing sides compromising.

5. Conflict must be resolved

Conflicts can be resolved in a several ways. These include: negotiation, mediation, arbitration, and litigation. Conflict resolution draws on the same principles of collaborative negotiation or deal making. Not all conflicts can be resolved peacefully.

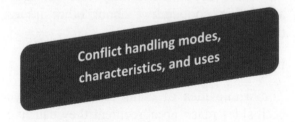

Conflict handling modes, characteristics, and uses

There are several conflict management styles.

1. Competing

Like a contest or race, competing involves opposing parties vying for the win.

a) Uncooperative and assertive

Competing is assertive and uncooperative. It's like a tug of war. There are winners and losers. Each side pursues its own concerns at the expense of the other side.

b) Power-oriented

Competition is a power struggle. Each side uses its resource to come out on top and gain more power.

c) Uses

Competition can spur greater work ethic. It can nurture more creative solution, better products and services. Competition is the reason for new technology, scientific breakthroughs, more efficient processes, and more innovative products. Competition increases economic growth and improved lifestyle.

2. Accommodating

The accommodating style makes sacrifices. Instead of being competitive, it stresses selflessness. It is low on assertiveness. Accommodating negotiators are willing to make major concessions to preserve the relationship. This works well when the issues in question are of little importance to one side.

a) Uncooperative and assertive

Those employing accommodation treat the other side with respect. They are cooperative and unassertive.

b) Self-sacrifice

Accommodators are willing to give major concessions to keep the other side happy.

c) Uses

As the owner of the facility or a manager of the nursing team if you want employees to take on a responsibility and learn from it, accommodating may be a good way to achieve this.

If, in negotiating the issue, one side has no wiggle room against the other and there is no room to compete, accommodation may be the only alternative. However, it leaves the other side bitter and disillusioned.

3. Avoiding

Just as it implies, avoiding means one side refuses to discuss the issue.

a) Uncooperative and unassertive

While like accommodating avoiding is an unassertive style, it is also as uncooperative as competition.

b) Not addressing conflict

Those who use avoiding fail to even discuss a conflict. It's as though the other side doesn't even recognize the problem.

c) Uses

When using avoiding, one side knows there is a conflict. However, that side has decided not to deal the issue. Tactics include ignoring the issue, sidestepping, being uncooperative, or withdrawing from interaction. Avoiding does not even acknowledge the needs, complaints, or issues of the other side. The goal is to avoid conflict as long as possible. It may buy time but it leaves the other side frustrated, dissatisfied, and angry.

4. Collaborating

This style is often called win/win. Collaboration attempts to ensure both sides are satisfied.

a) Cooperative and assertive

Collaboration requires open discussion. Both sides are assertive and honest about the issues and concerns. Both sides enter the negotiation with a spirit of cooperation. Both sides are willing to, explore alternatives to reach a solution. There is honesty and commitment on both sides.

b) Seeks mutual satisfaction

The goal of collaboration is to reach a settlement where both sides are satisfied with the outcome.

c) Uses

Collaboration works well when both sides are eager to make a commitment for their mutual benefit and for the good of the facility and its residents.

5. Compromising

Compromising is a style most used in negotiation. Compromising often comes down to haggling over issues and splitting the difference in a tit-for-tat ending that is half way between both side's beginning positions

a) Somewhat assertive and cooperative

Compromise involves both sides protecting the issues about which they feel strongest and being cooperative about other issues they care less about.

b) Mutual satisfaction

The whole idea of compromise is to have both sides reach an agreement they can live with.

c) Middle ground

Compromise in about meeting somewhere as close to the middle as both sides can get still keeping the things they feel strongly about. The theory is "give a little to get a little".

d) Uses

Early on, parents teach children about compromise. This technique is often a valuable in the workplace. Owners of a facility have to balance their concerns about profit and resident satisfaction against having employees who feel needed and respected for the job they do.

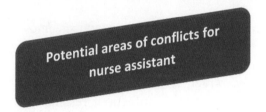

As employees of a long-term care facility, Nursing Assistants may be faced with areas of conflict with supervisors, with coworkers, and even with residents.

1. Attendance

The smooth running of a facility is dependent upon employees showing up for their shift. As professionals, Nursing Assistants are expected to be present and ready to work. If they have a legitimate reason for absence, Nursing Assistants need to let their supervisor know as far ahead as possible.

2. Punctuality

The smooth running of a facility is dependent upon Nursing Assistants showing up for their shift on time. Valuable resident information is shared by the outgoing shift before the incoming shift begins. As professionals, Nursing Assistants are expected to be on time and ready to work. If for some unavoidable reason they are going to be late, they need to let their supervisor

know. Habitual tardiness is not the sign of a professional.

3. Safety

When working in a long-term care facility, Nursing Assistants may encounter issues of personal or resident safety. They need to know the rules and regulations regarding workplace safety.

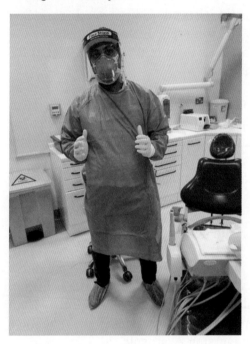

a) Personal

Viruses like COVID have, historically, been contracted by nursing staff and residents through lack of or inadequate Personal Protective Equipment. Better protective gear, stricter adherence to safety precautions, and better staff education and training is a must.

Other issues of physical, mental, and emotional safety for Nursing Assistants include working safely amid the lifting, moving, and repositioning of residents. Nursing Assistants should know and follow protocol for these physical demands. These protocols were put in place for staff safety and the safety of the residents.

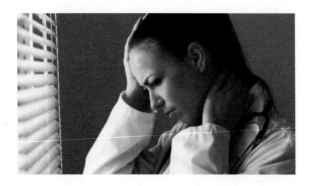

Nursing Assistants can't care for residents if they are not well. Ensuring safety of the workforce staff and in the facility is vital for patient safety.

Workplace safety includes both the physical and psychological safety of Nursing Assistants. According to the Occupational Safety and Health Administration reports hospitals and long-term care facilities are among the most dangerous places to work. There are high rates of musculoskeletal injuries and needle stick accidents.

There is intense psychological pressures from demanding residents, understaffing, disruptive behaviors, disrespect from residents and supervisors, and even violence against Nursing Assistants.

These issues impact Nursing Assistant health and have a direct impact on patient safety.

Nursing Assistants cannot perform at their best if their work environment is physically or psychological unsafe.

b) **Patient/resident**

Hospitals and long-term care facilities are charged with keeping patients safe from falls, injuries, and infections. Such issues as hand hygiene, medication errors, and environmental hazards often are a concern.

Healthcare-associated infections have been a long-time concern for healthcare facilities, both clinically and financially. Outbreaks like SARS, Ebola, and COVID-19 are always a nightmare in a patient/resident facility where many of the residents are fragile. Preparedness, the right equipment, and strict following of federal, state, and facility procedures can avoid many disasters. The Centers for Disease Control note that one in every 25 patients will contract an healthcare associated infection during a hospital stay. Long-term care facilities have the same problem.

In the current prescribing practices and a lack of new antibiotics, pathogens are becoming resistant at alarming rates. Presently, over two million Americans contract a bacterial infection resistant to antibiotics. The best defense against bacterial and viral infections is strict adherence to hand hygiene. Sadly, hand hygiene compliance is still only forty percent. Healthcare workers clean their hands less than half the time they enter resident/patient rooms. Although the recent COVID situation has changed this, estimates are that the situation will return to hand hygiene laxity.

Health IT is intended to speed up and make data more accessible in order to improve outcomes. Unfortunately, one of the outcomes is human error and patient safety mistakes. Communication around patient care is critical. It demands exact communicate of patient health information and changes in care to provide the next caregiver with vital information that will prevent diagnostic errors.

3. Medication errors occur more often than expected

The Institute of Medicine estimates that annually nearly one and a half million Americans experience a medication error. These are largely communication errors.

They occur most often between a resident and the pharmacist or the facility handing resident medication to the resident. These errors occur less than half as often when an electronic reconciliation tool is used. If this is unavailable, double checking medications in a two-Nursing Assistant approach is the next best safety precaution

Involving residents in the decision-making process regarding their healthcare and long-term care plans has greatly improved many safety issues. Technology has also improved fall and injury incidents.

When residents, the nursing team, and the facility make an ongoing, concerted effort aimed at resident safety, the results are gratifying.

4. Professional behavior

Being professional Nursing Assistant involves delivery of resident care ethically, competently, knowledgeably and empathetically. Nursing Assistants are bound by the professional code of their profession as well as the agreement they signed with their employer. They are legally obligated to fulfill their duties as outlined in federal and state law.

5. Attitude

Nursing Assistants need a have a caring, compassionate attitude towards residents. Many under their care are elderly and medically fragile people who
Need help with daily living activities. Nursing Assistants can greatly improve residents' quality of life with a cheerful, helping, empathetic attitude.

Willingness to work as part of a nursing team sets a happy, productive tone in the facility, making it a safer, more pleasant place to work.

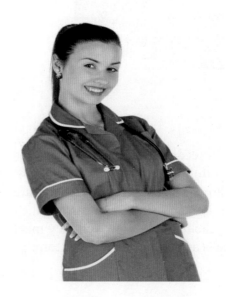

6. Appearance and hygiene

Neat, clean, professional attire and good personal hygiene are signs of a dedicated Nursing Assistant.

7. Performance

Nursing Assistants provide primary care to patients in hospitals or residents of long-term care facilities. Nursing Assistants work under the supervision of a nursing supervisor. They follow care instructions provided by doctors, outside service professionals through the direction of their immediate supervisor.

8. Confidentiality

Resident confidentiality involves the resident's right to his/her privacy of personal, identifiable medical information. These data should be available only to the healthcare professionals who serve this resident. Patient confidentiality is protected by federal, state regulations, and by the facility's policy on confidentiality.

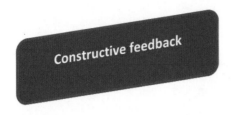

1. Definition

Constructive feedback in the workplace is supportive information given to employees. It reveals how well Nursing Assistants are doing their job, the skills and talents they bring to the facility, and how well they meet resident needs as part of the nursing team.

2. Use

Constructive feedback is designed to applaud Nursing Assistants' skills and effort. It also points out areas of potential improvement and helps to identify solutions.

The 4 "E's" of giving constructive feedback

1. Engage

Constructive feedback seeks to engage employees. Its goal is not to nitpick, lecture, or demoralize. Sneak attacks where employees are caught off guard are seldom productive. The evaluator should set up a specific time for feedback.

a) Prepare

Before giving feedback it is important to list areas for comment. Next, the evaluator should collect specific information, employee examples of those behaviors, organize it, and prepare to meet with the Nursing Assistant.

b) Link feedback with goals

Feedback should be linked to the goals of the facility as stated in its policy and mission statement.

c) Focus discussion

Generalizations are unproductive. Instead, the evaluator should provide specific demonstrated strengths and provide the Nursing Assistant with examples. In preparing for the meeting, the evaluator should compile a list of examples of employee strengths and weaknesses in action. The follow up should include suggestions for employee improvement.

2. Empathize

It is important to let Nursing Assistants know you are aware of and sensitive to their workplace pressures.

a) Environment

The time and place of the constructive feedback meeting are important. The evaluator should choose a quiet, private place that is not intimidating to the employee.

b) Timing

Evaluators should schedule meetings at a time when Nursing Assistants aren't feeling pressured to get back to their shift or to meet home responsibilities. There may be a long list of things the evaluator would like to see improvement. However each item raises stress and anxiety. To avoid overwhelming to Nursing Assistant, the evaluator should keep sessions short and focused.

3. Educate

Part of constructive feedback is aimed at teaching the Nursing Assistants where they are successful and where areas for improvement exist. Moreover, suggestions for improvement should be specific and helpful.

a) Describing observations

In preparation for the meeting, the evaluator prepared a list of areas for discussion. He/she then collected examples of Nursing Assistant behaviors. This is the time for sharing these observations.

b) Identifying impact of behavior

Besides identifying the Nursing Assistants behaviors, it is important for the evaluator to note the positive and/or negative effects these behaviors have on the individual, residents, colleagues, and the reputation of the facility.

c) Remaining objective

Constructive feedback is not a personal attack. It is important for the evaluator to stick to the identified areas and observed behaviors. There is no room in constructive feedback for opinions, feelings, conjecture, second-hand information, or biases.

4. Enlist

For constructive feedback to achieve its goals, it is important for the evaluator to encourage Nursing Assistant involvement.

a) Elicit response

The evaluator should ask the Nursing Assistant to comment on his/her observations. The evaluator might even turn the tables, asking the Nursing Assistant to comment on the evaluator's performance

b) Guiding toward solution

Criticism is actually low on Maslow's hierarchy of needs. It can feel like physical pain or a threat to security. Feedback sends those who are being evaluated into protective mode. Nothing is achieved toward a solution at this stage. That is why it is vital to point out strength and positive observation as well.

In moving toward solutions to an area for improvement, evaluators can map out doable actions and elicit Nursing Assistant ideas as well.

Objective of constructive feedback

Badly delivered feedback may create animosity, anger, resentment, lack of respect, and permanently damaged employer-employee relations. However, there are some important benefits.

Employee feedback can improve performance. If Nursing Assistants are not told how they are doing, they work in limbo. Feedback provides guidance, motivation and a clear sense of purpose.

Feedback nurtures growth. It shows Nursing Assistants the actions they can take to become even better at their job. It gives them an opportunity—and even impetus to learn and refine techniques.

Constructive feedback can improve employee/employer relations. If feedback is honest, fair and constructive, it can actually help further engage worker commitment and enthusiasm for the job and the facility.

Affection is as powerful as a drug. It nurtures feelings of self-worth, self-confidence, trust and connectedness. Touch has been shown to reduce cortisol—the stress hormone. Even as little as twenty seconds of hugging, massage, back rubs, or gentle stroking can trigger the release of oxytocin.

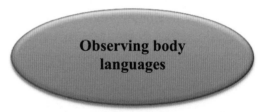

Cultural beliefs regarding touch

Touch can have profound meaning in some cultures and a far different effect in others. In Middle Eastern cultures and in Orthodox Jewish cultures, touching between men and women is avoided. Asians don't like being touched. Physical contact is infrequent in the Asian cultures. Most Hispanics are comfortable with hands-on care.

In Japan, Australia, New Zealand, Portugal, and Scandinavian countries, touch is considered rude. However, in Turkey, France, Italy, Greece, and Spain, touch is encouraged.

Long-term care facilities emphasize the importance of touch for all its therapeutic properties. However, they caution Nursing Assistants to be sensitive to cultural differences.

1. Modesty

In some cultures, it is considered improper to appear in public with the face, head, arms, and/or legs exposed. Nursing Assistants should be sensitive to this, note it, and respect resident wishes.

2. Gender of caregiver

Some residents are uncomfortable being bathed or other touch activity by a member of the opposite sex. Nursing Assistants should be sensitive to this, note it, and respect resident wishes.

3. Touching of body after death

Every culture has different ideas about touching the body of a loved one after death.

Some bathe, dress, and prepare a body for burial. Others hold vigil, holding the hand and stroking the forehead of a loved one.

In India in some cultures, the dead are paraded through the streets, dressed in colors that highlight their virtues. In Zoroastrian tradition, a dead body is believed to defile everything it touches.

Nursing Assistants should be sensitive to cultural differences about touching the dead, note it, and respect resident wishes.

4. Hugging and kissing

Hugging is not very common in Asia including China and Vietnam. Even the parent-child relationships lack physical intimacy. Many Arabian and Asian cultures view physical contact between unmarried couples or opposite sexes as unacceptable.

Even in North America, kissing across different cultures varies widely. In some cultures, children may kiss on the mouth when they are young. They are discouraged from kissing when they reach puberty.

Nursing Assistants should be sensitive to cultural differences about hugging and kissing, note it, and respect resident wishes.

Observing body languages

Different cultures read different meaning from body language. For example, direct eye contact may be expected in one country, but be inappropriate in another. Some other important nonverbal cues to pay attention to are hand gestures, personal space, and even posture.

1. Hands and extremities

Nursing Assistants should pay attention to how residents' arms and feet are positioned while speaking. In some cultures, folding arms across the chest is standoffish or even insulting.

Sitting positions are also very important. Feet positioning so the soles show while sitting is considered as rude in Middle Eastern countries.

2. Eyes

In some cultures, direct eye contact is expected. It is seen as a sign of trust, honesty, acceptance, and belonging. In other countries, eye contact is inappropriate.

3. Gestures

Some cultures are very demonstrative. They make use of gestures to express love, acceptance, anger, or threats.

4. Posture

Posture is also a key in understanding body language. Erect, straight posture indicates leadership, dominance, control, and self-confidence. Poor posture indicates low self-esteem, lack of control, fear, and inferiority.

Nursing Assistants need to pay attention to their posture and that of colleagues and residents.

5. Regression to child-like postures or behaviors

When mentally or physically ill, threatened, depressed, traumatized, or grief stricken, residents may revert to child-like behaviors like assuming the fetal pose, rocking, thumb sucking, or weeping uncontrollably.

Personal space

It is important for Nursing Assistants to pay attention to how residents feel about personal space during conversation is vital. Standing too close may be seen as a sign of aggression in some cultures. Stand too far away may seem insincere in others.

Japanese prefer more of distance. In Latin American cultures, people are very touchy and affectionate. Latin Americans stand very close to the other person.

Common psychological defense mechanisms

Defense mechanisms are psychological strategies. These are used unconsciously to protect against unacceptable, traumatic thoughts, feelings, ideas, or situations.

A. Denial

Often referred to as "the ostrich approach" denial is a commonly used defense mechanism. An individual is said to be in denial if he/she refuses to accept reality. Instead, he/she block facts, medical proof, or circumstances, refusing to deal with it. Denial is commonly used to avoid the emotional impact of abandonment, pain, death, financial ruin, or disease.

B. Projection

Projection occurs when an individual projects thoughts or feelings about a person to the other person. Here is an example. If a Nursing Assistant dislikes a resident but feels uncomfortable admitting it, she/he might say the resident dislikes him/her instead.

C. Anger

Feeling hurt, lonely, rejected, abandoned, the individual expresses these emotions as anger. The goal is to mask the hurt so no one will show pity.

D. Rationalization

Individuals may attempt to explain their own undesirable behaviors with invented "facts." The aim is to feel comfortable with the choice. Here is an example: Nursing Assistants who are angry because co-workers for not being on time are habitually late themselves.

E. Regression

When individuals feel threatened or anxious they may return to an earlier stage of Maslow's hierarchy. Residents struggling to cope with situations may return to a fetal position, rocking, singing to themselves, sleeping a doll or a stuffed animal. They might binge eat or drink, finding comfort in basic human needs.

F. Displacement

Displacement involves taking out feelings of anger on people, things, or objects that are less threatening. Those with rage at work take their feelings out on racing their car, punching a wall, chopping wood, kicking the dog, yelling at the neighbor, or slapping their child.

G. Conversion

Negative feelings like anxiety or stress resulting from a bad experience manifest themselves in physical symptoms and illnesses like migraines or ulcers or aching muscles, or a disease like MS.

H. Repression

Strong feelings are bottled up. This is a dangerous defense mechanism. Pent up emotions breed ulcers, stress, and migraines. Eventually, like a pressure cooker, the individual blows up

I. Sublimation

Those who choose this defense mechanism redirect strong emotions or feelings into an object. Here's an example: Instead of striking out at a combative resident, the Nursing Assistant runs, jogs, hits a punching bag, or does kickboxing to wear off pent up anger.

J. Substitution/compensation

In substitution, an unattainable goal is replaced by an attainable one. Those who wanted to be doctors opted to become Nursing Assistants.

K. Identification

Identification with the aggressor is a defense mechanism. The victim adopts the behaviors of the aggressor. That's why those who are bullied bully others.

Family communication/interaction patterns and the role of the Nurse Assistant

General principles when communicating with patient/resident families

Nursing Assistants have daily, face-to-face contact with residents. Frequently, they are also present when friends or relatives visit

1. Showing respect for all family structures and members

When interacting with family members, Nursing Assistants should be pleasant, respectful, polite, and nonjudgmental.

2. Listening to family members

Family members frequently want to voice concerns, vent frustrations, express anxiety, or ask questions. Nursing Assistants should offer a listening ear but avoid commenting, making promises, or offering information.

a. Showing courtesy, respect, and support

In discussion with residents' family, Nursing Assistants should be courteous, empathetic, and supportive.

b. Allowing uninterrupted time

Friends and family should be allowed and even encouraged to have visiting time uninterrupted by facility activities and routines as much as possible.

c. Providing privacy as indicated

If the resident's room does not provide privacy, the Nursing Assistant might suggest an alternative location.

3. Avoiding involvement in family matters

It is unprofessional and legally dangerous for Nursing Assistants to offer opinions, suggestions, or advice on family matters.

4. Maintaining patient/resident confidentiality

Nursing Assistants are bound by their professional code of conduct, the rules of the facility, as well as state and federal laws to protect resident confidentiality.

5. Encouraging family to participate in care planning and care as allowed by facility policy

The guidelines of the facility encourage residents and their families to be part of the resident's long-term care plan. In conversation, Nursing Assistants might remind them of that.

Providing information about the facility

While providing resident information to family and friends is a breach of professional conduct, Nursing Assistants are encouraged to share this facility information including:

1. Telephone numbers
2. Cell phone regulations
3. Visiting hours
4. Location of cafeteria/vending machines
6. Gift shop
7. Public restrooms
8. Orient to patient/resident activities
9. Social Services
10. Chaplain

Encouraging family members to provide information about patient/resident preferences

Whenever there is an opportunity to learn more about residents' preferences, hobbies, interests, skills, hopes, and dreams Nursing Assistants should welcome this information. Family and friends can be a valuable resource.

Social and cultural factors influencing communication

Social determinants of health may include physical conditions in our environment. Social conditions can influence health and well-being of individuals and communities. One of these is culture.

Culture

1. Shared, learned customs, beliefs and values of a group of people

Humans are social animals. From the group that reared them, humans learn a set of customs, beliefs and a value system. This is passed on by modeling, mentoring, and oral tradition.

2. Beliefs, religion, values, attitudes, likes and dislikes, rituals, foods, celebrations, and language

Cultural groups develop a common set of attitudes and religious beliefs. Tied to that is a common language, preferences for foods, rituals, and cultural celebrations.

3. Influence of culture on the reaction of residents and families to health and health care services

A resident's culture colors how he/she views healthcare, healthcare providers, traditional medicine, and ill health.

4. Rituals

Some cultures espouse alternative medicine and cultural beliefs about healing.

Physical and psycho-social reactions to illness and disability

1. Stress responses

Many have a stressful response to illness or disability. On the other hand, research has shown that many illnesses are triggered or exacerbated by stress. Examples include MS, ulcers, irritable bowel syndrome, heart disease, type 2 diabetes, and some cancers.

a. Variation of common physiological responses with each individual

Individuals deal with stress differently and common physiological responses may vary with each individual.

b. Pattern of responses based on experiences

Stress reactions often become a common response. Even symptoms will be the same.

c. Desirable and undesirable effects

While stress often spurs excellence of product, it can also create things like writer's block, performance anxiety, avoidance, erosion of confidence, mental or physical breakdown, and severe illness.

2. Physical loss or disability

When residents enter a long-term facility, their lives have undergone dramatic and sometimes traumatic change. Nursing Assistants who have daily contact with residents can bridge these changes with friendly, kind, caring, professional support.

a. Loss of spouse, friends, or family

Residents may have moved to the facility because of the loss of a spouse. Friends or family may no longer be close by.

b. Loss of homes, employment, security, or economics

Because of an illness, an injury, a disability, or a change in medical condition, the resident may have been forced to give up his home and/or his job. His economic security may now be in jeopardy.

c. Loss of control of life, independence, driving

Residents may have lost their ability to do daily living activities. They may no longer be able to drive anywhere they want to go. This loss of control and independence is frustrating and depressing.

d. Loss of control and function of body and mind

Some illnesses and medical conditions leave residents unable to think and/or control bodily functions. This is embarrassing and demoralizing.

e. Fewer choices and options

Now in a facility the resident has fewer social choices. He/she may have had to give up hobbies, pastimes, church, social get togethers, and even family holidays.

3. Emotional reactions

Faced with loss, lack of independence, loss of control, and inability to do daily living activities, it is little wonder residents react with strong emotions that include:

- Anger
- Uselessness
- Fear
- Grief
- Feelings of damage
- Dependency
- Depression
- Suspicion
- Sense of helplessness

- Loneliness
- Anxiety
- Guilt
- Frustration

Helpful Nurse Assistant actions

Nursing Assistants can play a vital role in helping residents work through these emotions.

1. Observing patient/resident for indications of emotional stress

As primary caregivers, Nursing Assistants are in a position to observe and hear indicators of resident stress and anxiety. This information should be documented in the resident's chart and shared with the nursing team,

2. Being a good listener

Nursing Assistants can improve residents' mental, emotional, social, and physical health by taking the time to visit with residents and listen to their concerns and joys.

3. Being patient and understanding

Nursing Assistants should strive to meet doable resident requests as quickly and efficiently as possible. A pleasant, patient attitude is a professional response.

4. Helping patient/resident function as independently as possible

Many residents, through aging and/or illness will have challenges to complete their daily living activities. Nursing Assistants should focus on things residents are able to accomplish independently and those that can be supported with technology and mobility aids.

5. Letting patient/resident know that staff cares about his or her wellbeing

By word and deed, Nursing Assistants should do whatever they can to let residents know the nursing team is committed to supporting their good health.

6. Being non-judgmental

Making judgments about cultures unlike their own is not the sign of a professional

7. Always treating all patients/residents with dignity

Regardless of race, culture, religion, disability, or age, every resident deserved respect.

8. Being respectful of all cultures and belief systems

Nursing Assistants can respect and learn about belief systems different from their own.

9. Taking time to learn about cultures and practices

When Nursing Assistants take an interest in the beliefs and practices of the residents' cultures, it adds a depth of understanding to the resident/healthcare professional relationship.

Communication between the members of healthcare team

Health care communication

In fulfilling their professional duties, Nursing Assistants use communication every day. Communication is absolutely necessary. Through oral and written communication, Nursing Assistants share resident information with the nursing unit. Using verbal and nonverbal communication Nursing Assistants seek and share information with residents. Communication helps professionals build relationships, share ideas, and form bonds with residents.

Learning and developing good communication skills is vital to providing competent resident care. It aids professionals in building a network.

Nursing Assistants use four main types of communication on a daily basis. These include: Verbal, nonverbal, written, and visual.

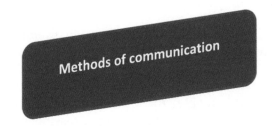

Methods of communication

1. Verbal

Verbal communication uses language to give information by speaking or using sign language. Verbal communication is used in speeches, lectures, oral reports, and presentations. Video conferences, phone calls, meetings, and conversations use verbal communication. This is a fast and efficient communication mode.

Nonverbal and written communication often provides backup or further clarification to a verbal message.

Good verbal communication skills include:

- **A strong, clear speaking voice.** Everyone should be able to hear and understand what the Nursing Assistant is saying.

- Ideas should be in easy-to-understand language.

- **Good verbal communicators are also active listeners.** When attending a meeting, Nursing Assistants should be listening intently and asking clarifying questions.

- **Good verbal communicators avoid filler words like** "um", "er", "so", or "yeah". Good communicators replace those filler words by taking a breath instead.

2. Non-verbal

Nonverbal communication uses body language, gestures, and facial expressions. Sometimes these information sharing techniques are intentional. At times, they are unintentional. Nonverbal communication is useful when Nursing Assistants are attempting to probe residents' thoughts, feelings, and motivations.

Closed or negative body language like crossed arms, a scowl, a frown, a shaken fist, or hunched shoulders may indicate fear, anxiety, anger, or nervousness. Open or positive body language communicates satisfaction, happiness, willingness to listen, confidence, and/or a sense of self-worth. Nursing Assistants can develop body language by:

- Noticing how their emotions feel. If they are angry, happy, worried, or excited how it does feel? How does it look to others? Developing self-awareness gives Nursing Assistants greater control over body language.
- Being intentional about nonverbal communications uses body language to support verbal communication. This might include facial expressions, arm movements, or gestures. When Nursing Assistants combine verbal and nonverbal communication, it sends a more powerful message.

- If they find certain nonverbal communicators like facial expressions, nodding, pats on the back or high-fives beneficial, Nursing Assistants can use them to improve communication with the nursing team or residents.

3. Written

Written communication is writing, typing or printing information. Written can provide a record of information for reference. Writing is commonly used to share information through books, pamphlets, blogs, letters, memos and more. Emails and chats are a common form of written communication in the workplace.

Here are a few steps that a nurse assistant can take to develop the written communication skills:

- Written communications should strive for simplicity and clarity. Nursing Assistants should consider the intent of the written communication and the intended audience.
- Nursing Assistants should try to keep their writing as simple and plain as possible and follow up with verbal communications, adding flair.
- Nursing Assistants should review written communications, identifying mistakes or opportunities to revise for greater clarity. It's also a good idea to get a trusted colleague to review written communication.
- Nursing Assistants should work to improve their written communication by reading the work of others, emulating their style.

4. Electronic

Nursing Assistants are responsible for sending and receiving messages and filling out forms using computers, tablets, fax machines, smart phone, and intercom systems. They need finely developed technological skills to communicate and receive information electronically.

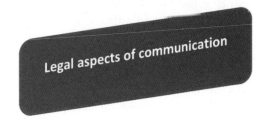

Nursing Assistants are expected to know when to document, what to document, and how to document. They are guided by state and federal laws and by the Nursing Assistant's code of conduct. They are also responsible for complying with the policies of the facility for which they work.

1. **Documentation for what has been reported verbally to licensed nurse**

It is the responsibility of Nursing Assistant to report resident observations to their immediate supervisor.

2. **Document for statements heard from the patient/resident and family**

In addition to reporting Nursing Assistant observations about the resident's medical condition, Nursing Assistants are required to share with their supervisor statements made from the resident and family members pertaining to the resident's medical condition.

Rules for effective communication

Nursing Assistants require effective communication skills to receive and give information to and from residents and other healthcare professionals.

With good communication skills, Nursing Assistants will be able to

- Express their thoughts, ideas, and resident data so they are understood
- Enjoy more meaningful interpersonal relationship with residents and medical professionals
- Do their job competently and receive recognition for doing so
- Increase self-esteem and resident confidence
- Work effectively and competently as part of a medical team
- Assist other healthcare workers in meeting resident needs

1. **Identifying self by name and title in any form of communication**

Nursing Assistants should have a thorough understanding of how effective communication works in its many varied forms. They should also know which form works best in each situation.

2. **Characteristics of Verbal reports**

Nursing Assistants are often called upon to provide oral reports to their nursing team, their supervisor, and occasionally to other medical caregivers. They also share with residents clearly and simply what they are doing, how, and why.

a) **Brief verbal reports**

At the end of a shift, Nursing Assistants share with their supervisor and the incoming nursing staff medical information and observations about the residents. It is important that these data be succinct as there are several residents and a short period of time to accomplish this task.

b) Organized verbal reports

Nursing Assistants share with their supervisor and the incoming nursing staff medical information and observations about the residents. The resident data should be organized in a logical manner. It is important to be organized in sharing these oral reports so that no important information is omitted or misunderstood.

c) Appropriate and focused reports

As healthcare professionals, Nursing Assistants share with their supervisor and the incoming nursing staff medical information and observations about the residents. These data should be focused on resident medical information. The language should be professional and the information appropriate to meeting the residents' unique needs.

▪ Diagnosis

Medical professionals are much better equipped to make accurate patient diagnosis with accurate, detailed information about patient symptoms and behavior. Nursing Assistants, as front-line caregivers, have a wealth of vital information from their observations and their communication with the residents.

▪ Allergies

Nursing Assistants are trained to be keen observers of resident behaviors. So front-line caregivers, have a wealth of vital information from their observations and their communication with the residents concerning food, medication, and/or environmental irritants.

▪ Activity and tolerance

Nursing Assistants who interact closely with residents on both individual and group settings have an awareness of activities residents prefer and their tolerance for social groups.

▪ Elimination

Elimination is a basic human need. When it doesn't occur normal, residents can become sick or die. In their providing primary care for residents, Nursing Assistants observe and report any irregularities in resident elimination.

▪ Special needs

Nursing Assistants provide care for residents with special needs. Some of these are physical. Residents may need assistance with daily living activities like eating, bathing, dressing, and walking. Some residents have difficulty with language. Interpreters may be required. Others are unable to speak. Signing or speech boards may be required. Some residents have physical challenges of sight and/or hearing. Nursing Assistants are trained to accommodate communication and care necessities of residents with special needs.

▪ Diet and appetite

Food and water are basic human needs. Without sufficient nutritious food and water, residents will become ill. They could even die. As primary caregivers, Nursing Assistants have a role to play in ensuring residents are eating and drinking enough. Nursing Assistants aid in resident feeding and drinking where necessary. When residents' eating or drinking patterns change, this information is shared with the nursing team.

▪ Vital signs and weight

Nursing Assistants observe and assess a patient's physical appearance, vital signs, and weight daily. They are noting patterns and trends like changes in health, reaction to medications, food, allergies, and other factors. They watch for signs and resident complaints of discomfort and anxiety. Nursing care is individualized. It is adjusted according to the reporting nurse's observations. Concerns are shared with the nursing assistant's supervisor who passes concerns on to the resident's doctor.

- **Code status**

Code status refers to the type of emergent treatment a person would or would not receive if their heart or breathing were to stop. As professionals, Nursing Assistants should know the code status of the resident for whom they provide care. Unfortunately, too often, code status is not discussed fully until there is a crisis with the resident's health status.

d) Timely

Nursing Assistants' communication needs to be current both in verbal reports to the nursing team and in resident chart notations. If the information isn't up to date changes in health may be lost.

e) Respectful of patient/resident confidentiality

Nursing Assistants can respect and protect resident confidentiality by recording and using only the information necessary to communicate resident health. Each medical professional should have access only to needed information. Both written and electronic resident records should be stored and accessed in a secure manner.

As professionals, Nursing Assistants never discuss resident cases in public places or with unauthorized personnel.

3. Telephonic communication

Normally in a long-term care facility Nursing Assistants do not answer phone calls. If friends or relatives wish to discuss a resident's health or care, he needs resident permission. These types of calls are normally referred to the resident's doctor. It is unwise and may even be illegal to share resident's health information with anyone except the nursing team.

If for some reason a Nursing Assistant picks up the phone, he/she should adhere to these guidelines for professional etiquette.

a) Taking notes during the call

Nursing Assistants should identify themselves and their title. They should take notes identifying the caller, the time of day, and details of the message.

b) Naming of person the message is for

The receiver of the message should be clearly identified including any details about resident room number or staff department.

c) Verifying correct spelling of caller's name

Before hanging up the Nursing Assistant should verify the spelling of the caller's name.

d) Indicating time of call

When the call took place and how long it lasted should be noted beside the date.

e) Clarifying the message with the caller by repeating it and repeating the telephone number

Before hanging up, the Nursing Assistant should get the caller's number and repeat the message to ensure the details are correct.

f) Clearly signing full name and title to the message

Finally, the Nursing Assistant should write his/her name clearly and add a title to the message. Messages should be delivered to the person for whom it is intended as quickly as possible.

4. Answering a patient/resident call signal

One of the tasks of Nursing Assistants is responding to resident call buttons.

a) Answering promptly, quietly, and in a friendly manner

Nursing Assistants should answer a resident's call as quickly as possible. The response should indicate the Nursing Assistant's name and title. When answering, the Nursing Assistant should respond in a pleasant, professional, clear voice.

b) Using an intercom

If the call system identifies the caller, the Nursing Assistant should call the resident by name and ascertain the reason for the call.

c) Making sure the patient/resident can always reach the call light

In providing primary care for residents, it is important to ensure that the resident's call button is easily accessible.

Helpful Resources

American School of Nursing. "Communication Tips for Nurses and Nursing Assistants" https://www.americannursinged.com/communication-tips-for-nurses-and-nursing-assistants/

CAN Plus Academy. "How to Improve Communication Skills" https://cna.plus/guidelines-to-improve-communication-skills/

Huitt, W. (2007). Maslow's hierarchy of needs. *Educational Psychology Interactive.* http://www.edpsycinteractive.org/topics/regsys/maslow.html

Martin, D., & Joomis, K. (2007). *Building teachers: A constructivist approach to introducing education.* Belmont, CA: Thomson/Wadsworth.

Maslow's Hierarchy. http://changingminds.org/explanations/needs/maslow.htm

National Commission on Correctional Healthcare. "Therapeutic Communication and Behavioral Management" https://www.ncchc.org/cnp-therapeutic-communication

Nurses Choice. "10 Essential Nurse Communication Skills for Success" https://www.nursechoice.com/traveler-resources/10-essential-nurse-communication-skills-for-success/

NurseKey.com. "Stereotypes, Judgement, and Communication" https://nursekey.com/stereotypes-judgement-and-communication/

VeryWellMind.com. "The 5 Levels of Maslow's Hierarchy of Needs" https://www.verywellmind.com/what-is-maslows-hierarchy-of-needs-4136760

VitalSource.com. *Nursing Assistant: A Nursing Process Approach* (8th ed.) https://www.vitalsource.com/en-ca/products/nursing-assistant-a-nursing-process-approach-barbara-acello-barbara-hegner-v9781305178007?duration=365&gclid=Cj0KCQjwtsv7BRCmARIsANu-CQccyxYfjABAyOFyXrARMIssN2NJyqXhxhrZsFxGNvKmK5cRbUeN7o8aAuGrEALw_wcB

VitalSource.com. *Assisting in Long-Term Care.* https://www.vitalsource.com/en-ca/products/assisting-in-long-term-care-mary-jo-mirlenbrink-gerlach-v9781285633008?duration=365&gclid=Cj0KCQjwtsv7BRCmARIsANu-CQe4CywcW_crzUs71SCLzqhNPtFAgCxXRDXAw69GOSB0ygoLmxOGI-8aAukLEALw_wcB

Winner, J. *Take Stress out of Your Life.* https://www.amazon.ca/Take-Stress-Out-Your-Life/dp/0738211745

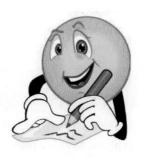

Chapter Four:

Prevention and Management of Catastrophe and Unusual Occurrences

Outline

I: The Nurse Assistant role in emergency, disaster, and fire situations

II: Common emergency codes used in healthcare facilities

III: Two major safety issues i.e. falls and burns for the patients/residents and common interventions to prevent these issues

IV: An overview of bioterrorism

V: Safety rules for the patient/resident receiving oxygen therapy

VI: Safe application of postural supports and the implication for their use

VII: The legal and psychological implication for the use of postural supports

VIII: Major causes of fire and general fire prevention rules

IX: General rules for providing a safe environment for the Nurse Assistant

X: General rules for providing a safe environment for the patients/residents

What is a Disaster or Catastrophe?

A disaster or catastrophe is any unexpected event or incident which leads to significant destruction or/and adverse consequences. More specifically, a catastrophe is an incident in which needs exceed the available resources. It is important to recognize that each catastrophe is unique in the way it affects communities, families, and individuals. Although most Americans when hear the term catastrophe or disaster, they immediately think any terrorist attack; however, in reality the most common forms of disaster are manmade or natural (e.g. major fires, floods, hurricanes, and tornadoes).

The role and responsibility of the Nurse Assistant in disaster, emergency, and fire situations

An emergency is a condition that arises suddenly and needs immediate intervention to keep an individual safe. Nurse Assistants must know how to respond in the event of an emergency to keep the patients or residents in their care safe.

The following major steps guide a Nurse Assistant's actions in an emergency and ensure his/her own safety and the safety of the patients/residents:

A. Emergency Preparedness

The main goal of emergency preparedness is to plan an emergency response from the Nurse Assistant that will minimize the damage and support the possible recovery from a disaster. Emergency preparedness

for the Nurse Assistant consists of understanding three basic components i.e. Knowledge of emergency color codes, knowledge of fire and disaster plans, and knowledge of fire exit, extinguishers, and alarms.

B. Emergency Preparedness

Each healthcare facility may have different emergency color codes; however, the Nurse Assistant should be well familiar with following emergency codes:

1. Code Red: It indicates fire emergency
2. Code Blue: Code Blue usually shows an adult medical emergency (e.g. cardiac/pulmonary)
3. Code Yellow: It is for a bomb threat
4. Code Gray: It is an indication of a combative person
5. Code Silver: It shows a person with weapon or hostage
6. Code Orange: Code Orange indicates any hazardous waste spill or release

STAT is a term used as a directive to nursing assistants and medical personnel during an emergency situation, is originated from the Latin word *statim,*" which means to respond at once or there is an immediate or instant need.

C. Fire and Disaster plans

Nursing Assistants should have an adequate knowledge of fire and disaster plans for dealing any emergency situation.

THE DISASTER PLAN
A healthcare facility's disaster plan demonstrates actions to take in a disaster. The disaster plan is usually activated when an emergency condition or disaster produces so many casualties that routine methods for patient care are inadequate. All employees including nursing assistants must know how to access the specific facility's disaster plan.

THE FIRE PLAN

Fire is a main emergency condition that can be caused by improper management of flammable gases or materials, frayed electrical wiring, careless smoking, or faulty equipments. The fire plans strongly forbid smoking in and around any healthcare facilities. Nursing assistants must know how to access the specific facility's fire plan along with the particular dangers of smoking when oxygen is in use, and safety hazards.

D. Knowledge of fire exits, extinguishers, and alarms

Nursing Assistants should also have an adequate knowledge of fire exits, extinguishers, and alarms while dealing any fire emergency.

Fire exits

There should be a minimum of two independent exit routes for every location on every floor. It is generally recommended that any room or suite of rooms of 230 square meters or more must have at least two independent exits. Exit routes must be located as far away from each other as possible because in case if one exit route is blocked with fire or smoke, the other alternative route can be used. The width of the corridor for the emergency exits should be at least 7.9 feet to permit the smooth transportation of hospital mattresses, beds, and the evacuation of non-ambulatory patients. Exit routes should be clearly mentioned with below internationally accepted identifying signs:

Fire extinguishers

There are three main fire types, classified as type A, B or C. Most of the fire extinguishers used are ABC fire extinguishers to manage all three types of fire effectively. In case when an ABC fire extinguisher is not accessible or available, the Nurse Assistant should use an extinguisher specific to the fire type, or take other measures per facility's policies.

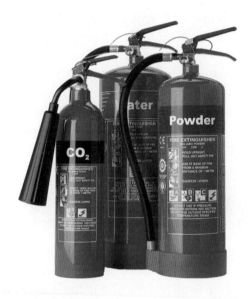

Fire alarms

There are various ways for the detection of fires. Fire alarms system is the most commonly used to detect fire. A variety of heat and smoke sensors can be installed as part of a fire alarm system for the detection of fires that begin in low-traffic areas away from personnel/staff. These sensors trigger an automatic alert system with visible strobe lights and audible bells to indicate that a fire was detected. The sensors are also able to pinpoint the fire-detected location at which the fire was detected. Nursing assistant should be well familiar with the location of these alarms, which is a part of their emergency preparedness.

E. Staying calm and controlling the nerves

It is one of the major roles of the Nurse Assistant to stay calm while dealing an emergency situation or any disaster. The Nurse Assistant should remain calm and should not shout the words like "fire" or "cardiac arrest", etc. Initial response of the Nurse Assistant should check the scene and then the patients/ residents under his or her care. There should be ensured that there is nothing that could hurt the Nurse Assistant or cause further injury to the patients/residents e.g. a downed wire in that area or any other dangerous equipment. Next, the Nurse Assistant should look for clues that may help him/her to understand what happened. And then finally, it should be checked the patient/resident (if possible) by tapping their shoulder or hand to confirm consciousness.

F. Using Emergency calling system for assistance

After initial assessment, the next step should be call for help. Nursing assistants should be well aware about the scope of their practice and should not act beyond level of their knowledge. In a healthcare facility, there is usually an emergency code can to call for help within the facility. In almost every health care setting, a registered nurse (RN) or nursing supervisor may be required to activate the EMS (Emergency Medical System) by dialing 9-1-1. The Nurse Assistants should know their employer's policies and procedures regarding calling for help in an emergency.

F. Application of "RACE" and "PASS" approaches

Nursing assistants should clearly understand the healthcare's fire plan and follow the "RACE" and "PASS" approaches per their facility's policies and procedures. If a fire start, the Nursing Assistant should act very fast. RACE is an acronym that may help a nursing assistant to remember the general order of procedures for dealing a fire:

R – Remove the patients/ residents from area of danger immediately

A – Activate the fire alarm system

C – Contain the fire, if possible (close doors)

E – Extinguish, if possible

All fire extinguishers should be checked on a regular basis to ensure that they are fully functional and ready to use in case of an emergency situation. Nursing assistants should remember the acronym P-A-S-S to use a general order for fire extinguisher:

P – Pull the pin

A – Aim at the base of the fire

S – Squeeze the handle

S – Sweep back and forth at the base of the fire

G. Moving patient/resident if in immediate danger

The Nurse Assistant should first of all look around and make sure that the patient/resident is not in an immediate danger. In case the patient/resident in immediate danger, the nurse assistant should move the patient/resident to a safe place. The simple approach for this initial scene safety assessment can be done through the mnemonic S-A-F-E:

S – Stop: The nurse assistant should always stop at the initial scene for a while and plan for how to act or respond.

A – Assess: The nurse assistant should make an initial assessment about safe approach to handle the patient/resident, scene safety, ventilation assessment, and assessment for other possible hazards.

F – Find: The next step should be to look for the first aid kit, AED unit, and oxygen if possible.

E – Exposure protection: The nurse assistant should always try to use barriers such as gloves and mouth-to-mask devices (if possible) to prevent the spread of infections.

H. Staying with patients/residents and keeping them calm and comfortable

The nursing assistants should stay with the patients/residents under their care and provide appropriate care (according to their level of training and situation) until advanced help arrives. They should help the patients/residents to rest comfortably, and should provide reassurance because the patients/residents are likely to be upset and frightened.

I. Evacuation of patients/residents to safety per facility's disaster and fire plans

Evacuation is a crucial component that aims to save more lives during an emergency situation in hospitals. A comprehensive evacuation plan should be established and all staff members including nursing assistants should be well aware and experienced in carrying out that plan. Evacuation time frames may differ depending on the nature of the threat and the amount of time required preparing the patients/residents for evacuation. Fire and bomb threats, for example, may require an immediate or rapid evacuation depending on the level of danger. However, natural disasters such as hurricanes and floods, with adequate warning periods, may require only a gradual evacuation of the health care facility. The following actions should be taken by the Nursing Assistant when the "prepare only" instruction is issued:

- If nursing assistant hears the fire alarm or see flashing lights, he/she should close all fire doors in that area.
- Nursing assistants should ensure that exit corridors are clear to allow movement of patients/residents and equipment.
- They should locate and secure patients' medical records and medical supplies.
- They should ready the evacuation transport equipment such as blankets, wheelchairs, and gurneys.
- Nursing assistants should await further instructions and do not start evacuation unless given the authorization to do so.

Movement

The movement of patients/residents for evacuation is based on nature of emergency situation. The movement may be horizontal, vertical, and shelter in place (SIP).

Horizontal: This is the primary mode of evacuation, which involves movements of patients in immediate threat away from the danger but keeping them on their same floor.

Vertical: It generally involves the complete evacuation of a specific floor in the hospital. Patients/residents and staff out of the hospital should only be evacuated if necessary.

Shelter in Place: Nursing assistants and other staff may be instructed to "shelter in place," i.e. staying in their units and waiting for further instructions.

Level of Evacuation

The level of evacuation may include complete evacuation or partial evacuation:

Partial evacuation: Evacuation of a subset of facility residents/patients. This may involve general evacuation of the areas of the hospital nearest the fire incident.

Complete evacuation: Complete evacuation of a healthcare facility due to an unsafe environment of care that may involve facility shutdown actions.

In most emergency situations, a complete evacuation will not be required. Due to the unstable condition and complex needs of many hospital patients, evacuation is usually considered as a last resort. If a complete evacuation of the facility is instructed, patients should be moved in the following order:

- Patients/residents are to be evacuated horizontally by wheelchair, stretcher, or other method of transportation to an adjacent safe compartment as per facility policies and procedures. Patients/residents in immediate danger (due to smoke or fire) should be evacuated first.
- Ambulatory patients should be directed or accompanied to an adjacent safe compartment.
- Non-Ambulatory patients should be evacuated using stretchers or wheelchairs when available to an adjacent safe compartment.
- Critical patients/residents, who require the more resources to transport, can be remained in their closed patient room until they can be moved safely. These patients/residents may be the last to be evacuated, if they are not being directly affected by an immediate danger (fire or smoke).
- Patients/residents evacuations should be coordinated with nursing assistants to make sure patients/residents needs are met at the location to which they are being relocated.

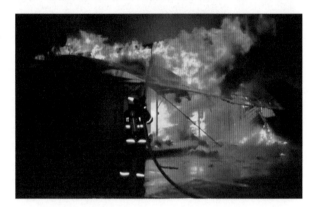

The following emergency conditions may warrant evacuation:

- Smoke, fire, and/or toxic fumes
- Structural damage to the facility
- Potential exposure to hazardous materials
- Terrorism or armed, violent visitors
- Credible bomb threat

J. Moving visitors or family to facility's designated area

The staff members including nursing assistants of the facility should be well aware of hospital's fire and disaster plans. They should have knowledge about the exit areas and several locations surrounding the hospital building that could be used as holding areas, assembly points, and/or discharge sites. Visitors or families of the patients/residents should be moved to the facility-designated area or assembly points as quickly as possible.

Common Emergency Codes Used in Healthcare Facilities

These are color-coded indicators used in healthcare facilities to alert all staff members for potential emergency issues arising in a facility. Emergency codes include unique criteria for how nursing assistants and other staff members should respond to a specific situation, ranging from an active shooter threat to cardiac arrest.

Depending on healthcare facility's size and level of care, designation of emergency codes may vary. There are no standard conventions or definitions for the use of code designations. While code blue means a cardiopulmonary arrest at many hospitals; however, it doesn't necessarily mean the same thing everywhere. It should keep in mind that every healthcare facility or hospital has its own conventions and policies for notification of emergencies. Doctors, nursing assistants, and other staff should be trained to recognize and respond appropriately to these emergency notifications.

These emergency codes can be categorized into three main groups of codes i.e. facility alerts, security alerts and medical alerts.

1. Facility alerts

Facility alerts provide safety and security of patients, visitors, and employees at all times, including the management of essential utilities.

Types of facility threats

- Evacuation
- Fire (Code Red)
- Hazardous spill (Code Orange)

Code red: Fire

Code red provides an appropriate emergency response in the event of an actual or suspected fire to protect life, property and vital services. Due to the non-ambulatory nature of many patients/residents and devastating effects of fire, all employees including nursing assistants have a responsibility to respond quickly to an actual or suspected fire.

Code Red should be initiated immediately in case of any one of the following indications:

1. Watching smoke, sparks or a fire.
2. Smelling smoke or other burning material.
3. Feeling unusual heat on a door, wall, and other surfaces.
4. In response to any life/fire safety system alarm.

The Code red task force including nursing assistants performs only basic fire response operations for initial stage of fires that can be extinguished by portable fire extinguishers without the usual need for self-contained breathing apparatus or protective clothing. All employees including nursing assistants should complete an annual safety training that includes appropriate life/fire safety procedures according to their facility policies.

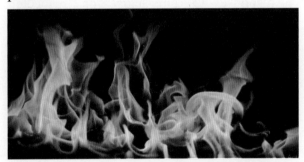

Upon discovery of suspected or actual fire:

At fire origin, R.A.C.E approach should be initiated in which first of all patients, visitors and personnel from the immediate fire area are removed from an immediate threat. Activation of the fire alarm and notification for others in the affected area to obtain assistance is the next step. Nursing assistants should follow their organizations' emergency reporting instructions. Smoke and fire should be contained by closing all doors and finally the fire should be extinguished if it is safe to do so.

S.A.F.E. Approach

S— Safety of life

A— Activation of the alarm

F — Fighting with fire (if it is safe to do so)

E — Evacuation (as necessary or instructed)

Code orange: Assistance needed or Hazardous Spill

Code Orange is the emergency code that may have facility-specific meanings. Joint Commission standards for hospitals (JCA) define code orange as an exposure to a hazardous substance or material within a health facility. However, it may also be used to indicate "attention needed" for violent patient conditions or other emergencies.

The main purpose of code orange is to provide an appropriate emergency response to an actual or suspected hazardous material spill in a manner that is safe for patients, staff, and visitors. Nursing assistants and other employees should be well familiar with the products they are using, understand how to use the products, and aware the spill precautions they should take. The clean-up of a hazardous material spill should only be done by appropriate knowledgeable and experienced nursing assistants and other personnel who have received proper training.

2. Security alerts

Security alerts protect employees including nursing assistants, patients, and visitors from an emergency situation or person posing a threat to the safety of any individual(s) within the healthcare facility.

Types of security threats

- Active shooter
- Armed, violent intruder
- Hostage situation
- Person with weapon or hostage (Code silver)
- Need for security personnel (Code Gray)
- Bomb threat (Code Yellow)

Code silver: Active shooter

Code silver provides an appropriate emergency response in the event involving a person with a weapon or who has taken hostages within the health facility (including an active shooter incident). The hospitals usually take all possible measures to minimize the negative impacts of a situation involving a hostage condition or person with a weapon.

Nursing assistants or anyone encountering a person brandishing a harmful weapon should:

a. Seek cover and warn others about the situation.

b. Notify the facility management of the incident with all information.

c. Provide the location in building, floor, area, and room number.

d. Describe the number of suspect(s) and any physical descriptions.

e. Provide information about any known hostages or victims.

Code gray: Combative person

Code gray provides an appropriate emergency response to situations involving a hostile, aggressive, combative, or potentially combative person. Aggressive, abusive, or combative behavior can be displayed by anyone like a patient, a patient's family member, staff, staff family members, or friends of patients and employees. Nursing assistants and other staff should effectively respond to ensure the security and safety of all persons on hospital property and minimize the number of potential injuries and assault victims.

Code yellow: Bomb threat

Code yellow provides an appropriate emergency response in the incident of a bomb threat or the finding of a suspicious device.

A code yellow denotes a bomb threat to the facility. It may include the identification of an actual bomb within the facility or just receiving a bomb threat.

If a threat is received through phone to the facility, it should be tried to get as much information as possible about the caller. Relevant questions about the threat should be asked, and share the information to other employees to activate the code yellow.

It is important to remain calm and not get angry at the person phoning in a threat. Upon the arrival of law enforcement security, the call should be turned over to them. Code yellow can be categorized into low-risk, medium risk, or high-risk threats:

A low-risk threat has the following features:

- The threat may be looking vague.

- Information is inconsistent or implausible.

- The caller may be identified easily and already has made multiple calls.

- The threat was discovered such as finding a package, not receiving an actual threat.

Medium-risk threats may have the following characteristics:

- A medium-risk threat is feasible.

- Wording may indicate the perpetrator has a possible plan for the bomb or threat.

- Time and place indications for the bomb to detonate.

- A lack of strong indicators that the perpetrator has taken preparation steps for completing the treat.

- Indications of the bomb's composition.

- There is an increased emotional state of the perpetrator, such as saying, "I'm serious," or "I'm going to do this."

High-risk threats are extremely specific and realistic. The perpetrator may give names, causes for why he/she is doing this, information about plans to indicate the bomb. The perpetrator may provide his or her identity.

Nursing assistants and other staff should follow these steps in the interim:

1. First step should be removing individuals in imminent danger from a suspected bomb or package. This may include evacuating the unit or floor if the bomb is located in a unit.

2. Contacting to authorities as soon as possible and activation the code yellow is the next step.

3. Unlike code silver, "shelter in place" is not an option in the code yellow.

4. If the threat not found to be valid by law enforcement, an evacuation order may be overturned.

3. Medical alerts

Medical alerts provide medical care and support to patients/residents while maintaining clinical care and safety of patients, employees and visitors within a healthcare facility during an emergency situation or incident.

Types of medical threats

- Emergency Operations Plan Activation
- Medical decontamination
- Medical emergency (Code Blue)

Code blue: Medical Emergency (Adults)/Code white: Medical Emergency (Pediatrics)

Code blue or code white provides an appropriate emergency response to an eminent or suspected cardiopulmonary arrest or a medical emergency situation for an adult or pediatric patient. Code blue or code white is initiated for patients who do not have an advance healthcare directive indicating otherwise. Code blue is to be activated immediately whenever a patient eight years of age or older is found in a medical emergency or cardiac/respiratory arrest (per facility protocol). Code white is to be activated immediately whenever a patient eight years of age or younger is found in a medical emergency or cardiac/respiratory arrest (per facility protocol).

Code blue or code white is among the most easily recognized emergency codes in existence. While these codes are mostly associated with the cardiac arrest of a patient; however, these may be used to indicate any medical emergency in a health care facility, including medical emergencies of patient family members.

Depending on health facility's policies, all available staff members including nursing assistants from floors adjacent to the affected floor may be called to assist with the code blue or code white.

It is also important to make sure that nursing assistants should have the appropriate credentials for responding during a code blue. It may include ACLS (Advanced Cardiac Life Support), PALS (Pediatric Advanced Life Support), BLS (Basic Life Support) and CPR & First Aid training.

Fall Risk Assessment

A major goal in all healthcare settings is the prevention of falls. A fall may be defined as an unplanned descent to the floor, with or without any injury. Falls may occur in almost any patient; however, older adults are more susceptible to falling. Falls are the common occurrence in older adults, both in the community and in healthcare settings. Approximately one-third of all older adults living in the community may experience of fall at least once a year and one-half of these people are more likely to fall more than once.

Routine fall prevention includes ensuring wheelchairs are locked when the patient/resident is transferring, assisting with ambulation when required, and ensuring all spills are cleaned up immediately. It is estimated that falls are 70% of all patient/resident-related accidents in healthcare facilities. Falls are the most common cause of injury for sedated, disabled, confused, and older adults.

Often falls occur during 4:00pm and 8:00pm and during shift changes when the patient/resident tries to get needed items.

The patient/resident has to reach too far and falls out of a chair or bed. Or the patient/resident tries to get up without help.

All patients/residents in the healthcare facility (except those in active labor or in the newborn ICU) should be assessed regularly for the risk for falling. The nurse assistant should document the Fall-Risk Assessment on the client's record at regular intervals. In the event of a fall, immediate action should be taken to determine any injury and ensured the patient/resident is protected from future falls.

Prevention of falls

Preventing falls is a major challenge and there should be a considerable amount of attention directed towards finding solutions. Fall prevention can effectively work if they include measures to address patient/resident, environmental, and staff issues that contribute to falls.

Patient issues and fall prevention

1) Modifiable risk factors: Gait instability, balance problems, and muscle weakness can be improved by using targeted exercise programs. Fear of falling can be relieved by different exercises and psychological interventions. The patient/resident's medication regimen should be checked to determine if any prescribed medication, or combination of medications, may increase the risk of falling.

2) Non-modifiable risk factors:

These risk factors cannot be significantly changed; however, accommodations and adaptations can be made. These accommodations and adaptations may include patient/resident education, environmental manipulations, maintaining good control of chronic medical conditions such as dementia, diabetes, orthostatic hypotension, and Parkinson's disease.

Environmental issues and fall prevention

Environmental issues that can cause falls may include loose rugs or loose carpet edges, poor lighting, uneven/worn stairs, exposed electrical cords, ill-fitting footwear, slippery floor surfaces, absence of supportive devices (handrails), and poorly fitted or broken assistive devices such as canes, wheelchairs, and walkers.

The Nurse Assistant should know why falls occur, who is likely to fall, and then applying that knowledge to prevent falls. Falls can be caused by anything mental or physical that affects sensory perception, strength, balance, or orientation to the environment. The patient/resident's assessment should include age, fall history, presence of any medical or psychiatric conditions that would predispose to a fall (Dementia, Depression, Diabetes, Inner ear disorders, Muscle weakness, Obesity, Osteoarthritis, Parkinson's disease, Peripheral neuropathy, Sleep disorders, Stroke, Vision impairment), cognitive status, presence of urinary frequency, the use of medications that are known to contribute to fall risk (Antihistamines, Anti-depressants, Anti-hypertensives, Antipsychotics, Anxiolytics, Anti-diabetics, Hypnotics and soporifics), and mobility status.

General preventive measures of falls

- Fluid needs should be met.
- Eyeglasses and hearing aids should be worn as needed. Reading glasses should not be worn when up and about.
- Tasks should be explained before and while performing them.
- Help should be provided with elimination needs (Assistance should be provided the patient/resident to the bathroom or providing the bedpan, urinal, or commode).
- The bedpan, urinal, or commode should be within easy reach of the patient/resident.
- A warm drink, back massage, or soft lights should be used to calm the patient/resident who is agitated.
- Barriers should be used to prevent wandering.
- The patient/resident should be properly positioned in chair, bed, or a wheelchair. Pillows, seats, wedge pads, or other positioning devices should be used as per the nurse and care plan directives.
- Showers and tubs should have non-slip surfaces or non-slip bath mats along with safety bars in showers.
- Carpeting (if used) should be wall-to-wall or tacked down.
- Floors should have non-glare, non-slip surfaces.
- Electrical and extension cords should be out of the way.
- Furniture should be placed for easy movement.
- A phone, lamp, and personal belongings should be kept within the patient/resident's reach.
- The bed should be at the correct height for the patient/resident.
- The bed should be in the lowest horizontal position, except when giving bedside care.
- Bed rails should be used according to the care plan.
- A mattress, special mat, or floor cushion should be placed on the floor beside the bed. This minimizes the chance of injury if the patient/resident falls or gets out of bed.
- Wheelchairs, canes, walkers, and crutches must fit properly. They should be in good repair.
- Canes, crutches, and walkers should have non-skid tips.
- Wheel locks on beds, stretchers, and wheelchairs must be in working order.
- Rooms, stairways, and hallways should have good lighting.
- Light switches including those in bathrooms must be within reach and easy to find.
- There should be night-lights in bedrooms, hallways, and bathrooms.
- Non-skid footwear should be worn. Socks, long shoelaces, and bedroom slippers should be avoided.
- Shoes should be fitted well. They should not slip up and down on the patient/resident feet. All shoelaces and straps should be fastened.
- Clothing should be fitted properly and not loose. It should not drag on the floor. Belts should be tied or secured in place.
- The patient/resident should be taught how to use the call light.
- The patient/resident should be checked often. This may be every 15 minutes or as directed by the care plan.
- There should be hand rails on both sides of stairs and hallways. The patient/resident should use these hand rails when walking or using stairs.
- Family and friends should be asked to visit during busy times. Shift changes and meal times are examples. They are asked to visit during the evening and night shifts.

- Wheelchairs, carts, stretchers, and other wheeled equipment should be pulled (not push) through doorways.

Assistive Devices

An assistive device is a product that aides to make the activities of daily life easier for the older or disabled patients/residents. There are multiple products which may be used as assistive devices, and keep the risk of accidents at a minimum level. Most common assistive devices include following:

1. Cane

Canes is a type of assistive devices that may help to redistribute weight from a painful or weak lower extremity, improve stability by improving the base of support, and give tactile information about the surface to improve balance. Canes may also improve self-reported functional ability and confidence.

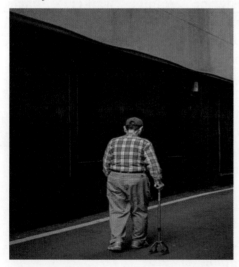

Types of Canes

There are various categories of canes on the market today, providing a slightly different amount of assistance. The cane should fit well with the patient/resident's current needs and functional level. Using a cane that isn't right for the patient/resident may cause to develop poor walking postures and may lead to injury from a fall.

A. Standard canes

A standard cane or straight cane is a single-tip cane generally made from wood or aluminum. These are inexpensive and lightweight. An aluminum cane has the benefit of an adjustable height. A standard cane may aide with balance of a patient/resident who does not need the upper extremity to bear weight.

B. "C" cane

The C cane is a single straight walking cane with a C-shaped curve forming a handle at its top. "C" cane is the most simple of all canes. Straight canes should be used by the patient/resident needing only slight assistance with balance or only minimal unweighting of the opposite leg.

C. The functional grip cane

These canes are similar to the C canes except for the handle. They have a straight grip handle rather than a smooth curve that allows for a better grip by the patient/resident and an improved grip allows for better cane control. Therefore, it offers more support than the C cane. Functional grip canes are suitable for the patient/resident who requires slightly more assistance than the C cane provides.

D. Quad cane

It is a walking cane with a rectangle base with four small supports that contact the floor. The large base of the quad canes provides more support than the above canes. Quad canes are available in two varieties depending on the size of the rectangle base i.e. small base and large base quad canes. The quad cane is helpful for patients/residents require much more balance support than provided by the above canes. These are often used by a patient/resident with hemiplegia or paresis. The large base of the quad cane and its four feet allow it to stand on its own.

E. The hemiwalker

The hemiwalker combines the features of a walker and quad cane. Its base is much larger than any of the canes described above, thus providing the most ideal support for the patient/resident. These also provide an additional amount of lateral support. Patients/residents with severe hemiplegia or those transferring from using a walker to a cane will benefit from the use of a hemiwalker.

2. Walker

A walker is a type of **assistive device** that offers support and stability while walking. Walkers are more stable than canes or crutches. They have a wider base of support that gives more stability front to back and side to side. There are also special pediatric walkers available for younger children. Walkers may be available with or without wheels.

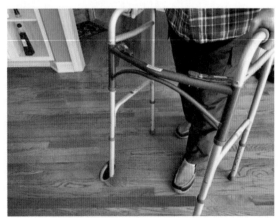

Types of Walkers

A physical therapist or licensed nurse will assess the patient to identify the best style of walker. Each walker is unique to needs of the patient/resident. Walkers may have different types with no wheels, 2 wheels, or 4 wheels. Different accessories, such as pouches, baskets and seats, may be added to make it easier to do daily activities.

A. Standard walkers

A standard walker consists of 4 straight legs and no wheels. The width and height can be adjustable to fit the patient. It is important to ensure that all 4 legs of the walker are on the floor before taking a step. Caps or gliders may sometimes be added to the legs of the walker (glider walker) to make the walking pattern to be more natural.

B. Rolling walkers (wheeled walkers)

For a smoother walking pattern or more natural gait, wheels can be used on the front of the walker. Wheels may also be placed if patients/residents are unable to lift and move the walker. Rolling walkers/wheeled walkers are designed with the support in back (posterior walker) or in front (anterior walker). A physical therapist or licensed nurse can help decide which is best for the patient/resident.

- **Anterior rolling walkers (front support)**: An anterior rolling walker provides support in front of the body. The base of support is broader to make it more stable for walking. Anterior rolling walker usually has 4 wheels and is used by pushing the walker forward.

- **Posterior rolling walkers (back support)**: A posterior rolling walker provides support behind the body. This type of walker may have 4 wheels (2 front and 2 back legs) or 2 (front legs only). The back legs have ratchet wheels or rubber tips to prevent backward rolling. This type of walker can assist with balance and posture during walking and standing. Posterior walker is used by standing in the middle of the walker with the support in the back. Holding the side handles, the walker is pulled from behind while stepping forward.

- **Rollator walkers**: It is a type of wheeled walker. Rollator walker has 3 or 4 wheels, handlebars with hand brakes, and a seat. A rollator walker can easily turn easily and move faster, which makes it more natural. However, it requires more balance and coordination to use. Rollator walker is used by standing behind the walker and pushing it forward by using the handlebars.

3. Gait Belt

A gait belt is an assistive device that can be used to help a safe transfer of a patient/resident from a bed to a wheelchair, assist with standing and sitting, and help with walking around. It is fastened around the waist to allow a caregiver or nurse assistant to grasp the belt, in order to provide assistance in lifting or moving a patient/resident. When used properly, the gait belt protects the patient/resident from falling and also protects from injuring his/her back as they move or lift the patient/resident accordingly. A gait belt is generally 1.5 to 4 inches wide, and 54-60 inches long. The belt may be made out of nylon, canvas, or leather with a buckle at one end.

A standard gait belt has a metal buckle with teeth and loops. Threading should be done through the teeth of the buckle and then belt should be put through the loop to lock it. A quick-release gait belt contains a plastic buckle that snaps into place to clip the two ends together.

A gait belt should be used if the patient/resident is partially dependent and has some weight-bearing capacity. Nursing assistants should be extra careful if the patient/resident has a catheter, feeding tube, or medical issues involving their abdominal area. There should always proper consultation with a physician about proper lifting under these conditions to find out if using a gait belt is safe.

4. Wheelchair

A wheelchair is an assistive device with straight-backed chair mounted on wheels with locking mechanisms, utilized for transporting the injured, ill, or patients/residents who suffer from limited mobility.

Types of wheelchairs

There are different types of wheelchairs, each with unique properties that might benefit a specific type of patient/resident.

A. Standing wheelchairs

Standing wheelchairs allow the patient/resident to raise the chair from a standing or seated position. The mechanism to raise the chair can be powered manually or electrically. The manual systems to raise the chair may have hydraulics in place to assist the patient/resident. Some standing wheelchairs may be driven in both seated and standing positions, while others can be operated just in the seated position.

Benefits of a standing wheelchair

A standing wheelchair allows the patient/resident to interact with others at the eye level, which may have various psychological advantages. It may raise patient/resident's self-esteem and sense of independence. From a physical standpoint, a standing wheelchair may promote better blood circulation, muscle tone, and kidney function.

Although standing wheelchairs can be suitable for a variety of different users; however, they are often used by those patients/residents affected by a spinal cord injury. They are also used by patients/residents who have multiple sclerosis, muscular dystrophy, or those who might have suffered from a stroke.

B. Reclining wheelchairs

These wheelchairs have a high back that can be reclined, either manually or electrically. The most important feature of reclining wheelchairs is that the back reclines independently of the rest of the chair. How much a backrest reclines depends on the specific type of wheelchair, with some wheelchairs reclining far enough to the point where they become a lie-flat bed.

Benefits of reclining wheelchairs

Besides the advantage of comfort, one of the most prominent benefits of a reclining wheelchair is that it permits the patient/resident to open up the hips (Sitting in one position for long periods may cause discomfort). With the reclining feature of these wheelchairs, the patient/resident can switch it up and get a good stretch.

Some other benefits of reclining wheelchairs may include:

- The patients/residents may be able to fall asleep in the reclining wheelchair when they need rest.
- It provides more accessible personal care, such as diaper changing or catheterization, if necessary.
- It also avoids pressure sores by adjusting how body weight is distributed.
- It relieves hypotension, if the reclining wheelchair has a feature of leg rest elevation.

C. Tilting Wheelchairs

Unlike a reclining wheelchair, the entire frame of the tilting wheelchair tilts back, thus it does not open up the hip angle when the patient/resident tilts the chair back. These wheelchairs may vary in how far they tilt back.

Benefits of tilting wheelchair

The primary advantage of tilting wheelchairs is that they permit for posture control. Just like a reclining wheelchair, the periodic change in position might bring comfort to the patient/resident. These wheelchairs also make it easier for patients/residents to get in and out of bed.

Some of the other benefits of a tilting wheelchair may include:

- **Edema management**: For patients/residents with edema, it is critical to have their legs elevated at the level of the heart or above, which may not be possible with a reclining chair. A tilting wheelchair permits the legs to be elevated adequately.
- **Relief of back pain**: A natural spine position may give rise to additional pressure for patients/residents experiencing back pain that can be relieved with a tilting wheelchair.
- **Promoting stability**: A tilting wheelchair may provide more stability with an added advantage of sense of security.

D. Bariatric wheelchairs

Bariatric wheelchairs are used for larger patients/residents dealing with mobility challenges. Patients/residents above a certain weight might feel constrained in a conventional wheelchair, which may limit their ability to move around safely and freely.

A bariatric wheelchair is manufactured with heavy-duty materials and has wider seats to accommodate larger individuals.

The primary aim of these bariatric wheelchairs is to increase the patient/resident's comfort, safety, and independence.

> ## Benefits of bariatric wheelchairs
>
> The main advantage of a bariatric wheelchair is that it prevents the slowing down of wheelchair due to extra load, as in the case of a conventional chair.
>
> Additional benefits of bariatric wheelchair may include:
>
> - Patients/residents who are more than 100 lbs.
> - Patients/residents suffering from a cardiovascular condition.
> - Patients/residents with weight-related joint health issues.

E. Lightweight wheelchairs

Lightweight wheelchairs are simple and easy to use, as well as being easily portable. Although these lightweight wheelchairs are light in weight; however, they are still stable, and they can handle a standard load.

> ## Benefits of lightweight wheelchair
>
> These wheelchairs are more comfortable to operate for the patient/resident. These lightweight wheelchairs can move relatively quickly without putting too much stress on the patient/resident's muscles and joints.
>
> Although these wheelchairs might not be ideal for all patients/residents, lightweight wheelchairs may be a great option for those looking to increase independence and mobility in a convenient, hassle-free manner.

F. Electric wheelchairs

Electric wheelchairs are a broad group of all types of wheelchairs, which are powered electrically, rather than manually.

Electric wheelchairs may include different types of wheelchairs i.e. a lightweight wheelchair, a standing wheelchair, or a reclining wheelchair can all be powered electrically. Electric wheelchairs may be available in rear-wheel drive, mid-wheel drive, and front-wheel drive.

Electric powered wheelchairs are ideal for patients/residents with conditions that may cause muscle weakness, which could make them more prone to fatigue with a manual wheelchair. Electric wheelchairs can also benefit those who have cardiovascular problems and need to avoid strenuous activities. Being adjustable positions in wheelchair may have various benefits like improving circulation, relieving back pain, and preventing pressure sores.

Burns

Burns are one of the most commonly occurring household injuries, especially among children. Burns are tissue damage results from heat, electrical contact, or overexposure to the sun, radiation, or chemicals.

Symptoms of burns may vary depending on how deep the skin damage is. It may take a day or two to develop the signs and symptoms of a severe burn.

- **1st-degree burns.** These are minor burns affects only the outer layer of the skin (epidermis). They may cause pain and redness.
- **2nd-degree burns.** These burns affect both the epidermis and dermis (the second

layer of skin). 2nd-degree burns cause swelling and redness, and white or splotchy skin. Blisters may be developed along with severe pain. Scarring can be caused by deep second-degree burns.

- **3rd-degree burns.** These burns reach to the fat layer beneath the skin. Areas of burned may be black, white, or brown and the skin may look leathery. Third-degree burns may destroy nerves, causing numbness.

Causes

Burns are generally caused by:

- Steam or hot liquid and steam
- Glass, hot metal, or other objects
- Fire
- Electrical currents
- Sunlight or other sources of ultraviolet radiation, such as a tanning bed
- Radiation
- Chemicals such as strong acids, paint thinner, or gasoline

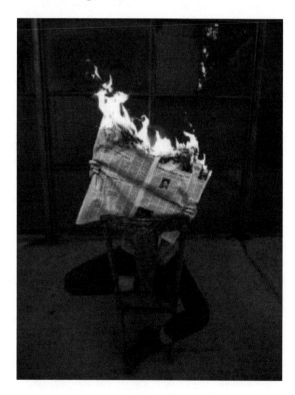

Types of Burns

A. Thermal Burns

Thermal burns occur when someone comes in contact with something hot such as:

- Flames or fire
- Hot, molten liquid or steam
- Hot objects, such as irons, cooking pans, or heated appliances

B. Chemical Burns

Chemical burns may occur if skin and/or eyes come in contact with an irritant, such as acid, chlorine, ammonia, bleach, battery acid, strong or harsh cleaners.

The symptoms of chemical burns may vary, depending on how the burn occurred. A burn due to a chemical swallowed has different symptoms than burns occurred on the skin contact. The symptoms of a chemical burn usually depend on:

- the length of time for which the skin was in contact with the chemical
- whether the chemical was swallowed or inhaled
- whether the skin had open cuts or wounds or was intact during contact
- the location of contact
- the amount and strength of the chemical used
- whether the chemical was a gas, solid, or liquid

C. Electrical Burns

Electrical burns occur when the body comes in contact with an electric current. Human internal body systems are not resistant to electricity, which may be injured if a strong jolt enters into the body. The main cause of electrical burn is coming in contact with an extension cord where the insulation material has worn away. Low-voltage electrical burns may also occur in the mouth, especially when young children place noninsulated cords in their mouth.

D. Friction Burns

A friction burn occurs when skin is scraped against a hard surface or repeatedly rubs against another surface. Most of the friction burns are first degree and often heal on their own within 3 to 6 days. These can be prevented by using moisturizing creams; however, medical care is needed for more serious friction burns.

E. Radiation Burns

Cancer patients receiving radiation therapy may experience an injury known as radiation burn. High-energy radiations are generally used to kill or shrink cancerous cells, and when these pass through the body, skin cells may be destroyed. If anyone frequently receiving radiation therapy, the skin cells may not have enough time to regenerate, and ulcers or sores may develop.

Preventing Burns

Spilled hot liquids, electrical items, smoking, and very hot water (sinks, showers, and tubs) are common causes of burns. Burns can be prevented by:

- Assisting with drinking and eating as needed. Spilling hot fluids or food can cause burns.
- There should be careful carrying of hot food and fluids, especially when near patients/ residents.
- Keeping hot food and fluids away from table and counter edges.
- Hot liquids should not be poured near a patent/resident.
- Turning on cold water first, then hot water and turning off hot water first, then cold water.
- Measuring bath or shower water temperature. Checking it before a patent/resident gets into the tub or shower.
- Checking for "hot spots" in bath water.
- Not permitting the patient/resident to sleep with a heating pad or an electric blanket.
- Following safety guidelines when applying heat and cold.
- Providing safety measures for patients/residents who smoke.
- By ensuring people smoke only in smoking areas.
- Not leaving smoking materials at the bedside.
- Supervising the smoking of persons who cannot protect themselves.
- Not allowing smoking in bed.
- Not allowing smoking where oxygen is stored or used.

Management of Major Burns

The three major goals for treating any burn are to **relieve pain and discomfort, prevent shock**, and **reduce the risk of infection**.

Nursing assistants should take following steps until advanced emergency help arrives:

- **Burned person should be protected from further harm.** It should be ensured that the victim is not in contact with the source of the burn e.g. for electrical burns, the power source should be turned off if possible.

- **Making sure that the person burned is breathing.** If needed, rescue breathing should be provided.

- **Removing jewellery, belts and other restrictive items,** especially from around the neck and burned areas. Burned areas swell rapidly.

- **Covering the area of the burn** by using a cool, moist bandage or a clean cloth.

- **Not immersing large severe burns in water.** Doing so may cause a serious loss of body heat (hypothermia).

- **Elevating the burned area.** There should be raised the wound above heart level, if possible.

- **Watching for signs of shock.** Signs and symptoms include pale complexion, fainting, or breathing in a notably shallow fashion.

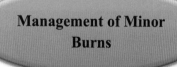

Management of Minor Burns

For minor burns:

- **Cooling the burn.** Burned area should be held under cool running water or a cool and wet compress should be applied until the pain eases.

- **Removing rings or other tight items from the burned area.** It should be done quickly and gently, before the area swells.

- **Not breaking blisters.** Fluid-filled blisters generally protect against infection. If a blister breaks, the area should be cleaned with water (mild soap is optional). An antibiotic ointment may be used; however, if a rash appears, the ointment should not be used anymore.

- **Applying lotion.** Once a burn is completely cooled, a lotion or moisturizer should be applied, in order to provide relief and prevent drying.

- **Bandaging the burn.** Burn should be covered with a sterile gauze bandage (not fluffy cotton). It should be wrapped loosely to avoid putting pressure on burned skin. Bandaging usually keeps air off the area, minimizes pain, and protects blistered skin.

Bioterrorism

Bioterrorism is the result of the release of a biologic agent into a specified environment. Some biologic attacks are covert or unannounced, and the onset of symptoms is delayed by an incubation period.

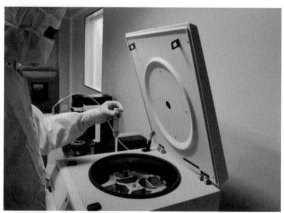

1. Biological threat/attack

Biological attack occurs as a result of the release of a biologic agent into a specified environment.

According to the CDC (Centers for Disease Control and Prevention), there are three major categories of biological agents that could potentially be used in a

biological attack i.e. Category A, B, and C agents:

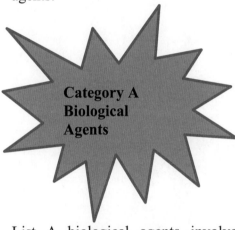

List A biological agents involve high-priority organisms that can be easily transmitted or disseminated from person to person, result in high mortality rates, might cause social disruption and public panic, and require special action for public health preparedness.

Following are the diseases that are caused by category A biological agents, along with the causative organism:

- Anthrax (Bacillus anthracis)
- Botulism (Clostridium botulinumtoxin)
- Smallpox (variola major)
- Plague (Yersinia pestis)
- Tularemia (Francisella tularensis)
- Viral hemorrhagic fevers, including Filoviruses and Arenaviruses

Anthrax

It is caused by the Bacillus anthracis bacterium. The incubation period of anthrax usually ranges from 1 to 6 days, although it is up to two months for inhalation anthrax. There are three types of anthrax i.e. cutaneous anthrax, gastrointestinal anthrax, and inhalation anthrax.

Symptoms of cutaneous anthrax may include the presence of painless skin lesions that are at beginning vesicles, then ulcers and finally eschar. Gastrointestinal anthrax is linked to the ingestion or exposure to meat from infected animals. Symptoms of inhalation anthrax may include flu like symptoms and upper respiratory symptoms such as rhinorrhea and congestion.

Anthrax can be diagnosed by the presence of Bacillus anthracis in blood cultures, cutaneous lesions, and in some cases the cerebrospinal fluid. Management of anthrax may include vaccination, antibiotic therapy (doxycycline or ciprofloxacin) and supportive care.

Smallpox

It is caused by the Variola major virus. At the times of the Revolutionary war, blankets and other objects that contained the smallpox virus were used as a biological weapon by the British soldiers against their enemies.

The incubation period for smallpox may range from 7 to 19 days after exposure. Initial symptoms of smallpox may include malaise, rigors, fever, headache, vomiting, and backache. After 2 to 3 days of the initial symptoms, lesions appear on the mouth and tongue, and then a rash appears on the arms, face and legs, later progressing to the trunk and lower extremities. The initial diagnosis of smallpox depends upon symptoms and the clinical presentation. Management for smallpox focuses on supportive care (hydration, antipyretics, analgesics, and management of secondary infections). Vaccination with the smallpox vaccine is most effective if it is administered within four days of exposure.

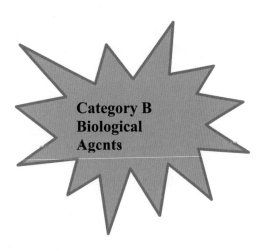

Category B
Biological
Agents

Second highest priority biological agents include those which are moderately easy to disseminate, result in low mortality rates and moderate morbidity rates, and require specific diagnostic capacity and enhanced disease surveillance.

Following are the diseases that are caused by category B biological agents, along with the specific causative organism:

- Brucellosis (Brucellaspecies)
- Ricin toxin from Ricinus communis (castor beans)
- Epsilon toxin of Clostridium perfringens
- Food safety threats (Salmonella species, Escherichia coliO157:H7, Shigella)
- Melioidosis (Burkholderia pseudomallei)
- Psittacosis (Chlamydia psittaci)
- Glanders (Burkholderia mallei)
- Q fever (Coxiella burnetii)
- Staphylococcal enterotoxin B
- Typhus fever (Rickettsia prowazekii)
- Water safety threats (Vibrio cholerae)

<u>Ricin</u>

Ricin is a poisonous substance found naturally in castor beans. If castor beans are swallowed or chewed, the released ricin may cause injury. Ricin can also be prepared from the waste material left over from processing castor beans. It can be in the form of a mist, powder, or a pellet. It can be dissolved in weak acid or water.

As a bioterrorist act, it may take a deliberate act to make ricin and use it to poison people. If manufactured into a partially purified material or refined into a warfare or terrorist agent, ricin can be used to expose people through the air, water, or food. Death from ricin poisoning may occur within 36 to 72 hours of exposure, depending on the route of its exposure (ingestion, inhalation, or injection) and the dose received.

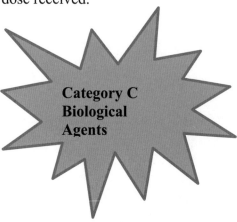

Category C
Biological
Agents

Third highest priority biological agents include emerging pathogens that can be engineered for mass dissemination in the future because of easy availability, ease of production and dissemination, and potential for high morbidity and mortality rates.

According to the Centers for Disease Control and Prevention, category C biological agents may include emerging infectious diseases, such as Nipahvirus and Hantavirus.

2. Chemical threat/attack

Chemical attack occurs as a result of the release of a chemical agent into a specified environment.

Chemical agents are poisonous vapors, liquids, aerosols, and solids that have toxic effects on people, plants, or animals. They can be released by bombs or sprayed from vehicles, aircraft, and boats. Some chemical agents may be tasteless and odorless. They may have an immediate fatal effect (a few seconds to a few minutes) or a delayed effect (2 to 48 hours).

A chemical attack may come with or without any warning. Signs of a chemical release may include individuals having difficulty breathing, eye irritation, losing coordination, becoming nauseated, or having a burning sensation in the throat, nose, and lungs. Additionally, the presence of many dead birds or insects may indicate a chemical agent release.

The use of chemicals as a chemical attack may include wide variety of chemicals such as:

- Disinfecting and sterilizing agents
- Cleaning agents
- Anesthetic agents
- Laboratory chemicals
- Medical gases
- Cytotoxic drugs and pharmaceutical substances

3. Incendiary/Fire and Explosive Threat

The threat of both incendiary devices and explosions is the most commonly used by terrorists. In the event of an explosion, shelter should be taken against a desk or a sturdy table. Concussive explosive devices are easily available worldwide. Explosives can easy be transported and operated without special training. They tend to be cheap, efficient, and effective. An explosive usually consists of any material that when induced into a chemical reaction converts rapidly from a liquid or solid into an expanding gas. The damage is mainly due to the tremendously increased atmospheric pressure, which is forced outward from where the original substance has expanded.

Explosive devices are commonly used as dispersal mechanisms for weapons of mass destruction. An explosive may rupture chemical storage tanks, biological agents, fling chemicals, or radioactive materials into the air and surrounding environment.

4. Nuclear threat/attack

Nuclear weapons are weapons of mass destruction that are used during a nuclear attack. Nuclear warfare can produce mass destruction in shortest time with a long-lasting radiological result. If a nuclear attack occurs, it can result death of millions of people on spot followed by deaths from starvation and severe injuries.

There are two types of nuclear weapons: fission and fusion.

Fission weapons

All existing nuclear weapons attain some of their explosive energy from a nuclear fission reaction. Those weapons whose explosive output is specifically from fission reactions are referred to as atom bombs or atomic bombs.

Fusion weapons

These nuclear weapons produce a large proportion of energy in nuclear fusion reactions. Those weapons whose explosive output is especially from fusion reactions are referred as thermonuclear weapons or hydrogen bombs. All these weapons derive a significant part of their energy from fission reactions to "trigger" fusion reactions. The major pathologic effect of nuclear reactions may cause damage to DNA.

5. Radiation threat/Radiological attack

Radiation attack occurs as a result of the exposure of radiological weapons of mass destruction in a specified environment.

Radioactive and nuclear agents are categorized separately, nevertheless are closely related. Nuclear weapons are instruments of mass destruction that have a main focus relevant to explosive impact and physical damage. Radioactive weapons of mass destruction differ in that they are all about radiation fallout. With radioactive agents, the major focus is to threaten and sicken people while preparing buildings or land unusable for extended periods of time.

Radiological dispersion devices (RDDs) can be used specifically for the spread of radiation emitting material over a wide area. A radiological dispersion device may not directly kill large numbers of people; however, yet the degree of terror and societal disruption due to its use would be almost indescribable. A radiological dispersion device is often referred to as a "dirty bomb," and usually consists of conventional explosives wrapped in some kind of container having low-grade radioactive waste or fissionable material.

Explosions may not be necessary for radioactive weapons of mass destruction. Radiation-emitting material can also be distributed by means of a passive dispersion device. These devices are usually as simple as hand sowed radioactive powders or waste products used to contaminate anything, such as a playground or a batch of cosmetics.

Radiation attacks may be intentional or unintentional. Unintentional radiologic attacks include Nuclear Reactor Accidents and Transportation Accidents like a spill of radioactive material from a train or truck.

Intentional acts may include:

- Contaminating water and food with radioactive material
- Spreading radioactive material into the environment
- Using conventional explosives such as dynamite (dirty bomb)
- Using wind currents or natural traffic patterns

- Destroying or bombing a nuclear reactor
- Causing nuclear material to spill while in transit
- Exploding a nuclear weapon

Oxygen therapy

Oxygen is a gaseous element, essential for life. If a person is deprived of oxygen, death may occur within minutes. Normally, all people get sufficient amount of oxygen from the air they breathe. Supplemental (therapeutic) oxygen is necessary only when an individual is unable to get sufficient oxygen for the body's needs due to a breathing or blood deficiency. Excess oxygen is not beneficial; in fact, it can be dangerous. Therefore, oxygen is prescribed just like medication that should be administered under controlled conditions.

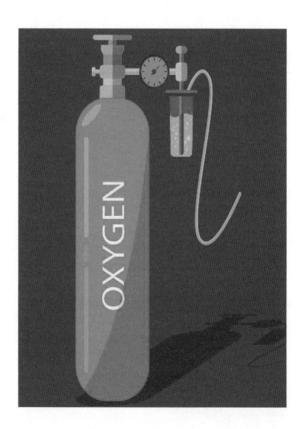

Oxygen administration

Oxygen may be administered to a patient with carbon monoxide poisoning, severe asthma, pneumonia, heart failure, or myocardial infarction, or after abdominal or chest surgery. It provides comfort for the patient/resident and permits him/her to breathe more easily.

Goals of oxygen therapy

Increasing the oxygen concentration (or percentage) the patient inhales accomplishes three major goals:

- Reverses hypoxemia (low concentration of oxygen in the blood)
- Decreases the work of the respiratory system
- Decreases the work of heart in pumping blood

Hazards of oxygen therapy

As with all medications, oxygen should be administered carefully and safely. Oxygen administered in high concentration over a long period can result in oxygen toxicity, manifested as changes in lung tissue. In some patients, increased oxygen concentrations may also affect their ventilatory drive control mechanisms, which can weak the stimulus to breathe. Therefore, oxygen should be considered just like a medication and it should be administered with the same care used in administering any medication. A physician evaluates the patient's need for oxygen and prescribes a specific order for oxygen therapy with the appropriate dosage.

Administration of oxygen by using a mask or cannula is generally expressed in liters per minute (L/min or LPM); however, some devices may control the specific oxygen concentration to be administered. When using mechanical ventilators, concentration of oxygen can be controlled more easily.

Assisting with oxygen therapy

Disease, surgery, and injury often interfere with breathing and the amount of oxygen in the blood may be less than normal (hypoxemia). If so, the physician prescribes oxygen therapy. Oxygen should be treated just like a drug. The physician orders when to give oxygen, the amount, and the device to use. Some patients/residents need oxygen constantly. Others need it for symptom relief (shortness of breath or chest pain). The nurse assistant usually does not administer oxygen. The nurse and respiratory therapist administer and maintain oxygen therapy. The nurse assistant just helps provide safe care.

Sources of oxygen

Large healthcare facilities generally use the large bulk storage tank, with its convenient in-room piping system. Most of the healthcare facilities have smaller oxygen tanks (cylinders) and oxygen strollers available to provide emergency or portable oxygen supplies. Some smaller facilities that require oxygen supplies less frequently have small cylinders. Most common source of oxygen may include:

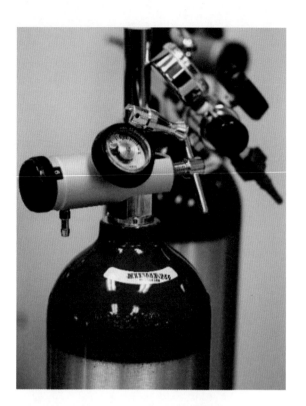

A. Wall outlets

A wall outlet with bulk storage and in-room piping systems is generally installed next to each bed. Adapters and wall outlets vary, not only in terms of type of gas they supply, but also in terms of color, shape, and connection method. The nurse assistant should be familiar with the wall outlet system used in the healthcare facility. Nursing assistants should also practice inserting the adapter into the outlet so that it can be done easily and quickly during an emergency.

B. Oxygen cylinders

Oxygen cylinders may be available in many sizes, but they are grouped into two major categories: large and small. A large oxygen cylinder is identifiable not only in terms of its size, but also by the presence of a metal cap screwed onto its top in order to protect the valve from damage. The valve itself also contains an attached handle and threaded connection site. Large cylinders are generally required when high oxygen flow rates are essential or when a patient/resident needs oxygen for an extended period of time. A small cylinder can be identified by its rectangular valve with no handle along with presence of three holes on one side. Small cylinders are used when transporting clients or for short-term emergencies. These small cylinders can be used at home.

C. Oxygen strollers

Portable oxygen can also be supplied by a liquid-oxygen stroller, also terms as a "walker" or "companion". The liquid-oxygen portable unit consists of a thermos-type vessel in a small carrying case or shoulder bag. Liquid oxygen is generally denser than the gaseous oxygen, so a portable oxygen stroller can carry more oxygen and yet be more compact and lighter than a steel gas cylinder.

D. Oxygen concentrators

Oxygen concentrators are widely used in extended care settings and home. Oxygen concentrators compress room air and extract oxygen with an oxygen flow of 1 to 5 LPM. An oxygen concentrator is safer and more convenient to use than an oxygen tank or oxygen stroller. An oxygen concentrator also does not need to be refilled; however, it requires periodic maintenance to operate, and may not be portable.

Oxygen delivery systems

A. Nasal canula

The nasal cannula is a device which is used to deliver small to moderate increases in oxygen concentration. The nasal cannula has two short tubes each fitting into the nostrils. This low-flow device can provides an oxygen concentration in the 24% to 44% range, with flow rates of 1 to 6 LPM. Most patients/residents prefer cannulas as they are less confining and do not interfere with talking, eating, or talking.

B. Simple mask

It is a transparent mask with a simple nipple adapter that fits over the patient/resident's nose, mouth, and chin. It is a low-flow device that can deliver 40% to 60% oxygen, with a flow of 6 to 10 LPM.

C. Partial-rebreathing mask

The partial-rebreathing mask (PRM) is a low-flow device that can be identified by the absence of valves and presence of a bag. This low-flow device can provides an oxygen concentration in the 60% to 90% range, with flow rates of 8 to 11 LPM.

D. Non-rebreathing mask

The nonrebreathing mask can be distinguished from the partial-rebreathing mask by the presence of valves on the outside of the mask, as well as valves between the mask and bag. It can provide oxygen in the 90% to 100% range, with flow rate of 12 LPM.

Oxygen safety

Everyone, including the patient/resident, visitors, nursing assistants, and others in the unit must know and follow the necessary instructions when oxygen is administered. If oxygen comes in contact with any flammable or combustible material, even a little spark can ignite an explosive or fire. Following are some precautionary measures that should be followed when providing oxygen:

- Oxygen device should not be removed immediately.
- It should be ensured that the oxygen device is secure but not tight.
- Signs of irritation from the device should be checked. Back of the ears, underneath surface of the nose (cannula), and surrounding areas of the face (mask) must be thoroughly evaluated. Also check the cheekbones.
- The face should be kept clean and dry when a mask is used.
- Oxygen flow should not be shut off. However, it must be turned off with removal of oxygen device if there is a fire.
- The supervised nurse should be informed at once if the flow rate is too high or too low.
- The supervised nurse should be informed at once if a humidifier is not bubbling. Humidified (moist) oxygen prevents dryness of the airway's mucous membranes. Bubbling in the humidifier indicates that moisture is being produced.
- An adequate water level should be maintained in the humidifier.
- Secure tubing should be in place.

- It should be ensured that there are no kinks in the tubing.
- It should be ensured that the patient does not lie on any part of the tubing.
- It should be ensured that the oxygen tank is secure in its holder.
- Any signs and symptoms of respiratory distress, hypoxia, or abnormal breathing patterns should be reported to the nurse at once.
- Oral hygiene should be provided as directed in the care plan.
- It should be made sure that the oxygen device is clean and free of mucus.
- Continuous observation of the patient/resident's respirations and proper bag deflation are essential.
- Cardiac monitoring with alarms is recommended strongly. As nonrebreathing mask produces extremely high oxygen concentrations, oxygen toxicity can occur in as little as 72 hours. Therefore, the patient/resident wearing an NRM should not be left alone.

Postural supports/Restraints/Soft protective devices

Postural supports

These are devices that help to keep the patient/resident in the correct posture and position when in a chair or bed.

Restraints

A restraint is any device that inhibits an individual's freedom of movement. Restraints can be chemical or physical. Chemical restraints are medications used to subdue a patient/resident; so that the patient is unable to function normally. A physical restraint is attached near or on a patient's body to limit his/her freedom of movement or ability to reach part of his/her body. Examples of physical restraints may include wrist restraints, jacket restraints, mitt restraints, and vest restraints. Devices like side rails and lap trays may also be considered physical restraints, if the patient/resident is unable to move them out of the way independently.

Soft protective device

Soft protective device is a device that serves as a reminder to the patient/resident of safety issues such as a waist device or Posey (also called safety device reminders-SDR).

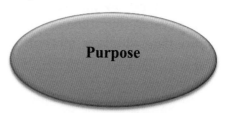

Purpose

Postural supports/Restraints/Soft protective devices may help to keep patient/resident safe by preventing them from getting up without assistance and falling or wandering away from the healthcare facility. These are also used to prevent the patient/resident from harming self or others around them. In various healthcare settings, they are an essential part to prevent patient/resident from

- Falling out of bed or chair
- Crawling the end of the bed or over side rails
- Hurting themselves or others
- Controlling behavior and can be used only in extreme measures like limb devices

Restraint alternatives

Often there are reasons and causes for harmful behaviors. Knowing and managing these reasons can prevent restraint use. It should be tried by asking following questions to find out what the behavior means.

- Is the patient/resident in pain, ill, or injured?

- Is the patient/resident short of breath?
- Is the patient/resident afraid in a new setting?
- Does the patient/resident need to use the bathroom?
- Is dressing or clothing tight or causing other discomfort?
- Is the patient/resident's position uncomfortable?
- Are body fluids, excretions, or secretions causing skin irritation?
- Does the patient/resident have problems communicating?
- Is the patient/resident confused or disoriented?

Restraint alternatives may be a part of the care plan. Restraint alternatives may not protect the patient/resident; however, restraints should be used as a last option before the following alternatives to restraints:

- Diversion like TV, videos, music, and games should be provided.
- Life-long habits and routines should be included in the care plan e.g. showers before breakfast, reads in the bathroom, walking outside before lunch, watching TV after lunch etc.
- Family and friends should make videos of themselves for the patient/resident to watch.
- Time should be spent in supervised areas (lounge, dining room, and near the nurses' station).
- Wedge cushions, pillows, and posture and positioning aids should be used.
- The signal light should be within reach.
- Signal lights should be answered promptly.
- Hygiene, food, fluid, and elimination needs should be met.
- The bedpan, commode, or urinal should be within the patient/resident's reach.
- Back massages should be given.
- Friends, family, and volunteers visit.

- The patient/resident should have companions or sitters.
- Time should be spent with the patient/resident.
- Extra time should be spent with a patient/resident who is restless.
- A calm, quiet setting should be provided.
- Exercise programs should be provided.
- Outdoor time should be planned during nice weather.
- Warning devices should be used on beds, chairs, and doors.
- Knob guards should be used on doors.
- Padded hip protectors should be worn under clothing.
- Floor cushions should be placed next to beds.
- Roll guards should be attached to the bed frame.
- Falls should be prevented.
- The patient/resident furniture should meet his/her needs (lower bed, reclining chair, rocking chair).
- Walls and furniture corners should be padded.
- Observations and visits should be made at least every 15 minutes or as often as noted in the care plan.
- The patient/resident should be moved to a room close to the nurses' station.
- Procedures and care measures should be well explained.
- Frequent explanations should be given about equipment or devices.
- Light should be adjusted to meet the patient/resident's basic needs and preferences.
- Staff assignments should be consistent; patient/resident's sleep should not be interrupted, and noise levels should be reduced.

Types of restraints

Restraints are made of leather or cloth. Leather restraints are used for agitation and combativeness and mostly applied to the ankles and wrists. Cloth restraints are also termed as soft restraints that may include mitts, belts, straps, jackets, and vests. They are applied to the wrists, hands, ankles, waist, and chest.

A. Wrist restraints

Wrist restraints (limb holders) limit and hold the arm movement. They are generally used when the patient/resident:

- Is at risk for pulling out tubes placed for life-saving treatment (feeding tube, intravenous infusion).
- Is at risk for pulling out devices placed for monitoring of vital signs.
- Scratches/pulls/peels the skin, a wound, or a dressing to damage the skin or the wound.

B. Mitt restraints

A mitt restraint prevents the patients/residents from being able to grasp things, but they are still able to move their arms. Hands are placed within mitt restraints to prevent finger use. They permit hand, arm, and wrist movements. Most of mitts are padded and they have the same goal as wrist restraints.

C. Belt restraints

A belt restraint can be used when there is increased risk of injuries from falls or when there is need for proper positioning during a medical treatment. The patient/resident cannot get out of bed or out of a chair. However, a roll belt may allow the patient/resident to turn from side to side or sit up in bed. The belt can be applied around the waist and secured to the chair or bed (lap belt). It is usually applied over a garment.

D. Vet restraints and Jacket restraints

Vest and jacket restraints are placed to the chest and have the same purpose as belt restraints. The patient/resident cannot turn in bed or get out of a chair. A jacket restraint is placed with the opening in the back, whereas, for a vest restraint, the "V neck" is in front along with the vest crossing in the front. Vest and jacket restraints should never be worn backward. Strangulation or other injuries are major risks if the patient/resident slides down in the bed or chair. The restraint should always be applied over a garment. Vest and jacket restraints may have life-threatening risks and death can occur from these restraints due to strangulation. If caught in the restraint, it can become so tight that the patient/resident's chest cannot expand to inhale air. The patient/resident quickly suffocates and dies. Therefore, correct application is critical. Nursing assistants are advised to only assist the nurse in applying them. The nurse should take full responsibility for applying a vest or jacket restraint.

Role of Nurse Assistant in the use of postural support

1. Patient/resident should be approached in a calm manner to reduce anxiety and agitation during application.
2. All details should be explained to the patient/resident and their family thoroughly in a non-threatening manner.

3. It should be used only on a patient/resident in a bed or chair that has wheels in case of an emergency.
4. Patient/resident should be placed in a good body alignment and position.
5. "Quick release" bow-tie knot should be used to secure postural support, in order to ensure easy removal in an emergency.
6. It should be tied securely with some space of slack movement (two-finger check between support and skin).
7. Circulation, sensation, and movement should be checked every two hours
8. The support should be removed, patient/resident should be repositioned and ROM should be performed to the joints every two hours for at least ten minutes or more as per facility policy.
9. Fluids, bedpan, or urinal should be offered on a frequent and regular basis to the patient/resident.
10. Vest device should be applied with the open area of the vest in the front to prevent strangulation or choking.
11. Type of device, reason for device, Circulation, sensation, and movement, effectiveness, and nursing care should be documented.

Legal support regarding the use of restraints

Legal aspects and laws applying to restraint use are followed:

- Restraints must protect the patient/resident. They should not be used for staff convenience or to discipline a patient/resident. Applying restraints is not easier and there should be properly supervising and observing the patient/resident. A restrained patient/resident needs more staff time for supervision, care, and observation.
- A physician's order is always required for restrained application. The physician provides the reason for the restraint, what to use, what body part to restrain, and how long to use it. This information should be on the care plan and nursing assignment sheet.
- The least restrictive method should be used to allow the greatest amount of movement or body access possible. Some restraints attach to the patient/resident's body and to a non-movable object. They restrict body access or freedom of movement e.g. vest, jacket, wrist, ankle, hand, and some belt restraints. Other restraints do not directly attach to the patient/resident's body (bed rails or wedge cushions) and do not totally restrict freedom of movement or body access. Thus, it should always prefer less restrictive restraints if possible.
- Restraints should be used only when other measures fail to protect the person.
- Unnecessary restraint is considered as false imprisonment. If applied an unneeded restraint, false imprisonment charges can be applied as legal aspect.
- Informed consent is always required before applying restraints. The patient/resident must understand the reason for the restraint. The patient/resident should be explained how the restraint will help the planned medical treatment. The patient/resident should be informed about the risks of restraint use. If the patient/resident cannot give consent, his/her legal representative should be given the information. It should be remembered that consent must be given before a restraint can be used. The physician or nurse provides needed information and obtains the consent.

The restrained patient must be kept safe. The use of restraints can rob a patient/resident of his or her own dignity. Consequently, restraint use is decreasing in all healthcare settings. Currently, many healthcare facilities, especially nursing homes, strive to be restraint free.

Following safety measures should be remembered while caring a restrained patient/resident:

- Patient/resident should be observed for increased confusion and agitation as restraints may increase agitation and confusion. Patients/residents are aware of restricted movements. They may struggle to pull at the restraint or try to get out of it. Some restrained patients/residents beg others to free or to help release them. These behaviors should be viewed as signs of confusion. Not understanding what is happening to them can significantly increase their confusion. Therefore, restrained patients/residents need repeated explanations and reassurance. Spending time with these patients/residents has a calming effect.

- The quality of life of a restrained patient/resident should be improved and protected. Restraints should be used for as short a time as possible. The care plan should show how to reduce restraint use.

- The patient/resident's needs should be met with as little restraint as possible. Nursing assistants should meet physical, emotional, and social needs of the patient/resident. They should visit with the patient/resident and explain the reason for the restraint.

- Manufacturer's instructions should be followed to ensure the safe and secure application of the restraint. The restraint must be firm and snug, but not tight. Tight restraints may affect breathing and circulation. The patient/resident must be comfortable and able to move the restrained part to a safe and limited extent. • The patient/resident should be observed at least every 15 minutes or as often as directed in the care plan.

- Restraint should be removed or released for at least 10 minutes and the patient/resident should be re-positioned periodically as directed in the care plan, Basic needs should be met at least every 2 hours or as noted on the care plan.

General rules for providing safe environment for nursing assistants may include:

- Nursing assistants should have a proper knowledge regarding body mechanic principles and should also applied these principles practically

- They should also have a clear understand and practical knowledge of ergonomics

- They must know the procedures and policies regarding OSHA safety laws on use of equipment and secure handling of hazardous material.

- It is necessary for nursing assistants to wipe up spills immediately and identify wet floors with the appropriate signs

- They should walk, instead of running in halls and should watch carefully at intersections

- The nurse assistant should use contents of containers only if they have proper labels/dates and he/she knows how to use them correctly and safely

- Nursing assistants should tag and report broken equipment
- They should also report unsafe situations as quickly as possible.
- They should use 3-pronged plugs on electrical equipment
- The nurse assistant should refuse to do any task that is beyond his/her knowledge and out of scope of practice.
- They should know proper operation of commonly used routine equipment
- They should watch linen and garbage cans for safety hazards (sharps) and should report immediately if sharps container is over half full.
- They should also know procedure to follow in case of personal injury such as:
  - Immediate reporting the injury to the supervisor
  - Filling out an incident report/unusual occurrence form as per facility procedure and policy
  - Seeking medical help as necessary

General rules for providing a safe environment for the patient/resident

General rules for providing safe environment for the patient/resident may include:

- Nursing assistants should have proper knowledge regarding the National Patient Safety Goals.
- They should check name tags/wrist bands before performing any task on a patient/resident
- Patients/residents should use side rails when appropriate. Nursing assistants should have clear understanding of facility policy and procedure on side rails.

- Nursing assistants should ensure that the patient/resident must use handrails/appropriate assistive device when unstable
- They should also ensure that the patient/resident wear non-skid footwear when ambulatory
- Nursing assistants should place the call signal light within the easy reach of the patient/resident and must instruct them on its correct use
- They should always lock wheels on bed/wheelchair/gurney when transferring the patient/resident
- The nurse assistant must answer call lights promptly
- Nursing assistant should make sure that patient/resident is using night-lights for good lighting and to reduce obstacle hazards
- They should keep the bed of the patient/resident in the lowest position except when tending to the patient/resident
- They should always check bed/chair alarms and ensuring that these are in working condition
- They should keep the environment clutter free
- A patient/resident may slide out of a wheelchair. The nurse assistant should position the patient/resident correctly in the chair.

Fire safety

A fire in a healthcare facility can have devastating effects. Many patients/residents who are receiving clinical care may have limitations in hearing, mobility, vision or understanding (all of which can interfere with their positive response to react to a fire). A nurse assistant must be well aware of how to prevent a fire from occurring, and how to respond if a fire does occur.

For a fire to occur, the following stimulants must be present:

2. Fuel (something that burns)
3. Heat (something to ignite the fuel)
4. Oxygen

Removing any one of these stimulants will inhibit a fire from increasing. Many patients/residents who receive clinical care require oxygen therapy that increases the risk for fire. Following precautions should be taken to prevent fires:

- Patients/residents should always be supervised by the nursing assistants in their care whenever they smoke.
- Employer's rules and policies must be followed about smoking. It should be ensured that if patients/residents are smoking, they should smoke only in appropriate places and their smoking materials should safely extinguish. It should also be ensured that the patient/resident uses any protective equipment (such as a smoking apron) as per employer's policy.
- Materials such as matches and lighters should be placed in a secure place, and out of reach from children and confused people.
- Patient/resident should never be permitted smoking around a person who is using oxygen.
- Nursing assistants should report to their supervisor about any electrical equipment that is not properly working or is not well-maintained.
- Safety measures should be followed to prevent burns.
- Flammable liquids should be stored outside in their original containers.

- Any frayed electrical cords, smoke or burning smells should be reported immediately.
- There should be avoided from using too many electrical devices on one wall socket. 3-pronged grounded plugs are the best options to prevent electrical fires.

If a fire does break out, the nurse assistant must know how to respond. Each facility has a fire emergency plan to specify the procedure used to alert others to fire (e.g. a phone number to call or the location of fire alarm pull boxes). The fire emergency plan also specifies when and how to evacuate the patients/residents in the facility, as well as any special measures to prevent a fire from spreading. The nurse assistant should be familiar with facility's fire emergency plan and should participate in the periodic drills that are held to practice putting the plan into action.

The acronym "RACE" may help the nurse assistant to remember how to react during a fire emergency:

■ **R—Rescue**

All routine activities should be stopped and patient/resident in immediate danger should be removed from the fire to a safe area as quickly as possible. If the exposure to poisonous gases, heat or flames will be less, the safer everyone will be.

■ **A —Alarm**

The nearest fire alarm pull station should be activated (if applicable). It should be dialed 9-1-1 (or another number, per employer's policy) in order to report the location and current extent of the fire.

■ **C — Contain**

All doors and windows should be closed to contain the fire. As the nurse assistant leaves an area, he/she should close the door behind him/her.

■ E —Extinguish

Only attempt to extinguish the fire should be made if it is safe for anyone to do so. If the fire is relatively small and contained, the nurse assistant may be able to put it out using a fire extinguisher.

All fire extinguishers should be checked on a regular basis to ensure that they are fully functional and ready to use in case of an emergency situation. Nursing assistants should remember the acronym P-A-S-S to use a general order for fire extinguisher:

P – Pull the safety pin out
A – Aim the hose at the base of the fire
S – Squeeze the handle
S – Sweep back and forth at the base of the fire

There are three main types of fires, which are classified as type A, B or C. Most fire extinguishers are ABC fire extinguishers that are effective against all types of fires.

Helpful Resources

1. *Bioterrorism.* (2019, February 21). Emergency Preparedness and Response | CDC.

    https://emergency.cdc.gov/bioterrorism/

2. *Classification of burns - Health encyclopedia - University of Rochester Medical Center.* Welcome to URMC - Rochester, NY - University of Rochester Medical Center.

    https://www.urmc.rochester.edu/encyclopedia/content.aspx?ContentTypeID=90&ContentID=P09575

3. *A definitive guide to emergency codes used in health care.* (2020, January 29). NHCPS.com. https://nhcps.com/emergency-preparedness-response-health-care-guide-emergency-codes/

4. *Disaster preparedness plan*. American Red Cross | Help Those Affected by Disasters. https://www.redcross.org/get-help/how-to-prepare-for-emergencies/make-a-plan.html

5. *Disaster preparedness*. International Federation of Red Cross and Red Crescent Societies. https://media.ifrc.org/ifrc/what-we-do/disaster-and-crisis-management/disaster-preparedness/

6. *Emergency action plan*. Amherst College. https://www.amherst.edu/offices/enviro_health_safety/fire/fire-emergency/emergency_actionplan

7. Feder, G. (2000). Guidelines for the prevention of falls in people over 65. *BMJ*, *321*(7267), 1007-1011. https://doi.org/10.1136/bmj.321.7267.1007

8. *Home fire safety*. American Red Cross | Help Those Affected by Disasters. https://www.redcross.org/get-help/how-to-prepare-for-emergencies/types-of-emergencies/fire.html

9. Lee, A. (2013) Preventing falls in the geriatric population. *The Permanente Journal*, 37-39. https://doi.org/10.7812/tpp/12-119

10. *Oxygen therapy*. (2020, March 24) American Lung Association | American Lung Association. https://www.lung.org/lung-health-diseases/lung-procedures-and-tests/oxygen-therapy

11. *Oxygen therapy* NHLBI, NIH. https://www.nhlbi.nih.gov/health-topics/oxygen-therapy

12. *Restraints* Azure Prod. https://nurses.ab.ca/standards-and-learning/restraints

13. Stander, M., & Wallis, L. A. (2011) The emergency management and treatment of severe burns. *Emergency Medicine International*, *2011*, 1-5. https://doi.org/10.1155/2011/161375

14. Theresa. (2017, July 12) *Assistive devices* Elderly Fall Prevention.

   https://elderlyfallprevention.com/assistive-devices/

15. *Types.* Stanford Health Care (SHC) - Stanford Medical Center | Stanford Health Care.

   https://stanfordhealthcare.org/medical-conditions/skin-hair-and-nails/burns/types.html

16. *What is RACE/PASS?* RACE/PASS Fire Safety. https://race-pass.com/aboutus.sc

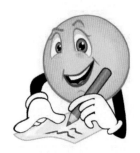

Chapter Five:

Body Mechanics

Outline

I: The purpose and rules of proper body mechanics

II: Comfort and safety measures used to lift, move, turn, and position patients/residents in bed

III: Body positions for bedridden patients/residents

IV: Patients/residents transfers

V: Appropriate body mechanics used for ambulation of a patient/resident

Purpose and Rules of Proper Body Mechanics

Purpose of proper body mechanics

Body mechanics is the coordinated and synchronized effort of the nervous and musculoskeletal systems to maintain posture, balance, and body alignment during moving, bending, lifting, and performing activities of daily livings (ADLs). Proper body mechanics also promotes body movement so a person can perform a physical activity without consuming excessive muscle energy. Many patients/residents need limitations in activity recommended by their treatment plan or have problems resulting in immobility. It is therefore an important responsibility for the nursing assistants to safely move and position patients/residents, in order to minimize the risks related to immobilization. Appropriate positioning patients/residents to maintain accurate body alignment is significant in preventing complications. These complications may include pressure sores (which can develop in less than 24 hours and usually needs months to heal) and contractures (which usually develop within a few days when joints, muscles, and tendons become less flexible because of incorrect alignment and lack of mobility). Some patients/residents have greater risk for complications from incorrect positioning and have higher risk for injury during transfer such as patients/residents with poor nutrition, loss of sensation, poor circulation, alterations in joint mobility or bone formation, and impaired muscle development. The application of appropriate body mechanics,

alignment, and the use of safe positioning techniques and patient transfer may help patients/residents achieve an ideal level of independence without resultant injury to healthcare professionals.

Appropriate use of body mechanics may avoid the following:
- Muscle tears or strains
- Excessive fatigue
- Skeletal injuries
- Injury to the patient/resident
- Injury to assisting healthcare providers

Body mechanics moves around proper alignment, balance, and coordinated movement. When the body is correctly aligned, different body parts are in position to develop optimal balance. Perfect alignment reduces excessive stress and strain on the joints, muscles, tendons, and ligaments whether a person is standing, seated, or lying down.

Nursing Assistants often need to guide patients/residents the use of proper body mechanics for safe movements and walking. Therefore, a Nurse Assistant first needs to understand and practice appropriate body mechanics himself/herself. Both the patent/resident and nursing assistants differ in size, weight, and ability to move. The Nurse Assistant's physical strength is not as important as how efficiently he/she uses the body to support a patient/resident. Ultimately, efficient and proper use of one's body determines how safely and comfortably he/she is able to move patients/residents. It is significant to provide safety for both the Nurse Assistant and the patient/resident.

Proper body mechanics

Body mechanics is generally the use of the most effective and safest methods of lifting and moving, which means applying mechanical principles of movement to the human body.

Principles of proper body mechanics

The laws of physics regulate all motions. From these laws of physics, we derive the general rules and principles of body mechanics. In other words, some manners of carrying and moving and objects are more efficient than others. Rules underlying appropriate body mechanics usually involve three main factors:

- Base of support
- Line of gravity
- Body alignment

An individual's center of gravity is situated in the pelvic area. This means that almost half the body weight is distributed over this area, and half below it, when imagining of the body divided horizontally. Additionally, half the body weight is to each side, when imagining of the body divided vertically. Therefore, when object is lifted, the back should be kept straight along with bending at the knees and hips. By doing this, the center of gravity remains over the feet, providing extra strength and stability. It is therefore much easier to maintain balance.

Base of support

An individual's feet provide the base of support. The broader the base of support,
the more stables the object, within limits. The feet should be spread sidewise when lifting, to provide side-to-side stability. One foot should be placed slightly in front of the other to give back-to-front stability. The weight should be distributed evenly between both feet. The knees should be flexed slightly to absorb jolts. The feet should be moved to turn the object being moved (It is significant not to twist the body).

Line of gravity

An imaginary vertical (up and down) line is drawn through the top of the head, the base of support, and the center of gravity. This line is considered the line of gravity, or the gravital plane. The line of gravity is the direction of gravitational pull (from the head top to the feet). For highest efficacy and efficacy, this line of gravity should be straight from the head's top to the base of support, with uniform weight on each side. Therefore, if an individual stands with the head erect and back straight, the line of gravity will be almost through the center of the body, and appropriate body mechanics will be in place.

Body alignment

When walking, lifting, or performing any activity, correct body alignment is necessary to maintain the balance. When an individual's body is in proper alignment, all the muscles work together for the most efficient and safest movement (without muscle strain). Body stretching as high as possible produces correct alignment. This can be established through proper posture. When a person is in standing position, the weight is a bit forward and is held up on the outside part of the feet. Again, the back is straight, the head is erected, and the abdomen is tucked in (It should be remembered that the patient/resident in bed should be in almost the same position as if he/she were standing).

Basic rules of proper body mechanics

- It is easier to push pull, or roll an object than to lift it. The movement should be continuous and smooth, rather than jerky.

- Often less force or energy is needed to keep an object moving than to start and stop it.

- It takes less force to lift an object if the nurse assistant works as close to it as possible. The stronger arm and leg muscles should be used as much as possible. The back muscles, which are not as strong, should be used little as possible.

- The nurse assistant should rock forward or backward on the feet and with her/his body as a force for pushing or pulling.

- The nurse assistant should keep his/her body in good alignment with a wide base of support.

- An upright posture should be used, which involve bending the legs. The back should not be bent to maintain an upright posture.

- Heavy objects should be pulled, pushed, or slided rather than lifting them. Pushing is much easier than pulling.

- Widening the base of support to pull or push is an important component of proper body mechanics. A person should move his/her front leg forward when pushing and he/she should move his/her rear leg back when pulling.

- Both hands and arms should be used to carry, lift, or move objects.

- The whole body should be turned to change direction instead of twisting the body.

- The work should be done with smooth and even movements, without sudden or jerky motions.

- The nurse assistant should not lean over a patient/resident to provide care.

- The nurse assistant should get help from a co-worker to carry or move heavy objects. He/she should not move or lift them by himself/herself alone if possible.

- For lifting heavy objects from the floor, hips and knees should be bended to lift them. The back should be in straight position as the object reaches thigh level. The leg and thigh muscles should work to raise the object off the floor and to waist level.

- Objects should not be lifted higher than chest level or above the shoulders. A step stool or ladder should be used to reach an object higher than chest level.

- The nurse assistant should evaluate and assess the situation before acting so that he/she can plan to use proper body mechanics.

Legal and total quality improvement issues: Protecting the body from injury

Nurse assistants usually move and lift patients/residents and things all day long.

This can result a great deal of strain on their joints and muscles, causing skin abrasion and work-related musculoskeletal disorder (WRMD). Currently, many employers have "safe patient handling" or "no lift" programs, per OSHA (Occupational Safety and Health Administration) recommendations. These programs suggest minimizing on-the-job injuries by providing equipment (such as powered standing-assist devices and mechanical lifts), resources (such as extra staffing), and training to make repositioning and lifting patients/residents safer and easier for the health care worker. Nursing assistants should always follow their employer's policies and the patient/resident's care plan when they are determining how to assist a patient/resident with moving, and proper utilization of the equipment that is available. They should ask for assistance from their co-workers when they need it. Finally, nursing assistants should also learn and practice proper body mechanics and lifting techniques.

Practicing Good Body Mechanics: Comfort and safety measures used to lift, turn, move, and position patients/residents in bed

By practicing good body mechanics, the nurse assistant can use his/her body in an efficient and safe way to accomplish tasks such as pushing, lifting, and pulling. Proper body mechanics are all about balance, alignment, and coordination.

Balance is strength and stability obtained through the even distribution of weight.

The most important thing to stay balanced is having a wide base of support and keeping the heaviest part of the body (center of gravity) closer to the base of support. During standing position, feet and legs are the base of support, and torso is the center of gravity. Therefore, spreading the legs apart and bending knees to bring torso lower may help to remain stable on feet.

Alignment is basically all about good posture. If an individual have ever driven a car that is out of alignment, he/she knows that it's difficult to steer and it's extremely unsafe. Human bodies without proper alignment may have similar issues. Body parts can get pulled out of shape, leading to extreme discomfort and severe injury. Holding body in alignment can minimize strain on muscles and joints.

Coordination is generally the utilization of force and direction for purposeful action. For example, when the nurse assistant is moving a patient/resident up in bed, he/she will place one of his/her feet in front of the other. Shifting weight from the back foot towards the front foot may provide an additional power and assist him/her to move the patient/resident toward the head of the bed easily. Coordination also depicts working with someone, rather than against them. For example, when the nurse assistant is repositioning a patient/resident, he/she should encourage that patient for support as much as possible. Similarly, if a nurse assistant is working with another nurse assistant to reposition a patient/resident, they should use good communication to ensure that both performing the same actions at the same time. This will provide them twice the power and make the move much easier.

General guidelines and comfort measures for safe patient handling and movement

Patients/residents should be kept in good alignment and protected from any injury while being moved. Nursing assistants should follow these recommended guidelines when moving and lifting patients/residents:

- Initial Assessment of the patient/resident and knowledge about the patient/resident's medical diagnosis, capabilities, and any movement not allowed.
- Placing braces or any device the patient/resident wears before helping the patient/resident from the bed.
- Assessing the patient/resident's ability to support with the planned movement.
- Patients/residents should be encouraged to support in their own transfers. Encouraging the patient/resident to perform activities that are within his/her capabilities boosts independence.
- Reducing or eliminating unnecessary tasks by the nurse assistant reduces the risk of injury.
- Assessing the patient/resident's ability to understand instructions and support with the staff to achieve the movement.
- During any patient/resident transferring task, if a nurse assistant is required to lift more than 35 pounds of a patient/resident's weight, then the patient/resident should be considered to be fully dependent and there should be the recommendation of assistive devices for his/her safe transfer.
- Ensuring sufficient staff is available to move the patient safely.

- Assessing the area for clutter and availability of assistive devices. Any obstacles that may make moving and lifting inconvenient should be removed.
- Decision of which equipment to use. For reducing risk of injury to the nurse assistant and patient, handling aids should be used whenever possible.
- Careful planning for what will be done before moving or lifting a patient/resident. A nurse assistant may injure the patient/resident or himself/herself without well planning. If necessary, it should be enlisted the support of another nurse assistant. This minimizes the strain on everyone involved. There should be clear communication with staff and the patient/resident, to make sure coordinated movement.
- Explaining to the patient/resident about the decided plan and assessing his/her capabilities to participate in the plan. This technique usually reduces the effort required and the possibility of injury to the patient/resident as well as the staff.
- If the patient/resident is in pain, the prescribed analgesic should be administered in advance of the transfer to allow the patient/resident to contribute in the move comfortably.
- Elevation of the bed, as necessary, so that a nurse assistant can work at a safe and comfortable height.
- Wheels of the bed, stretcher, or wheelchair should be locked so that they do not slide while moving the patient/resident.
- The principles of proper body mechanics should be followed to prevent personal injury while working.

- Supporting the patient/resident's body well. Avoiding holding and grabbing an extremity by its muscles.
- Using friction-reducing devices, whenever available, especially during lateral transfers.
- Moving the body of the nurse assistant and the patient in a smooth, rhythmic motion. Jerky movements usually tend to put extra strain on joints and muscles and are uncomfortable for the patient/resident.
- Using mechanical devices, such as slides, lifts, gait belts, or transfer chairs, for moving patients/residents.
- It should be ensured that the nurse assistant must understand how the device operates and that the patient/resident is properly informed and secured of what will occur. Patients/residents who are afraid or do not understand may be not able to cooperate and may suffer any injury as a result.
- Ensuring equipment used meets weight requirements.
- Bariatric patients/residents (BMI greater than 50) require bariatric transfer aids and equipment.

Transferring and moving can be extremely painful after an injury or surgery. Many older patients/residents have painful joints. Thus, patients/residents should be provided comfort while moving and transferring.

Safe and secure patient/resident lifting

Nursing assistant usually require to lift patients/residents and equipment frequently. If they don't use appropriate techniques when lifting, they may put themselves at risk for injuring their back. Back injuries are extremely painful and difficult to treat. These back injuries can prevent the nursing assistants from participating in activities that they enjoy, and may even end their career in health care.

Encouraging comfort and safety

Comfort
To promote mental comfort when transferring or moving the patient/resident:
- The nurse assistant should explain about what he/she is going to do and how the patient/resident can help.
- Patient/resident should be screened and covered to protect the right to privacy.

To promote physical comfort when transferring or moving the patient/resident:
- Patient/resident should be kept in good alignment.
- Care should be taken for not hitting the patient/resident's head on the head-board when he/she is moved up in bed. If the patient/resident is without a pillow, it should be placed upright against the head-board.
- Pillows should be used to position the patient/resident as directed by the nurse supervisor and the care plan. If a pillow is allowed under the patient/resident's head, it should be positioned under the head and shoulders.
- Other positioning devices should be used as directed by the nurse supervisor and the care plan.

Encouraging comfort and safety

Safety

Many older patients/residents have fragile joints and bones. To prevent injuries:

- The rules of proper body mechanics should be followed.
- There should always have help to move a patient/resident.
- The patient/resident should be carefully moved to prevent pain.
- The patient/resident should be positioned in good alignment after the procedure.

It should be ensured that the nose, face, and mouth are not obstructed by a pillow or other device.

Proper and appropriate lifting technique involves utilizing the powerful muscles of the buttocks and legs for safe and secure lifting. It involves:

- Planning for lifting, and getting assistance as needed.
- Standing closer to the patient/resident or object for lifting and avoiding leaning over or reaching.
- Placing feet almost 12 inches apart along with one foot slightly in front of the other. This position allows a broad base of support in maintaining the balance.
- Avoiding bending over at the waist. Instead, bending should be on knees, keeping the back straight. The nurse assistance should keep his/her body closer to the patient/resident and drive himself/herself upward, using the muscles of his/her buttocks and legs.
- Avoiding twisting the body at the waist when the arms are loaded.

Body positioning for bedridden patients/residents

The patient/resident must always be properly positioned. Good alignment and regular position changes promote comfort and well-being. Breathing becomes much easier. Circulation is being promoted. Contractures and pressure sores are prevented. Whether in chair or bed, the patient/resident should be re-positioned at least every 2 hours. Some patients/residents are re-positioned more often. The nurse assistant should follow the recommendations of the nurse supervisor and the care plan. To safely position a patient/resident:

- Good body mechanics should be followed.
- A co-worker should be asked to help if needed.
- The procedure should be well explained to the patient/resident.
- A nurse assistant should be gentle when moving the patient/resident.
- There should be provided proper privacy to the patient/resident.
- Pillows should be used as directed by the nurse supervisor for support and alignment.
- Proper comfort should be provided after positioning.
- The call light and needed items should be placed within reach of the patient/resident after positioning.
- A thorough safety check should be completed before leaving the room.

A contracture is the deficient joint mobility due to abnormal shortening of a muscle.

Positioning devices and comfort pillows may support the body parts and keep the patient/resident in good alignment. This promotes patient/resident's comfort. Pillows should be placed and positioning devices should be used as directed by the nurse supervisor and the care plan. Older patients/residents may have limited range of motion in their necks. The sim's and prone positions are usually not comfortable for them. Therefore, the nurse assistant should check with the nurse supervisor before placing any older patient/resident in the prone or Sims' position.

Moving patients/residents

Moving patients/residents in bed

Some patients/residents may move and turn in the bed themselves. Others may require assistance from at least one person. Those who are weak, unconscious, in casts, or paralyzed may need help. When the bed's head is raised, it is comfortable to slide down toward the middle and foot of the bed. The nurse assistant should move the patient/resident up in bed for good alignment and comfort. Light-weight patients/residents can be sometime moved up in bed alone if they assist using a trapeze. However, it is usually recommended to take help and use an assist device for this purpose. For heavy and older persons, two or more staff members are recommended.

Moving patients/residents up in bed with an assist device

The nurse assistant can use assist devices to move some patients/residents up in bed. Such assist devices may include a turning pad, drawsheet (lift sheet), slide sheet, flat sheet folded in half, and large waterproof pad. With these assist devices, the patient/resident can be moved more evenly along with the reduction of shearing and friction. At least two staff members are recommended. This procedure is used for:

- Most patients/residents recovering from spinal cord surgery or spinal cord injuries.
- For older patients/residents.

Encouraging comfort and safety

It should be remembered that not all waterproof pads can be used as assist devices. Single-use, disposable underpads are usually not strong enough to hold the patient/resident's weight during the move. Re-usable underpads are much stronger. For safety purposes, the underpad must:

- Be strong enough to support the patient/resident's weight.
- Extend from under the patient/resident's head to above or below the knees.
- Be wider enough for the nurse assistant and other staff members to get a firm grip for the lift. It should be asked from the nurse supervisor if the patient/resident's underpad is safe as an assist device. To use a slide sheet, it should be placed under the patient/resident. After the procedure, the slide sheet should be removed. Otherwise the patient/resident can be in danger of sliding down in bed or off the bed.

Moving patients/residents to the side of the bed

Care and re-positioning procedures usually require moving patients/residents to the side of the bed. The patient/resident should be moved to the side of the bed before turning. Otherwise, after turning, the patient/resident may lie on the side of the bed, instead in the middle. At least two staff members are recommended. This procedure is used for:

- Most patients/residents recovering from spinal cord surgery or spinal cord injuries.
- For older patients/residents.
- For patients/residents with arthritis.

Assist devices used for this procedure may include a slide sheet, drawsheet (lift sheet), turning pad, flat sheet folded in half, and large waterproof pad. An assist device may prevent pain. It can also prevent skin damage and injury to the joints, bones, and spinal cord.

Turning patients/residents

Turning patients/residents onto their sides can prevent complications such as contractures and pressure sores. Several procedures and care measures also need the side-lying position. Many older patients/residents have arthritis in their hips, spines, and knees. Thus, less painful and logrolling is preferred for turning these patients/residents.

Encouraging safety and comfort
Safety

- Proper body mechanics should be followed to turn a patient/resident in bed.
- The patient/resident must be in good alignment. This helps prevent skin breakdown, musculo-skeletal injuries, and pressure ulcers.
- The patient/resident should not be turned away from the nurse assistant with the far bed rail down.
- The bed rail should be raised on the side near the nurse assistant.
- The patient/resident should be turned toward the nurse assistant.

Comfort

- After turning, the patient/resident should be positioned in good alignment.
- Pillows should be used as directed to support the patient/resident in the side-lying position.
- It should be ensured that the patient/resident's face, mouth, and nose are not obstructed by a pillow or other device.

Logrolling

Logrolling is turning the patient/resident as a unit, in alignment, with single motion. The spine should be kept straight. The procedure is often used to turn:

- Older patients/residents with arthritic spines or knees.
- Patients/residents recovering from hip fractures.
- Patients/residents with spinal cord injuries. The spine should be kept straight at all times after a spinal cord injury.

Encouraging comfort and safety

For logrolling, usually two or three staff members are required. If the patient/resident is heavy or tall, three staff members are recommended. Sometimes the nurse assistant may use an assist device like slide sheet, drawsheet, turning pad, and large waterproof pad. After spinal cord surgery or injury, the neck and spine should be kept straight. The nurse assistant holds the neck during re-positioning or moving. The nurse assistant should explain the patient/resident about what to do step by step. After spinal cord surgery or injury, usually a pillow is not allowed under the neck and head. The nurse assistant should follow the nurse supervisor's directions and the care plan to position the patient/resident and use pillows

Sitting on the side of the bed (Dangling)

Patients/residents usually sit on the side of the bed (dangle) for many reasons. They may become faint or dizzy when getting out of bed too quick. They may require sitting on the side of the bed for one to five minutes before transferring or walking. While dangling the legs, the patient/resident coughs and deep breathes. He/she may move the legs back and forth

in circles. This activity greatly stimulates circulation. Two staff members may be required to perform this procedure. Patients/residents with coordination and balance problems usually need support. If fainting or dizziness occurs, the patient/resident should be laid down.

Basic positions

Fowler's position

It is a semi-sitting position. The head of the bed is generally raised between 45 and 60 degrees. The knees can be elevated slightly. For good alignment:

- The spine should be straight.
- The head should be supported with a small pillow.
- The arms should be supported with pillows.

The nurse assistant may place small pillows under the thighs, lower back, and ankles of the patient/resident. Patients/residents with respiratory and heart disorders usually breathe much easier in Fowler's position.

Supine position

The supine position or dorsal recumbent position is the lying on the back position. In this position, the bed is generally flat. The patient/resident is on his/her back, with his/her head supported by a pillow. A small rolled towel or pillow is used to support the small area of the back. The patient/resident's arms are extended at his/her sides, with his/her palms down. If the patient/resident's arms are weak or paralyzed, they should be supported with small pillows. The patient/resident's thighs are extended in a straight line from his/her hips. If the patient/resident's feet tend to roll outward, pillows or rolled towels can be placed against the outer thighs to keep the legs in alignment. A foot board may be placed to prevent foot drop and to maintain the toes pointing upward. For keeping pressure off the heels, a small pad can be placed under the patient/resident's ankles and calves.

Prone position

In the prone position, the patient/resident lies on the abdomen with the head turned to one side. In this position, the patient/resident lies on his/her stomach, with his/her head turned toward the other side. The head is usually supported with a small pillow. The arm the patient/resident is facing is bent at a 90-degree angle, with the hand placed palm-down closer to the patient/resident's head. The other arm is generally extended straight along his/her side. A small pillow or folded blanket is tucked underneath the patient/resident's lower abdomen or pelvis to provide the patient/resident's chest room to expand when he/she breathes. A pillow is usually placed under the patient/resident's shins to raise his/her toes off the bed. The prone position is not frequently used because many individuals find it uncomfortable. If the prone position has been recommended for a patient/resident (or the patient/resident prefers the prone position), the nurse assistant should ask his/her co-worker to assist the patient/resident into the prone position.

Lateral position

In the lateral or side-lying position, the patient/resident lies on one side or the other. In the lateral position, the patient/resident is lying on his/her side, with his/her head supported by a pillow. The lower arm of the patient/resident is positioned so that he/she is not laying on it, and the top arm is supported on a pillow. A towel or rolled blanket is placed along the back to keep the patient/resident in the proper position. The bottom leg is generally straight, and the top knee is bent. A pillow is usually placed between the lower legs to assist the ankle and knee and to prevent the legs from resting on each other.

Sim's position

The Sims' position or semi-prone side position is a left side lying position. In Sims' position, the patient/resident is almost laying on his/her stomach. The right leg is sharply flexed so that it is not on the left leg. The left arm is behind the patient/resident. Sims' position is generally used for procedures such as giving an enema or taking a rectal temperature. It should be ensured that the patient/resident is not lying on the arm.

Lithotomy position

In lithotomy position, the patients/residents are on their back with the hips and knees flexed and the thighs apart. This position may be used for pelvic or perineal examination. It is also used for vaginal examinations and **childbirth**.

Trendelenburg's position

In the Trendelenburg's position or head-down position, the body is laid flat or supine on the back with the feet elevated above the head. The Trendelenburg position is often used in surgery, especially of the genitourinary system and abdomen. It permits better access to the pelvic organs due to gravitational pull of the intra-abdominal organs away from the pelvis.

Reverse Trendelenburg's position (head elevated)

In Reverse Trendelenburg's or head elevated position, head is kept higher than feet. Pillow should be placed between the patient/resident's feet and footboard of bed. This position is used to facilitate tube feedings, and emergency treatment in head injury and severe bleeding.

Semi-Fowler's position

It is position is a position in which patients/residents are lying on their back with the head and torso raised between 15 and 45 degrees. The most common and frequently used bed angle for this position is 30 degrees.

The Semi-Fowler's position is commonly used for purposes same to those of the Fowler's position, including lung expansion, feeding, cardiac or respiratory conditions, and for patients/residents with a nasogastric tube.

Patient/resident transfer

Patients/residents are moved to and from chairs, beds, wheelchairs, commodes, toilets, shower chairs, and stretchers. The amount of help required and the method used may differ, based on the patient/resident's dependency level. The room should be properly arranged to allow enough space for a safe transfer. The chair, wheelchair, or other device should be placed correctly.

Encouraging safety and comfort

Safety

The patient/resident should wear non-skid footwear for transfers. Such footwear generally protects the patient/resident from falls. Sliding and slipping should be prevented. Shoelaces should be tied securely. Otherwise the patient/resident can trip and fall. Long gowns and robes may also cause falls. Robes with long ties should be avoided. Wheels of bed, wheelchair, and other devices should be locked. This prevents the moving of bed and the device during the transfer. Otherwise, the patient/resident can fall.

Comfort

After the transfer, the patient/resident should be positioned in good alignment. The needed items should be placed within reach.

Bed to chair or wheelchair transfers

Safety is extremely important for wheelchair, chair, commode, and shower chair transfers. The patient/resident should be assisted out of bed on his/her strong side. If the right side is weak and the left side is strong, the patient/resident should be helped to out of bed on the left side. In transferring, the stronger side should move first. It should pull the weaker side along. Often, transferring a patient/resident from the bed to a chair or wheelchair can help him/her begin engaging in physical activity. Also, changing a patient/resident's position can prevent complications related to immobility. Safety and comfort are major concerns when assisting the patient/resident out of bed.

Transfers from the weak side are unsafe and awkward. Some patients/residents are able to stand and pivot. A pivot and stand transfer is used if:

- The patient/resident's legs are strong enough to bear some or all of his/her weight.
- The patient/resident is cooperative and can follow directions.
- The patient/resident can assist with the transfer.

Encouraging comfort and safety

Comfort

Most bedside chairs and wheelchairs have vinyl backs and seats. Vinyl usually absorbs body heat. The patient/resident may become warm and perspire more. If the nurse supervisor allows, the nurse assistant should cover the seat and back with a folded bath blanket. This may increase the patient/resident's comfort. Some people have positioning devices or wheelchair cushions. The nurse supervisor should be asked about how to use and place the devices. The nurse assistant should also follow the manufacturer's instructions.

Safety

- The wheelchair, chair, or other device must support the patient/resident's weight.
- The number of staff required depends on the patient/resident's abilities, size, and condition. Sometimes the nurse assistant may use a mechanical lift.
- The patient/resident must not put his/her arms around the nurse assistant's neck. Otherwise the patient/resident can pull the nurse assistant forward or may cause to lose his/her balance. Back, neck, and other injuries are possible.
- If not using a mechanical lift, a transfer belt can be used for wheelchair or chair transfers. It is safer for both the patient/resident and the nurse assistant.
- Putting the arms of the nurse assistant around the patient/resident and grasping the shoulder blades is another method. However, it may cause the patient/resident discomfort. And it can also be stressful for the nurse assistant. This method should only be used if instructed to do so by the nurse supervisor and the care plan.
- Wheels of the bed and wheelchair should be locked for a safe transfer.
- After the transfer, these wheels should be unlocked to position the chair as the patient/resident prefers. After positioning the chair, wheels can be locked or unlocked according to the care plan. Locked wheels are usually considered as restraints if the patient/resident cannot unlock them to move the wheelchair. However, falls and other injuries are risks if the patient/resident attempts to stand when the wheels are unlocked.

Wheelchair or chair to bed transfers has the same set of rules as bed to wheelchair transfers. The patient/resident should be assisted out of chair or wheelchair on his/her strong side. If the right side is weak and the left side is strong, the patient/resident should be helped to out of wheelchair or chair on the left side. In transferring, the stronger side should move first. It should pull the weaker side along. The chair or wheelchair should be positioned so the patient/resident's strong side should be near the bed.

Encouraging comfort and safety

- The number of staff required depends on the patient/resident's abilities, size, and condition.
- Sometimes the nurse assistant may use a mechanical lift.
- The patient/resident must not put his/her arms around the nurse assistant's neck. Otherwise the patient/resident can pull the nurse assistant forward or may cause to lose his/her balance. Back, neck, and other injuries are possible.
- If not using a mechanical lift, a transfer belt can be used for wheelchair or chair transfers. It is safer for both the patient/resident and the nurse assistant.
- Putting the arms of the nurse assistant around the patient/resident and grasping the shoulder blades is another method. However, it may cause the patient/resident discomfort. And it can also be stressful for the nurse assistant. This method should only be used if instructed to do so by the nurse supervisor and the care plan. Wheels of the bed and wheelchair should be locked for a safe transfer.

Using the bathroom for elimination generally promotes self-esteem, dignity, and independence. It is also more private than using a urinal, bedpan, or bedside commode. However, getting to the toilet is difficult for patients/residents who use wheelchairs.

Bathrooms are usually small. There is little room for a wheelchair. Therefore, transfers with wheelchairs are often difficult. Work-related injuries and falls are major risks. Sometimes mechanical lifts can be used for toilet transfers.

Encouraging comfort and safety

- It should be ensured that the patient/resident has a raised toilet seat. The wheelchair and toilet seat should be at the same level.
- There should be the grab bars in the toilet. Patient/resident should not be transferred to the toilet if grab bars are not secure.
- The nurse assistant should follow Standard Precautions and the Bloodborne Pathogen Standard.
- The nurse assistant should wear gloves if the patient/resident has incontinent of urine or feces or if contact with feces or urine is likely.

Assistive equipment used to transfer patients/residents

Transfer belts

Transfer belts also called as gait belts. They are used to:

- Support patients/residents during transfers.
- Re-position patients/residents in wheelchairs and chairs.

Encouraging safety and comfort

Safety

- To use a transfer belt safely, the nurse assistant should always follow the manufacturer's instructions.
- The belt buckle should be positioned where the patient/resident cannot reach and release it.
- Snugness should be checked by sliding an open, flat hand under the belt. The patient/resident should be asked if it feels too loose or too tight.
- The belt should be grasped from underneath. If the belt has handles, the belt should be grasped by the handles.
- The belt should be removed after the procedure.
- The patient/resident should not be left alone while he or she is wearing the belt.
-

Comfort

A transfer belt is generally applied over clothing. It should never be applied over bare skin. Also, it may be applied under the breasts; however, the breasts must not be caught under the belt. The belt buckle should never be positioned over the patient/resident's spine.

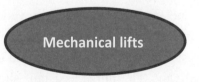

Mechanical lifts

Patients/residents who cannot help themselves can be transferred with mechanical lifts. They can be used to transfer patients/residents who are too heavy for the staff to transfer. Mechanical lifts are used for transfers to and from chairs, beds, stretchers, wheelchairs, tubs, shower, commodes, toilets, whirlpools, or vehicles. There are battery-operated, manual, and electric lifts. Some mechanical lifts are mounted on the ceiling.

Slings

The sling used in mechanical lifts depends on the patient/resident's size, condition, and other needs. Slings are unpadded, padded, or made of mesh. There are different types of slings, including:

- Standard full sling—for normal transfers.
- Extended length sling—for patients/residents with extra-large thighs.
- Bathing sling—to transfer the patients/residents directly from the bed or chair into a bathtub.
- Toileting sling—the sling bottom is wide and open. Each patient/resident has his/her own toileting sling.
- Amputee sling—for the patient/resident who has had both legs amputated.
- Bariatric sling—for use with a bariatric lift.

Using a Mechanical Lift

Before using a lift:

- The nurse assistant must be trained in its use.
- It must work.
- The sling, hooks, straps, and chains must be in good repair.
- The patient/resident's weight must not exceed the lift's capacity.
- At least two staff members are required. There are multiple types of mechanical lifts. The nurse assistant should always follow the manufacturer's instructions.

Lateral-assist devices

Lateral-assist devices minimize patient/resident-surface friction during lateral transfers. Roller boards, transfer boards, slide boards, inflatable mattresses, and friction-reducing lateral-assist devices are some common examples of these devices that make transfers comfortable and much safer for the patient/resident. An inflatable mattress is a flexible lateral-assist device that is placed under the patient/resident. An attached, portable air supply inflates the mattress, which produces a layer of air under the patient/resident. This air cushion permits nursing assistants to perform the transfer with much less effort. Transfer boards are the lateral-assist devices placed under the patient/resident. They provide a slick surface for the patient/resident during transfers, minimizing friction and the force required to move the patient/resident. Transfer boards are lateral-assist devices made of rigid, smooth, and low-friction material, such as coated wood or plastic.

Some lateral-assist devices have long handles that minimize reaching by staff, to improve safety and make the transfer much easier and comfortable.

Trapeze

The standard trapeze bar is a mobility assistive device which is a sturdy triangle trapeze, attached to an overhead metal frame. The hook of trapeze is positioned to be suspended over the bed and is either attached to the hospital bed frame or anchored to a stand-alone base with lengthy legs that extend under the bed. This mobility assistive device is indicated for use by patients/residents who are confined for long periods of time to the bed, or having very limited mobility and using a wheelchair to get around.

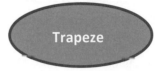

Ambulation

The act of walking is termed as ambulation. Some patients/residents are unsteady and weak due to any illness, injury, bed rest, or surgery. They need support for walking. After bed rest, activity increases gradually and in steps. Initially, the patient/resident sits on the side of the bed (dangles), followed by sitting in a bedside chair. Next the patient/resident walks in the room and then in the hallway. The nurse assistant should follow the care plan when helping a patient/resident walk. They should use a gait (transfer) belt if the patient/resident is weak or unsteady. The patient/resident may also use hand rails along the wall.

Walking increases flexibility of the most of the body's muscles and joints. It improves gastrointestinal and respiratory function. Ambulating also minimizes the risk for complications of immobility. However, even a very short period of immobility may reduce a patient/resident's tolerance for ambulating. If necessary, the nurse assistant should make use of appropriate equipment and assistive devices to assist in patient handling and movement.

Before helping with ambulation, the nurse assistant needs following information from the nurse supervisor and the care plan:

- How much help the patient/resident needs?
- Is the patient/resident using a walker, cane, crutches, or a brace?
- Areas of weakness—right leg or arm, left leg or arm?
- How far to walk?
- What observations to record and report?
- How well the patient/resident can tolerate the activity?
- Shuffling, limping, sliding, or walking on tip-toes?
- Complaints of discomfort or pain?
- Complaints of orthostatic hypotension—dizziness, weakness, spots before the eyes, faintness?
- The distance walked?
- When to report the recorded observations?
- What patient/resident concerns to report at once?

Helping the person to walk

The nurse assistant should follow the below procedure to assist a patient/resident walk:

1. The nurse assistant should knock before entering the patient/resident's room.
2. After proper introduction, explaining the procedure, and proper hand hygiene, following items should be arranged for further procedure:
   - Robe and non-skid footwear
   - Towel or paper to protect bottom linens
   - Gait (transfer) belt
3. The bed should be adjusted to a safe and comfortable level for the patient/resident. The nurse assistant should always follow the care plan. Bed wheels should be locked with lowering the bed rail if up.
4. Top linens should be fan-folded to the foot of the bed.
5. Paper or towel should be placed under the patient/resident's feet.
6. The nurse assistant should help the patient/resident to sit on the side of the bed (dangling).
7. It should be ensured that the patient/resident has put and fastened the shoes. The patient/resident's feet should be flat on the floor.
8. The nurse assistant should help the patient/resident to put on the robe.
9. The gait belt should be applied at the waist over clothing.
10. Proper support should be provided to the patient/resident in standing. The gait belt should be grasped at each side. If no gait belt, the nurse assistant should place his/her arms under the patient/resident's arms around to the shoulder blades.
11. The nurse assistant should stand at the patient/resident's weak side while he/she gains balance. The belt should be held at the side and back. If not using a gait belt, the nurse assistant

should place one arm around the back and the other at the elbow to support the patient/resident.

12. The patient/resident should be encouraged to stand erect with the head up and the back straight.

13. The patient/resident should be provided proper help and support to walk. The nurse assistant should walk to the side and slightly behind the patient/resident on his/her weak side. Support should be provided with the gait belt. If not using a gait belt, the nurse assistant should place his/her one arm around the back and the other at the elbow to support the patient/resident.

14. Patient/resident should be encouraged to use the hand rail on his/her strong side. He/she should also be encouraged to walk normally. The heel should strike the floor first. The patient/resident should be discouraged from shuffling, walking, or sliding on tip-toes.

15. The nurse assistant should walk at the required distance if the patient/resident tolerates the activity. The patient/resident should not be rushed during walking.

16. The patient/resident should be provided proper help in returning to bed. The gait belt should be removed and the head of the bed should be lowered down. The patient/resident should be assisted to move at the center of the bed.

17. Shoes and the paper towel over the bottom sheet should be removed.

18. Comfort should be provided to the patient/resident.

19. The call light should be placed within reach.

20. Bed rails should be adjusted at a safe and comfortable level.

21. The robe and shoes should be returned to their proper place.

22. The patient/resident should be unscreened and safety check of the room should be completed before leaving the room.

23. The nurse assistant at the end should report and record his/her observations.

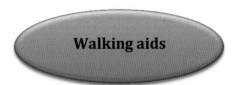

Walking aids

Walking aids provide support for the body. The type of walking aid depends on the patient/resident's condition, the disability, and the support needed. The physical therapist evaluates and trains the patient/resident to use the device.

Crutches

Crutches are the walking aids used when the patient/resident cannot use one leg or when one or both legs need to gain stability and strength. Some patients/residents with permanent leg weakness can use crutches. Falls are a major risk. The nurse assistant should follow these safety measures:

- The crutch tips should be thoroughly checked. They must not be torn, worn down, or wet. Worn or torn crutch tips should be replaced. Wet tips should be properly dried with paper towels.

- Crutches should be checked for any flaws. Wooden crutches should be evaluated for cracks and metal crutches for bends.

- All bolts should be tightened.

- It should be ensured that the patient/resident wear street shoes. The shoes must be flat with non-skid soles.
- It should be ensured that clothes of the patient/resident fit well. Loose clothes may get caught between the underarms and crutches. Loose skirts and long clothes can hang forward and may block the patient/resident's view of the feet and crutch tips.
- The nurse assistant should practice safety rules to prevent falls.
- Crutches should be kept within the patient/resident's reach. They should be placed at the patient/resident's chair or against a wall.

Walkers

Walkers provide more support than canes. Wheeled walkers are more common, which have wheels on the front legs and rubber tips on the back legs. The patient/resident pushes the walker about 6 to 8 inches in front of his/her feet. Rubber tips on the back legs usually prevent the walker from moving while the patient/resident is standing. Some walkers may have a braking action when weight is applied to the walker's back legs. Pouches, baskets, and trays are generally attached to the walker and can be used for needed items. This permits more independence and free the hands to grip the walker.

Encouraging comfort and safety

Walker wheels are usually located on the outside of the walker. With the wheels on the outside of the walker, the walker can be too wide for some doorways. The wheels should be moved to the inside of the walker. This minimizes the width of the walker. Some walkers may contain seats. The patient/resident sits when a rest is needed. The walker should never be pushed when the patient/resident is seated.

Transfer belts

Transfer belts also known as gait belts are most commonly used to:
- Support patients/residents during their transfers.
- Re-position patients/residents in wheelchairs and chairs.

Encouraging safety and comfort

Safety
- To use a transfer belt safely, the nurse assistant should always follow the manufacturer's instructions.
- The belt buckle should be positioned where the patient/resident cannot reach and release it.
- Snugness should be checked by sliding an open, flat hand under the belt. The patient/resident should be asked if it feels too loose or too tight.
- The belt should be grasped from underneath. If the belt has handles, the belt should be grasped by the handles.
- The belt should be removed after the procedure.
- The patient/resident should not be left alone while he or she is wearing the belt.

Comfort
.A transfer belt is generally applied over clothing. It should never be applied over bare skin. Also, it may be applied under the breasts; however, the breasts must not be caught under the belt. The belt buckle should never be positioned over the patient/resident's spine.

Canes

Canes are walking aids used for weakness on one side of the body. They usually help to provide support and balance. A cane should be held on the strong side of the body (i.e. if the right leg is weak, the cane should be held in the left hand). The size of the cane tip is almost 6 to 10 inches to the side of the foot. The grip should be on the level with the hip. The patient/resident walks as follows:

- **Step I:** The cane is moved ahead 6 to 10 inches.
- **Step II:** The weaker leg that is opposite to the cane is moved forward even with the cane.
- **Step III:** The stronger leg is moved forward and it should be ahead of the weak leg and the cane.

Braces

Braces are walking aids that support weak body parts. They also correct and prevent joint deformities or joint movement. Plastic, metal, or leather is used for braces. A brace is usually applied over the knee, ankle, or back. The skin and bony points under braces should be kept dry and clean. This may prevent skin breakdown. Nursing assistants should report redness or signs of skin breakdown at once. They should also report complaints of discomfort or pain. The nurse supervisor usually assesses the skin under braces every shift. The care plan suggests when to apply and remove a brace.

Prevention of injury if fall occurs during ambulation

Safety measures

- The nurse assistant should practice appropriate safety measures to prevent falls.
- The nurse assistant can use a gait belt to assist the patient/resident stand. Also he/she may use it during ambulation. Appropriate measures should be taken to protect the patient's/resident's head from hitting on the ground.
- The patient/resident should remind to walk normally.
- The patient/resident should be encouraged to stand erect with the back straight and head up.
- The nurse assistant should discourage sliding, shuffling, and walking on tip-toes.

Comfort

The fear of falling may greatly affect the mental comfort. Therefore, the patient/resident should explain the purpose of the gait belt. The nurse assistant should also explain how the help will be provided to the patient/resident if he/she starts to fall.

Helpful Resources

R. B. (2004). Intraoperative positioning and care of the obese patient. *Plastic Surgical Nursing, 24*(3), 118-122. https://doi.org/10.1097/00006527-200407000-00009

Hunter, S., Divine, A., Omana, H., Madou, E., & Holmes, J. (2020). Development, reliability and validity of the safe use of mobility aids checklist (SUMAC) for 4-wheeled Walker use in people living with dementia. https://doi.org/10.21203/rs.2.22127/v1

Jones III, H. (2014). Choosing the correct hysterectomy technique. *Vaginal Hysterectomy,* 337-337. https://doi.org/10.5005/jp/books/12309_34

Kang, S. (2017). The use of body mechanics principle, clinical-practice fatigue, and practice satisfaction of nursing students. *NursingPlus Open, 3,* 6-10. https://doi.org/10.1016/j.npls.2017.03.001

Lieber, S. J., Rudy, T. E., & Boston, J. R. (2000). Effects of body mechanics training on performance of repetitive lifting. *American Journal of Occupational Therapy, 54*(2), 166-175. https://doi.org/10.5014/ajot.54.2.166

MCCONNELL, E. A. (2002). Using proper body mechanics. *Nursing, 32*(5), 17. https://doi.org/10.1097/00152193-200205000-00012

Pihl-Thingvad, J., Brandt, L. P., & Andersen, L. L. (2018). Consistent use of assistive devices for patient transfer is associated with less patient-initiated violence: Cross-sectional study among health care workers at general hospitals. *Workplace Health & Safety, 66*(9), 453-461. https://doi.org/10.1177/2165079917752714

A review of patient lifting interventions to reduce health care worker injuries. (2015). *Workplace Health & Safety, 63*(6), 276-276. https://doi.org/10.1177/2165079915589941 Stethen, T. W., Ghazi, Y. A., Heidel, R. E., Daley, B. J., Barnes, L., Patterson, D., &

McLoughlin, J. M. (2018). Walking to recovery: The effects of missed ambulation events on postsurgical recovery after bowel resection. *Journal of Gastrointestinal Oncology, 9*(5), 953-961. https://doi.org/10.21037/jgo.2017.11.05

Teeple, E., Collins, J. E., Shrestha, S., Dennerlein, J. T., Losina, E., & Katz, J. N. (2017). Outcomes of safe patient handling and mobilization programs: A meta-analysis. *Work, 58*(2), 173-184. https://doi.org/10.3233/wor-172608

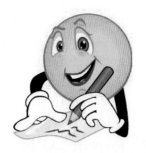

Chapter Six:

Medical and Surgical Asepsis

Outline

I: Common infectious agents and diseases they cause

II: Antibiotic resistant bacteria.

III: Conditions necessary for infectious agents to grow

IV: Chain of infection

V: Four lines of defense against infection in the body

VI: Signs and symptoms of infection

VII: Medical and surgical asepsis

VIII: Roles of Center for Disease Control (CDC) and Occupational Safety and Health

Administration (OSHA) in the prevention of infections.

IX: Standard precautions

X: Personal protective equipment (PPE) and proper use

XI: Transmission-based precautions

XII: Psychological effects of standard precautions and transmission based precautions on

patients/residents

Infection

Infection is a disease state resulting from the growth and invasion of microbes in the body. Infection is a main health and safety hazard. Minor infections usually cause short illnesses. A serious infection may cause serious complications and even death. Disabled and older persons are usually at risk. The healthcare providers including nursing assistants must follow certain procedures and practices to prevent the spread of infection (infection control). The main goal is to protect patients/residents, visitors, and staff from infection.

Microorganisms

A microorganism (microbe) is a micro (small) organism (creature). It can be seen only with a microscope. Microorganisms are everywhere—nose, mouth, stomach, respiratory tract, and intestines. They are on the skin and in the air, soil, water, and food. They are on animals, clothing, and furniture. Microorganisms that are dangerous and can cause infections are known as pathogens. Non-pathogenic organisms are microbes that do not usually cause an infection.

Microbes are tiny living things that are everywhere. They can only be seen using a microscope. Examples of microorganisms may include bacteria, viruses, fungi, yeasts, and molds. Most microorganisms grow rapidly wherever they have moisture, warm temperatures, food, and darkness. These features make the human body an ideal site for microbial growth. Many of the microorganisms that residue on and in human bodies are not harmful, and some even may perform useful functions. However, microbes that are even necessary and useful in certain areas of the body may cause disease if they spread to another area of the body where they are not normally found. For example, some bacteria in the stomach and bowel are helpful to digest food. But if these same bacteria are present in the bladder or kidney, they can cause an infectious disease. The human body has various natural defenses against pathogenic organisms. Healthy, intact skin and mucous membranes are considered as body's first line of defense that can help to prevent microbes from entering the body. Reflexes, such as sneezing and coughing, help to expel microorganisms from the body. Finally, WBCs (white blood cells) carried in the blood are able to destroy infectious organisms that enter the body. These natural defense mechanisms of the human body can help to keep the human beings healthy. In addition, modern medicine has developed some other tools available prevent and fight against infections, such as vaccinations and antibiotic medications. Even though human body has several ways of protecting from infectious agents and there are certain medications available to treat some infections, still prevention is the optimal goal. Some infectious diseases can be fatal, especially in individuals who are not otherwise healthy, and various infections cannot be treated with medications.

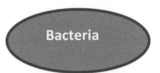

Bacteria are single-celled, microscopic organisms that thrive in diverse environments. These organisms can live in the ocean, soil, and inside the human gut.

Bacteria can be classified into five main groups according to their basic shapes: Cocci (spherical), bacilli (rod), spirilla (spiral), vibrios (comma), or spirochaetes (corkscrew). They may exist as single cells, in chains, pairs, or clusters.

Bacteria are usually found in every habitat on Earth: rock, soil, oceans and even arctic snow. Some bacteria live on or in other organisms including animals, plants, and humans. There are about 10 times as many bacterial cells as human cells inside the human body. A number of these bacterial cells are generally found lining the digestive system. Some bacteria may live in the soil or on dead plant matter where they can play an important role in the re-cycling of useful nutrients.

Harmful bacteria that can cause infectious diseases are called pathogenic bacteria. Bacterial infections may occur when pathogenic bacteria enter into the body and start to reproduce and grow in tissues that are normally sterile. Harmful bacteria may also release some toxins that can disrupt the body. Most common pathogenic bacteria and the resultant bacterial diseases may include:

- *Escherichia coli* can cause food poisoning and urinary infections.

- *Helicobacter pylori* usually cause gastritis and ulcers.

- *Staphylococcus aureus* causes a number of different infections in the body, including cellulitis, boils, abscesses, wound infections, food poisoning, and pneumonia.

- *Streptococcal bacteria* may cause multiple infections in the body,

including meningitis, pneumonia, ear infections, and strep throat.

Rickettsia

It can cause a variety of infections in the human body including itching (body, head and pubic) and scabies (skin rash).

Tuberculosis

TB is a bacterial infection in the lungs. It is spread by airborne droplets with sneezing, coughing, singing, speaking, or laughing. Nearby individuals can inhale the bacteria. Those who have close contact with an infected individual are at risk. TB is more likely to occur in crowded and closed areas.

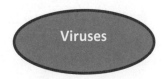

Viruses are the smallest amongst all the microorganisms. Viruses are unique because they are alive and able to multiply only within the cells of other living things. The cell they residue and multiply is called the host cell.

Viruses may cause a wide variety of diseases. Most pathogenic viruses cannot be destroyed or easily controlled. Immunization is considered the most effective tools for preventing viral infections, such as polio and measles. The most common viral infection is the common cold, caused by a viral infection of the upper respiratory tract (nose and throat). Viruses can affect every tissue and system of the body. One of the most deadly viruses is the HIV (Human Immunodeficiency Virus), which causes the AIDS (Acquired Immunodeficiency Syndrome).Other common viral infections may include:

- Chickenpox
- Herpes
- Human papillomavirus (HPV)
- Viral gastroenteritis (stomach flu)
- Infectious mononucleosis
- Mumps, measles and rubella
- Shingles
- Viral hepatitis
- Viral pneumonia
- Viral meningitis

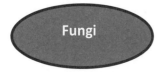

Fungi

Fungi are the microorganisms, including the single-celled yeasts and the multicellular molds. They are not belonged to the same cellular domain as bacteria. Fungi are eukaryotic microorganisms. Infection caused by a fungus is known as mycosis. Common fungal infections may include tinea capitis (a lesion of the scalp often found in children) and tinea pedis, also known as athlete's foot.

Another example of a common fungal infection is "Thrush" caused by Candida albicans. Thrush creates a white growth on a person's tongue and in the mouth. Candida albicans also causes about one third of cases of vaginitis (an inflammation of the vagina).

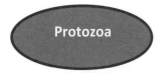

Protozoa

Protozoa are single-celled microorganisms that can be visible under an ordinary laboratory microscope. Two most common protozoa are the paramecium and amoeba. Although most protozoa are not harmful and non-pathogenic; however, there are some notable exceptions. Amoebic dysentery is a condition caused by Entamoeba histolytica, which develops ulcers in the colon and attacks red blood cells. Malaria is another example of protozoal infection, caused by a protozoan known as Plasmodium malariae. Plasmodium malariae reproduces in the Anopheles mosquito, and is transmitted to people through mosquito bites. Malaria causes huge number of deaths each year and the incidence is increasing because of resistant strains of the organism.

Multidrug-resistant organisms (MDROs)

Effective antimicrobial therapy generally destroys or significantly minimizes the number of microorganisms that cause disease. These medications stimulate and boost the body's natural defenses to take over and fight against harmful microorganisms. However, multidrug-resistant organisms (MDROs) are microorganisms that can resist the effects of antibiotics. Some pathogens can notably change their shapes and structures. This makes them very difficult to kill, thus they can live in the presence of antibiotics. Several microorganisms, including viruses, bacteria, fungi, and parasites, have a tendency to develop resistant strains to existing medications. The development of antimicrobial resistant strains may occur in several ways. The most common way for developing resistance is an unnecessary or incomplete use of antimicrobial therapy, allowing multiple invading microorganisms to survive. These invading microorganisms have the tendency to transfer their resistance to future generations. Therefore, future antimicrobial therapy may be not effective. These resistant microorganisms can be transmitted into the environment through sneezing, coughing, and direct contact. It is very important to educate these measures to patients/residents as well as general public:

- Antimicrobial drugs should be taken only as prescribed and only if these are absolutely necessary.
- Antimicrobial drugs should be taken for the entire period prescribed, even if symptoms of illness disappear.
- Antimicrobial drugs should not be shared with others or an individual should not take "leftover medications."
- Antibiotics should not be taken for viral infections.

Common multidrug-resistant organisms (MDROs) are:

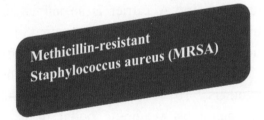

Methicillin-resistant Staphylococcus aureus (MRSA)

Staphylococcus aureus is a bacterium usually found on the skin and in the nose. MRSA is resistant to antibiotics that are often used for Staphylococcus aureus infections. MRSA can cause severe pneumonia and serious bloodstream and wound infections. Staphylococcus aureus that are resistant to the antibiotic methicillin are called as Methicillin-resistant staphylococcus aureus (MRSA).

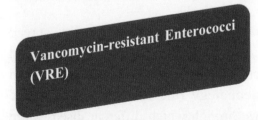

Vancomycin-resistant Enterococci (VRE)

Enterococcus is a bacterium generally found in the intestines and in feces. It can be transmitted to other people by contaminated hands, care equipment, toilet seats, and other items that the hands touch. When not in the intestines (their natural sites), enterococci can cause wound, pelvic, urinary tract, and other infections. Enterococci that are resistant to the antibiotic vancomycin are called as Vancomycin-resistant Enterococci (VRE).

Metabolism and growth: Conditions necessary for infectious agents to grow

Microbes are said to grow when their number at an individual site increases. At the initial stages of a bacterial infection, number of bacterial cells may be of only a few thousand. As the bacteria reproduce, they rapidly divide and form groups of many millions of individual bacterial cells, collectively named as colonies. Several environmental factors may affect the metabolism of microorganisms.

Oxygen

Most microorganisms need oxygen for their growth; these organisms are called obligate aerobes. Other microorganisms called as obligate anaerobes, cannot survive in the presence of oxygen. Some microorganisms can survive in either the presence or absence of oxygen and called as facultative anaerobes.

Nutrients

Organic (carbon-containing) nutrients are the major nutrients for microbial growth. Microorganisms also need other chemical elements, such as sulfur for manufacture of proteins and vitamins, and nitrogen for the synthesis of proteins. Some microbes prepare their own food from raw materials, such as carbon dioxide. Most of other microorganisms must find their nutrition ready-made. Microorganisms that residue on or within another living being (the host) are called as parasites. Saprophytes are the microbes that live off the organic remains of dead animals and plants.

Temperature

The specific temperature at which a microorganism shows its best growth is called as optimal temperature. Most pathogenic and infectious microorganisms flourish at normal body temperature. Some types of microorganisms prefer either extremely hot or cold environments. Cold temperatures usually slow the growth of microorganisms significantly, which is the basic reason for which refrigeration is used to control bacterial growth in food. High temperatures generally kill and destroy most microorganisms. Boiling water and steam sterilization are two most common techniques used to kill pathogenic microorganisms.

Moisture

All microorganisms require moisture or water for their proper growth. The matter on or in which they grow must contain some available moisture (for example jellies) or may be a liquid such as blood or milk.

pH

A substance's specific pH (hydrogen ion concentration; alkalinity or acidity) also affects growth. Microorganisms usually survive only in environments with a pH that is neither too alkaline nor too acidic.

Light

Some microorganisms need light for growth. Other microorganisms, however, flourish in darkness. Many microorganisms die when exposed to the sun's ultraviolet rays, although moderately diffused light does not affect them.

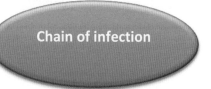

The chain of infection starts with a source—a pathogen. It must have a reservoir through which it can grow and multiply. Animals, humans, and objects are reservoirs. A carrier is an animal or human that is a reservoir for microorganisms but does not develop the infection. Carriers can transmit pathogens to others. To leave the reservoir, the pathogen must require a portal of exit. Exits are the gastro-intestinal (GI), urinary, respiratory, and reproductive tracts; breaks in the skin; and blood. After leaving the reservoir, the pathogenic microorganisms must be transmitted to another host. The pathogenic microorganism enters the body through a portal of entry. Portals of exit and entry are the same. A susceptible host is required for the microorganism to grow and multiply.

Communicable diseases usually spread very easily. Healthcare workers and scientists use knowledge gained in epidemiology (the study of methods and ways through which different diseases are transmitted to people) to establish methods for preventing the spread of pathogenic infections. The CDC (Centers for Disease Control and Prevention) in Atlanta, Georgia, is devoted to the study of pathogenic organisms and the control of communicable diseases. A disease can be prevented from spreading if the chain of infection is broken. The chain of infection consists of the following six components:

1. Pathogenic microorganism
2. Reservoir in which the infectious microorganism can live and grow
3. Portal of exit from which the microorganism can leave the reservoir
4. Vehicle to transmit the pathogenic microorganism
5. Portal of entry through which the pathogenic microorganism can enter the host.
6. Susceptible host

Some of these components are controllable and some are not. The below section explains each component of the chain of infection and measures at each stage to break the chain of infection.

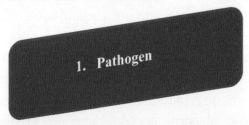

For an infectious disease to occur, a pathogenic microorganism capable of causing disease must be present.

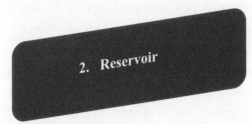

The word reservoir is originated from a French word that means "storehouse." Reservoir means a place where pathogens can grow and multiply. Possible reservoirs for microorganisms may include the bodies of animals and humans, water, and food.

As pathogenic microorganisms exist everywhere, therefore, reservoir can be any place where the pathogenic microorganism can survive before moving to a place where it can grow and multiply. Reservoirs may be living beings (people, wild or domesticated animals, and insects) or inanimate objects (soil, air, fluids, food, bedding, and utensils). Healthcare personnel including nursing assistants can break the chain of infection at this point by disrupting the pathogenic microorganisms or retarding their growth through the following measures:

- Sterilizing dressings and instruments used in the operating room and elsewhere.
- Disinfecting equipment and floors.
- Using bedpans or other personal items for one patient/resident only.
- Discarding disposable equipment such as catheters and thermometer probe covered in appropriate receptacles after their use; other equipment should be discarded, such as urinals, bedpans, and water pitchers, when the patient/resident is discharged.
- Baths should be given using water and soap or a special disinfectant solution, to remove drainage and dried secretions.
- Dressings should be changed promptly when they become wet as per nurse order.
- Placing contaminated articles, such as tissues, dressings, or linen, in moisture-proof bags; red, specially labelled biohazard bags should be used as indicated.
- Contaminated needles, syringes, and other sharps should be discarded in the

appropriate punctureproof and moisture-resistant container— they should never be thrown in the waste container.

- It should be ensured that collection bags and drainage tubes drain properly. They should be emptied according to agency policy.
- Any sterile package that has a broken seal or has become wet should never be used.
- PPEs (Personal protective equipments) should be used as needed.
- Hands should be thoroughly washed or sanitized frequently. In addition, healthcare personnel including nursing assistants should not work when they might become a source of infection for patients/residents.

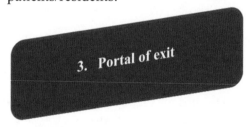

3. Portal of exit

Portal comes from the Latin word means "gate." For an infectious disease to occur, the pathogen must have a way of leaving the portal of exit or a reservoir. The portal of exit may vary depending on the pathogenic microorganism and the reservoir. When the reservoir is an animal or human body, the portal of exit may be the digestive tract, the genitourinary tract, respiratory tract, or breaks in the skin.

Pathogenic microorganisms must have a way of escape from their reservoir. Portals of exit in the human body may include all body openings (orifices). Pathogenic microorganisms may leave the human body in any of its natural discharges such as mucus, sweat, sputum, saliva, semen, feces, or urine. They may also leave the

body in drainage, vomitus, or blood from breaks in the skin.

Healthcare personnel including nursing assistants can break the chain of infection at this stage and prevent pathogenic microorganisms from escaping with thorough handwashing, proper waste disposal, and careful management of drainage and secretions. Gloves should always be worn when potential contact with body secretions. Patients/residents who have airborne infections may require wearing masks or receive medications that prevent coughing. Some patients/residents must be isolated to prevent the spread of infection.

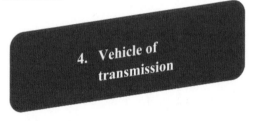

4. Vehicle of transmission

The way a pathogenic microorganism gets from one individual to another is called the pathogen's vehicle of transmission. The vehicle or method of transmission may be direct or indirect. In direct transmission, the pathogenic microorganism is passed from one individual to another through close physical contact, such as kissing, touching, having sex or breathing infected air. Indirect transmission means that pathogenic microorganisms are spread by way of a contaminated object or surface. Usually this condition occurs when an infected individual touches something and then someone else touches that same thing.

Airborne transmission of an infectious disease is usually accomplished by moisture or dust particles carrying pathogenic microorganisms or spores that blow from place to place. For instance, pathogenic infections can be transmitted by pathogen-containing moisture drops—produced by coughing or sneezing—that can be propelled far from the carrier. Common colds and other upper respiratory tract infections can be easily spread through droplet infection.

Healthcare personnel including nursing assistants can break the chain of infection at the vehicle of transmission level by burning all trash in non-residue incinerators. Linen should be removed without shaking it or allowing it to touch clothing. All infected wounds should be covered carefully. Food should be handled and prepared properly. Healthcare facilities should take appropriate measures including isolation of patients/residents with contagious diseases, sterilization of reusable supplies and equipment, proper disposal of trash and wastes, and control of airflow. Nursing assistants should be well aware of how specific infections are spread. For example, TB (tuberculosis) is spread through the air; thus, when treating patients/residents with TB, healthcare personnel including nursing assistants should use airborne precautions. If a patient/resident has a disease that can spread through body excretions, there should be proper disinfection of the toilet after use or having the patient/resident use a toilet in a separate room. All feces and urine must be carefully disposed of and urinals and bedpans should be carefully cleaned. Syringes and needles should be used safely. Nursing assistants should not recap or attempt to break needles. A needlestick from a contaminated needle may spread pathogenic infection to the nurse assistant. In all healthcare settings, patients/residents should have their own set of personal care items. Sharing items,

such as urinals, bedpans, and eating utensils, may lead to the transmission of infectious diseases.

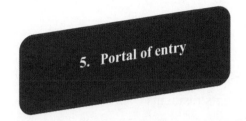

5. Portal of entry

Just as the pathogenic microorganism must have a way of exiting the reservoir, it must also have a way of achieving entry to a new reservoir. This is known as a portal of entry. In the case of person-to-person or animal-to-person transmission, potential portals of entry may include the digestive tract, the genitourinary tract, the respiratory tract, the eye and breaks in the skin.

Pathogenic microorganisms require a portal of entry to gain access to an individual's body. They can enter through the gastrointestinal, urinary, respiratory, and reproductive systems and through breaks in the mucous membranes or skin. Incisions, puncture sites from injections, open wounds, or body orifices into which catheters are inserted are common portals of entry. To prevent pathogenic microorganisms from entering a host, healthcare personnel including nursing assistant should take these measures:

- The patient/resident's skin should be kept clean and dry. Moisturizers should be applied to dry skin or lips, to prevent cracking.
- The nurse assistant should be very careful if clipping a patient/resident's nails. The patient/resident should be encouraged not to bite their fingernails or cuticles and not to pull on hangnails.

153

- The nurse assistant should avoid positioning patient/residents against tubes or objects that could cause skin breaks.
- There should be frequent repositioning of patients/residents who have impaired mobility.
- Patients/residents should have dry, clean, and wrinkle-free linen.
- It should be ensured that urine collection bags are lower than the patient/resident.
- Tubes and ports should be properly disinfected before collecting specimens from drainage tubes or intravenous lines.
- Appropriate sterile technique should be used when performing invasive procedures. As a healthcare worker, the nurse assistant is always at risk for infection. He/she should wear gloves to protect himself/herself when handling body substances, blood, or other potential pathogenic reservoirs (contaminated equipment). He/she should wear protective eyewear, gowns, masks, and shoe covers if any danger exists of spraying or splashing body substances. Procedures, such as proper handwashing and appropriate wound and catheter care, also help to break the chain of infection.

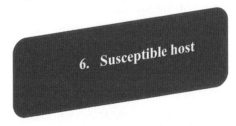

6. Susceptible host

Finally, the pathogenic microorganism must enter a susceptible host, or an individual who is capable of becoming infected with that particular pathogenic microorganism. Several factors may increase a person's susceptibility to infection, including poor general health, very old or very young age, and the presence of medical devices that are inserted in the body (such as urinary catheters).

Normally, healthy individuals have a variety of defense mechanisms against infection, both non-specific (skin as a barrier, phagocytosis, and fever) and specific (immunity). Healthcare personnel including nursing assistants are responsible for helping to reduce each patient/resident's susceptibility to infection by managing the patient/resident's underlying condition. They should provide adequate rest and skin care. Sufficient nutritional support should be given. Appropriate help should be provided to reduce anxiety. Adequate fluid intake should be encouraged. The nurse assistant should help with deep breathing and coughing when the patient/resident is immobilized. Proper immunization of older adults and children who are at great risk of acquiring communicable diseases should be encouraged. Appropriate infection control measures should be practiced. Preventing infectious diseases is the daily job of every healthcare worker.

Lines of defense against infectious agents

The human body has multiple natural defenses against infections. Healthy, intact skins along with mucous membranes help to prevent pathogenic microorganisms from entering the body. Reflexes, such as sneezing and coughing may help to expel pathogenic microorganisms from the body. Finally, WBCs (white blood cells) carried in the blood are able to disrupt pathogens that enter the body. These natural defense mechanisms are extremely helpful to keep human beings healthy.

The major four lines of defense against infection in the body include:
1. Intact skin
2. Mucous membranes
3. Normal flora
4. Immune system

1. Intact skin

The skin is dry, salty, tough, dry, oily, thick, and rich in fatty acids. It is considered as body's first line of defense. The sweat glands in the skin secrete a mixture of fatty acids and salts, which inhibit many pathogenic microorganisms. It also a home for normal flora that are antagonistic to potential pathogens.

2. Mucous membranes

Mucous membrane such as the lining of the nose, mouth, and eyelids is also an important line of defense that serves as an effective barrier for pathogenic microorganisms. Mucous membranes are typically coated with secretions that fight against pathogenic microorganisms. For example, the mucous membranes of the eyes contain tears, which consist of an enzyme called lysozyme that attacks several bacteria and helps to protect the eyes from infection.

The walls of the passages in the airways are coated with mucus. Pathogenic microorganisms in the air become stuck to the mucus and blown out or coughed up from the airways.

3. Normal flora

Normal flora are the microorganisms that residue on another organism (animal or human) or inanimate object without causing disease. Human body is usually not sterile and contains large population of these harmless microorganisms. There are almost one hundred trillion bacteria in intestines that form the normal flora of bodies. This normal flora is considered as body's significant line of defense and helps to prevent the body becoming colonized with more dangerous bacteria, which might lead to serious infectious diseases.

4. Immune system

The immune system is a line of defense that protects the body from outside invaders, such as viruses, bacteria, fungi and toxins (chemicals produced by microorganisms). Immune system is made up of different cells, organs, and proteins that work together to protect the body from invading microorganisms.

There are two major parts of the immune system. The innate immune system that is present from the time of the birth. The adaptive immune system is developed when the body is exposed to pathogenic microorganisms or chemicals released by microorganisms.

How to recognize an infection: Signs & Symptoms

An infection occurs when pathogenic microorganisms grow and multiply inside the body. Almost any of the body part can become infected. It can be recognized a possible infection in an individual's body by certain signs and symptoms. These signs and symptoms of infection may vary according to the type of pathogen and the site in the body where the infection is occurring. The nurse assistant should report his/her observations to the nurse supervisor if he/she observes these signs and symptoms in any patient/resident. It should be remembered that not all individuals with infections will show similar signs and symptoms of infection. Therefore, it is important to practice infection control with every patient/resident under the nursing care; even if he/she does not present any signs or symptoms of infection.

Common signs and symptoms of infection

- High body temperature (Fever)
- Chills
- Red or draining eyes
- Stuffy nose
- Coughing
- Headache
- Sore throat
- Flushed face
- Diarrhea
- Vomiting
- Cloudy or smelly urine
- Increased pulse rate
- Increased respiratory rate
- Pain or tenderness
- Fatigue and loss of energy
- Loss of appetite (anorexia)
- Joint pain
- Muscle ache
- Skin rash
- Sores

- Redness around a wound or incision
- Drainage from a wound or incision
- Swelling
- Heat or warmth in a body part
- Limited use of a body part
- Confusion

Asepsis

The condition of being free from disease-causing agents is called as asepsis. Asepsis actually refers to practices that eliminate or reduce pathogenic organisms. Asepsis may be broadly divided into two major categories: medical asepsis and surgical asepsis. _Medical asepsis is the minimization of the number of pathogenic agents and their spread._ On the other hand, _the absolute elimination of the pathogenic agents along with their spores from the surface of an object is known as surgical asepsis._

Basic principles of medical asepsis

The basic principles for the reduction of the number of pathogenic agents and their spread may include:

- The nurse assistant should practice good hand hygiene techniques.
- The nurse assistant should carry soiled items including equipment, linens, and other used articles, away from his/her body to prevent them from touching the clothing.
- Soiled bed linen or any other items should not be placed on the floor, which is grossly contaminated.
- The nurse assistant should avoid having patients/residents sneezing, coughing, or breathing directly on others. They should provide patients/residents the disposable tissues

and instruct them to cover their nose and mouth to prevent spread of infections by airborne droplets.

- The nurse assistant should move equipment away from him/her when dusting, brushing, or scrubbing articles.

- They should avoid raising dust by using a specially treated or a dampened cloth. Lint and dust particles may act as a vehicle by which pathogenic organisms can be transported from one place to another.

- There should be proper disposal of used or soiled items directly into appropriate containers.

- Liquids that are to be discarded, such as mouth rinse or bath water should be poured directly into the drain to avoid sprinkling in the sink.

- There should be proper sterilization of items that are suspected of containing pathogenic microorganisms. After proper sterilization, they can be managed as clean items if appropriate.

- Personal grooming habits that may help to prevent spreading pathogenic microorganisms should be encouraged.

- The nurse assistant should follow guidelines for infection control or barrier techniques as recommended by the agency.

Basic principles of surgical asepsis

The absolute elimination of the pathogenic agents and their spores from the surface of an object is called surgical asepsis. It is a more complex process than medical asepsis. The important factors to be taken care of when surgical asepsis is carried out may involve proper preparation and maintenance of the surgical equipment, environment, and personnel involved in the procedure along with the adequate cleaning of the surgical site. The basic principles of surgical asepsis include:

- Only a sterile thing can touch another sterile thing. Unsterile touching sterile depicts contamination has occurred.

- Spilling of any solution should be avoided on a paper or cloth used as a field for a sterile setup.

- The sterile objects should be held above waist level to prevent accidental contamination.

- It should be avoided coughing, talking, sneezing, or reaching over a sterile object or field. This prevents contamination by droplets from the mouth and nose.

- The nurse assistant should never walk away from or turn his/her back on a sterile field to prevent possible contamination.

- All objects must be sterile which are brought into contact with broken skin, used for skin penetration to inject substances into the body, or used to enter sterile body cavities. These objects include dressings used to cover incisions and wounds, catheters used to drain urine from the bladder, and needles for injection.

- Dry and sterile forceps should be used when necessary. Forceps that are soaked in disinfectant are usually not considered sterile.

- The outer 1-inch edge of a sterile field can be considered as contaminated.

The difference between surgical and medical asepsis may include:

Medical vs. Surgical Asepsis	
Medical asepsis is the minimization of the number of pathogenic agents and their spread.	Surgical asepsis is the absolute elimination of the pathogenic agents and their spores from the surface of an object.
Techniques	
The technique used for the process of medical asepsis is called clean technique.	The technique used for the process of surgical asepsis is called sterile techniques.
Occasions	
This technique is usually carried out in the administration of medications, enemas, and tube feedings, etc.	Sterile techniques are used in catheterization, changing dressings of a wound, and surgeries.

Roles of CDC and OSHA in the prevention of infections

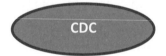

The United States CDC **(Centers for Disease Control and Prevention)** is the public health agency at the national level of the United States. It is a federal agency of the United States, under the Department of Health and Human Services (HHS), and is headquartered in Atlanta, Georgia.

The major goal of the CDC is to protect public health and safety through the prevention and control of disease, disability, and injury in the United States as well as at international level. The **Centers for Disease Control and Prevention** mainly focuses national attention on the development and application of disease control and prevention strategies. It especially focuses on infectious disease, occupational safety and health, food borne pathogens, health promotion, environmental health, and injury prevention and educational activities designed to improve the health and well beings of United States citizens. The CDC also widely conducts research and provides updated knowledge on non-infectious diseases, such as diabetes and obesity, and is a founding member of the International Association of National Public Health Institutes.

There are two major recommended precautions from CDC for the prevention of the spread of infections in healthcare settings: Standard Precautions and Transmission-Based Precautions.

Standard Precautions for All Patient Care

Standard precautions can be used for all patient care. They are generally based on an initial risk assessment and making use of personal protective equipment. Standard precautions protect healthcare providers from infectious diseases and prevent the infection spread from one patient to another. These precautions are the minimum infection prevention practices that should be used for all patient care, regardless of confirmed or suspected infection status of the patient/resident, in any healthcare setting where health care is delivered. Standard precautions may include:

- Proper hand hygiene
- Use of personal protective equipment (gloves, masks, eyewear)
- Respiratory hygiene / cough etiquette
- Sharps safety
- Safe injection practices (aseptic measures for parenteral medications)
- Use of sterile devices and instruments
- Disinfected and clean environmental surfaces

Transmission-based precautions

Transmission-based precautions should be used in addition to standard precautions for patients/residents with suspected or known infections. These precautions are the second most important recommendations of basic infection control and should be used in addition to standard precautions for patients/residents who may be colonized or infected with certain infectious agents to prevent infection transmission.

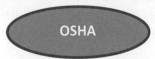

OSHA

In 1992, the OSHA **(Occupational Safety and Health Administration)** implemented some standards named as "Occupational Exposure to bloodborne pathogens (BBP)". This standard enforces the implementation of procedures, policies, and control measures that may prevent employee exposure to the body fluids and blood of patients/residents. Violations of these standards may cause a severe fine to the healthcare facility.

OSHA regulations require that healthcare employers should:

- Establish and enforce an infection control policy that conforms to OSHA guidelines. This policy should identify when PPE is required, how to clean up spills of body fluids or blood, how to send or take specimens to the laboratory, and how to dispose of infectious waste.
- Staff members should be educated about the policies.
- Free immunization should be provided for hepatitis B to the staff that might be exposed to body fluids or blood.
- Proper follow-up care should be provided to staff that is accidentally exposed to splashes of body fluids, blood, or needlesticks.
- Accessible PPEs should be readily supplied.
- Proper sharps disposal containers should be provided and should be replaced them regularly.

Standard precautions

Standard precautions should be applied for all patients/residents receiving care in hospitals, regardless to their presumed infection status or diagnosis. Standard precautions relate to blood; all secretions, body fluids, and excretions except sweat, regardless of the evidence of visible blood; nonintact skin; and mucous membranes.

Standard precautions minimize the risk of transmission of pathogenic microorganisms that cause infections in hospitals.

Healthcare personnel including nursing assistants should follow below standard precautionary measures while proving care to the patients/residents:

- The nurse assistant should always follow hand hygiene techniques.
- They should wear clean, nonsterile gloves when touching body fluids, blood, secretions, excretions, nonintact skin, mucous membranes, and contaminated objects. They should change gloves between tasks on the same patient/residents, as necessary, and should remove gloves promptly after their use.
- Nursing assistants should wear personal protective equipment, such as mask, face shield, eye protection, or fluid-repellent gown during procedures and care activities that have high risks to generate sprays or splashes of body fluids or blood. They should also use gown to protect skin and prevent soiling of clothing.
- Recapping of used needles must be avoided. If the nurse assistant must recap, he/she should never use two hands. There should always be used the one-handed scoop technique or a needle-recapping device. Needles, scalpels, and sharps should be placed in appropriate puncture-resistant containers after their use.
- The nurse assistant should carefully handle the used patient-care equipment that is soiled with body fluids, blood, excretions, and secretions to prevent transfer or spread of pathogenic

microorganisms. They should reprocess and clean items appropriately if used for another patient/resident.

- Nursing assistants should practice proper respiratory hygiene and cough etiquette. They should take measures to contain respiratory secretions that can spread pathogenic infections such as influenza. They should also encourage other people who enter the facility with signs of a respiratory problem to sneeze or cough into a tissue to contain respiratory secretions. They should dispose of these used tissues properly and clean their hands with water and soap or an alcohol-based hand rub after coughing, sneezing, or handling dirty tissues. Individuals with signs of respiratory problem may also be provided with masks or should be separated from other individuals to limit the spread of infections.

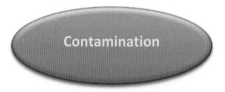

Contamination

It is the process of becoming unclean. In medical asepsis, an area or object is clean when it is free of pathogenic microorganisms. The area or object is contaminated when pathogenic microorganisms are present. Sterile means the absence of all microorganisms including pathogenic and non-pathogenic. A sterile area or object is contaminated when pathogenic or non-pathogenic microorganisms are present.

Asepsis means free of disease-producing microorganisms. Microorganisms are everywhere. Appropriate measures should be taken to achieve asepsis.

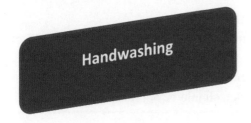

Methods to prevent contamination: Common aseptic practices

Proper aseptic practices break the chain of infection. To prevent the spread of microorganisms, following measure should be taken:

Handwashing

The CDC recommends routine handwashing for at least 15 seconds. The CDC recommends handwashing for healthcare personnel including nursing assistants in the following situations:

- At the start and end of each shift.
- When hands are visibly soiled.
- After contact with personal or another person's body fluids, blood, body fluids, excretions, or secretions. This includes vomitus, saliva, feces, urine, mucus, vaginal discharge, pus, semen, wound drainage, and respiratory secretions.
- Before and after contacts with all patients/residents.
- After contact with a source of pathogenic microorganisms (body fluids/blood, nonintact skin, mucous membrane, or contaminated objects).
- Before and after performing any invasive procedure.
- Each time after removing gloves.
- After elimination.
- After changing sanitary pads or tampons.
- After sneezing, coughing, or blowing the nose.

- Before and after preparing, handling, or eating food.
- After smoking.

Handwashing is the single most appropriate and effective measure to minimize the risk of transmitting infections. In general, the frequency and products for handwashing usually correlate to the type, duration, type, intensity, and sequence of the performed activities. For example, touching an object or area that is sterile does not require handwashing; however, touching something contaminated with body fluids or blood requires thorough handwashing. The nurse assistant should always follow his/her facility's guidelines.

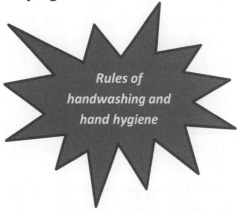

Rules of handwashing and hand hygiene

The nurse assistant should follow these rules for washing his/her hands with soap and water:

- Hands should be washed under warm running water.
- The nurse assistants should stand away from the sink. They should not let their hands, body, or uniform touch the sink as the sink is considered as a contaminated object.
- They should keep their hands and forearms lower than their elbows. Hands are dirtier than elbows and forearms. If anyone holds his/her hands and forearms up, dirty water that runs

from hands towards elbows may contaminate these areas.

- Palms should be rubbed together along with interlacing of fingers. The rubbing action aids remove dirt and microorganisms.
- There should be paid special attention to areas often missed during hand washing i.e. knuckles, thumbs, little fingers, sides of the hands, and under the nails.
- Fingernails should be cleaned by rubbing the fingertips against the palms.
- An orangewood stick or a nail file should be used to clean underneath surface of fingernails as microbes can grow easily under the fingernails.
- Hands should be washed for at least 15 to 20 seconds.
- Hands should be washed longer if they are dirty or soiled with body fluids, blood, secretions, or excretions. The nurse assistant should use his/her judgment and must follow agency policy.
- Clean and dry paper towels should be used to dry hands.
- Hands should be dried starting at the fingertips. The cleanest area should be dried first.
- A clean, dry paper towel should be used for each faucet to turn the water off. The paper towels prevent from contaminating clean hands.

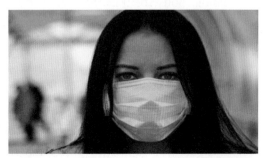

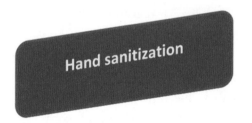

Hand sanitizers are fast and easy to use and are most commonly used in healthcare facilities. Everyone should be encouraged to "foam in/foam out" whenever having any contact with a patient/resident. Hand sanitization is sufficient if there is no visible soil on the hands and if the nurse assistant has not been in contact with patient/resident' blood and body fluids. Most healthcare facilities have containers in multiple handy locations. It should be remembered that a thorough handwashing should be done at the beginning and end of the shift, and any time when left the unit and returned.

Healthcare personnel including nursing assistants should follow these rules when decontaminating their hands with an alcohol-based hand rub:

- The product should be applied to the palm of one hand. They should always follow the manufacturer's instructions for the amount to use.

- Hands should be rubbed together.
- All surfaces of hands and fingers should be covered appropriately.
- Hands should be continued to rub together until hands are dry.
- Hand lotion or cream should be applied after hand hygiene. This prevents the skin from chapping and drying. Skin breaks may occur in dried and chapped skin. Skin breaks may act as portals of entry for pathogenic microorganisms.

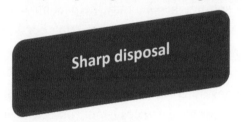

Needlestick prevention

The most common route of exposure to bloodborne pathogens for health care workers is from needlestick injuries. These injuries may occur when health care workers mishandle IV lines and needles, recap needles, or leave needles at a patient/resident's bedside.

A SESIP (sharp with engineered sharps injury protection) is a device that is effective in preventing needlesticks injuries. Healthcare personnel including nursing assistant should know the use of the SEPSIS to reduce their risk of needlestick injuries. Special leak- and puncture-proof containers are also available in health care agencies for the disposal of sharps. Containers are manufactured so only one hand needs to be used while disposing of an uncapped needle. In addition, containers should stand upright, and be labelled with a biohazard symbol or be colored red.

Equipment

Parenteral medications are administered by using a needle and a syringe. Most syringes come with safety needles or needleless systems that help prevent needlestick injuries. A number of electronic infusion pumps can be used to deliver IV or continuous subcutaneous infusions.

Syringes

Syringes are disposable, single use, and either Luer-Lok or non– Luer-Lok. Syringes are available with or without a sterile needle and also available with a needleless SESIP device. Syringes are available in a variety of sizes, ranging from 0.5 to 60 mL. Larger syringe should be used to administer some IV medications and for irrigation of drainage tubes. Most of syringes are packaged with their needle attached. Several other syringes require changing the needle based on the route of administration, size of the patient, and viscosity of the medication. The nurse assistant should follow the facility's policies and procedures for preventing needlestick injuries and safe disposal of sharps.

Needles

Several needles are attached to syringes. Most of the others are packaged individually to allow flexibility in selecting the right needle for a patient/resident. Needles are generally disposable, and most of these needles are made of stainless steel. The needle parts i.e. hub, shaft, and bevel must remain sterile at all times. To prevent contamination, a gentle force should be applied to place the needle onto the syringe with the cap intact. Some needles are available with filters for preparation of medications. Filters should never be used when administering a medication. Needles should never bend, broken or recapped by hand. The nurse assistant should dispose needles in appropriate sharps containers (biohazardous containers).

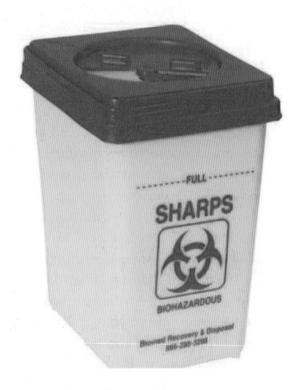

Environmental controls

The nurse assistant should always try to use Environmental Protection Agency (EPA) registered disinfectant on solid surfaces including furniture, floors, utility rooms, and bathrooms. Reusable equipment must always be disinfected or cleaned before reusing them. For resuscitation, appropriate mouthpieces should be readily available. Solid linen and waste should be kept in plastic bags and discarded according to agency policy. Separate containers should be used for regular wastes and biohazardous wastes (blood and body fluids containing blood). Body fluid spills should be wiped up immediately and area should be disinfected properly according to agency's policy.

Healthcare personnel including nursing assistants should follow the below protocols regarding **Environmental controls** for maintaining and improving the general environment of the workplace:

Keeping surfaces and objects clean

When a nurse assistant works in any health care setting, he/she may help control the spread of infectious diseases by understand exactly what is meant by dirty and what is meant by clean. Clean surfaces or objects are considered to be free of pathogens and dirt. Dirty surfaces or objects are considered contaminated because they contain pathogens or dirt. An unused object is considered to be clean until it comes in contact with an individual or his/her environment. One of the primary responsibilities of the nurse assistant is to help keep the patient/resident's environment clean. The nurse assistant may also be responsible for cleaning some types of equipment after their usage.

Healthcare providers use multiple strategies to remove pathogenic microorganisms from surfaces and objects. Simply washing the surface or object with water and soap will remove dirt and some microbes. Or any disinfectant can be used to kill microbes on the surface or object. The healthcare facility will recommend which disinfectant solution to use or it can be prepared by mixing a solution of 1½ cups bleach to 1 gallon of water. While using a bleach solution, it should always be ensured good ventilation along with wearing gloves and eye protection. The disinfectant or bleach solution should be allowed to stand on the surface for the recommended amount of time (10 to 15 minutes for a bleach solution, or 1 to 3 minutes for a disinfectant solution). When it must be necessary to disrupt and kill all of the microbes on a surface or object, sterilization is used. Objects that are needed to be placed inside a patient/resident's body (indwelling urinary catheters) must always be sterile. Sterilization can be achieved by using chemicals, gas, dry heat, or pressurized steam.

Equipment and supplies

Most health care equipment and supplies are disposable. They can prevent the spread of infectious diseases. Single-use items should be discarded after their single use. A patient/resident can use multi-use items many times. They may include urinals, bedpans, wash basins, and water mugs. These items should be labelled with the patient/resident's room and bed number. Such items should not be "borrowed" for another patient/resident. Non-disposable items should be cleaned and then disinfected. Finally, they should be sterilized.

- **Cleaning**

Cleaning minimizes the number of microorganisms present. It also removes organic matter such as body fluids, blood, excretions, and secretions. To clean equipment:

- The nurse assistant should wear PPE when cleaning items contaminated with body fluids, blood, excretions, and secretions. Personal protective equipment includes gloves, a gown, a mask, and goggles or a face shield.

- They should work from clean to dirty areas. If they work from a dirty to a clean area, the clean area also becomes dirty (contaminated). T

- The objects should be rinsed to remove organic matter. Heat makes organic matter sticky, thick, and hard to remove. Therefore, cold water should be used.

- **Disinfection**

It is the process of destroying pathogenic microorganisms. Chemical disinfectants are generally used to disinfect surfaces. Tubs, counters, and showers are examples. The process of disinfection can also be used to clean re-usable items, such as blood pressure cuffs, metal bedpans, commodes, wheelchairs, stretchers, and furniture.

- **Sterilization**

It is the process of destroying all microorganisms (pathogenic and non-pathogenic). Extremely high temperatures are used for the process of sterilization. Extreme heat destroys microorganisms. Boiling water, dry heat, radiation, liquid or gas chemicals, and steam under pressure are different sterilization methods. An autoclave is a device that is used as a pressure steam sterilizer. Surgical items, glass, and metal objects are autoclaved. High temperatures destroy and melt plastic and rubber items. Therefore, they are not autoclaved.

Cleaning up spills

It is very important to clean up biochemical or biohazardous wastes that are spilled in the healthcare facility properly. These may include any body fluids or discharge (blood, feces, urine, sputum, vomitus, wound drainage, and items such as used tissues and grossly soiled laundry). Each healthcare facility has its own written protocols and materials for safely cleaning up such spills. As biohazardous substances are highly contaminated, it is important to:

- Wear gloves
- Follow the protocols of the facility
- Disposal of contaminated material and supplies immediately
- Sanitization of the contaminated area
- Carefully washing hands

Labelling

Hazardous material containers must have manufacturer warning labels. Warning labels may identify:

- Health and physical hazards. Health hazards usually include potential health problems and the organs affected.
- Precautionary measures, such as "Do not use near open flame" Or "Avoid direct skin contact."
- Labelling for what type of personal protective equipment should wear such as mask, gown, gloves, goggles, and so on.
- Labelling for how to use the substance safely. There should be appropriate biohazard symbol for sharps and liquid blood.
- Labelling for storage and disposal information. If a warning label is damaged or removed from a substance, it should not be used. The nurse assistant should show the container to the nurse supervisor and explain the problem. The container should not be left unattended. Laboratory specimens

and specimen containers are potentially highly infectious. Therefore, agency policies should be followed for their labelling and properly transporting.

Personal protective equipment

Personal protective equipment (PPE) refers to specialized equipment or clothing worn by an employee for protection against infectious or hazardous substances. PPE is used in healthcare settings to improve personnel safety through their appropriate use of PPE. This equipment includes clean and sterile gloves, impervious aprons/gowns, N95 disposable masks, surgical and high-efficiency particulate air (HEPA) masks, face shields, and protective goggles/eyewear. It is the nurse supervisor's responsibility to enforce the proper wearing of PPE during patient/resident care for members of the healthcare team.

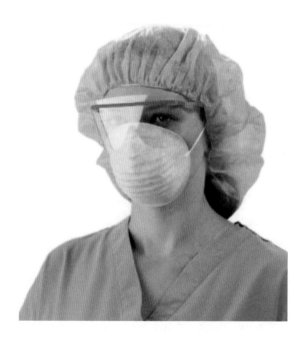

Personal protective equipment (PPE) is used to prevent infectious agents from contaminating uniform, skin or mucous membranes. Appropriate use of PPE eliminates a portal of entry for potential pathogenic microorganisms, and helps to keep healthcare personnel safe from infectious agents. PPE is usually worn outside of the patient/resident's room, and discarded and removed inside the patient/resident's room. When it is necessary to wear multiple types of PPE, items should be worn in the order as gown, mask, protective eyewear, and gloves. When it is necessary to remove the PPE, the order should be as gloves, protective eyewear, gown, and mask.

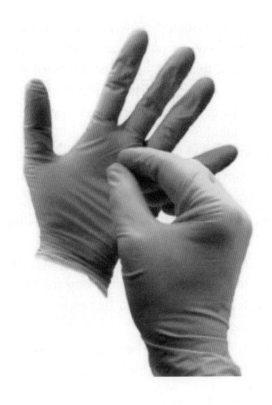

Gloves

Gloves are the most commonly used to reduce hand contamination by almost 70% and provide a protective barrier when touching body fluids or blood. It is important to use gloves in all patients/residents care involving potential exposure to blood or body fluids. Gloves provide protection from infectious agents and prevent the spread of microbes from one person to another. Disposable and clean gloves are usually available in all healthcare facilities, including community-based settings. The nurse assistant must always wear gloves if he/she has any breaks in the skin of the hands. Used gloves should be discarded in the appropriate receptacle.

Small skin breaks on the finders and hands are common. Gloves act as a protective barrier. They protect:

- From pathogenic microorganisms in the person's body fluids, blood, secretions, and excretions.
- The person from pathogens on his/her hands.

When using gloves:

- The outside of gloves should be considered as contaminated.
- These should be applied to dry hands. Gloves are generally easier to wear on dry hands.
- Gloves should not be torn when putting them on. Long fingernails, carelessness, and rings can tear gloves. Body fluids, blood, secretions, and excretions may enter into the glove through the tear and contaminate hands.
- There should be a new pair of gloves applied for every person.

- Gloves should be removed, discarded, torn, cut, or punctured at once. Proper hand hygiene should be practiced and then a new pair should be put on.
- Gloves should be worn once. They should be discarded after use.
- Gloves should be changed when moving from a contaminated body site to a clean body site.
- Gloves should be changed when touching portable computer keyboards or any other mobile equipment, transported from one room to another.
- It should be ensured that gloves cover the wrists.
- Gloves should be removed so the inside part is on the outside.

Removing Gloves
1. It should be ensured that glove touches only glove.
2. Glove at the palm should be grasped. It should be grasped on its outside.
3. The glove should be pulled down over hand so it is inside out.
4. The removed glove should be held with other gloved hand.
5. The first two fingers of the ungloved hand should be used to reach inside the other glove and should be pulled the glove down (inside out) over the hand. The gloves should be discarded as per agency policy.
6. Proper hand hygiene should be practiced.

Gowns or aprons

A gown is worn to protect the body and clothes from sprays and splashes of blood and body fluids. The gown must completely cover the body from the neck to the knees. A gown should be worn only once and then it should be placed in a laundry hamper (if it is made of fabric) or thrown away (if it is made of paper). Because a wet or damp gown cannot provide protection, it must be changed if it becomes wet.

The nurse assistant should follow these measures when using gowns or aprons:
- The inside of the apron or gown is clean; the outside is considered as contaminated.
- The apron or gown must be long enough to cover the clothing or uniform.
- The neck of the clothing is considered clean because the nurse assistant does not touch that part with contaminated hands.
- If the nurse assistant is wearing long sleeves, the sleeves should be rolled up above the elbows before putting on the apron or gown.
- A supply of clean aprons or gowns should be ready outside the patient/resident's room.
- After their use, they should be removed and disposed of inside out (contaminated side in), and placed in the receptacle. Reusable gowns should be placed in the linen hamper.
- After removing gowns or aprons, hands should be washed thoroughly.

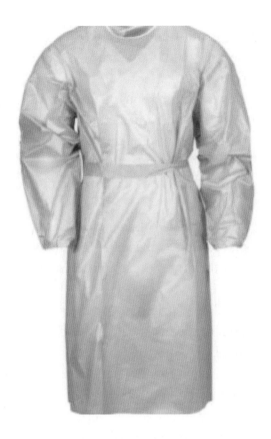

Donning and Removing a Gown

1. Watch and jewelery should be removed.
2. Sleeves of the uniform should be rolled up.
3. Proper hand hygiene should be practiced.
4. The hands and arms should be put through the sleeves.
5. It should be ensured that the gown covers the body from the neck to the knees. It must cover arms to the end of the wrists.
6. The strings should be tied at the back of the neck.
7. The back of the gown should be overlapped and must cover the uniform. The gown should not be loose.
8. The waist strings should be tied. They should be tied at the back or the side.

9. Other PPE should be put on as: Mask or respirator (if needed), Goggles or face shield, Gloves.
10. It should be ensured that gloves cover the gown cuffs.
11. Gloves should be removed and discarded after use.
12. Goggles or face shield should be removed and discarded if worn.
13. Lastly, the gown should be removed. There should be no touching at the outside of the gown. It should be removed as:

- The neck and waist strings should be untied at firs.
- The gown should be pulled down from each shoulder toward the same hand.
- The gown should be turned inside out as it is removed.
- The gown should be rolled and held away from the body and it should be kept inside out. The gown should not touch the floor. Lastly, it should be discarded as per agency policies.

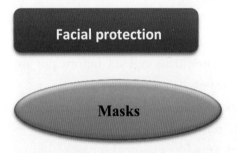

Facial protection

Masks

Masks help protect healthcare personnel and patients/residents from upper respiratory infections and various communicable diseases. The nurse assistant should use a mask when caring for patients/residents with respiratory disorders. For example, if a patient/resident is sneezing or coughing, a mask should be worn to cover the nurse assistant's mouth and nose. Healthcare facilities have established certain procedures and policies about types of masks and when to use them. In some cases, everyone who comes in contact with a patient/resident, including family members and visitors, wears a mask, or the patient/resident may wear a mask when outside his/her room. A surgical (face) mask that is most commonly used is effective for providing a protective barrier against large droplets. These simple surgical masks can only screen out large-sized particles. When a patient/resident is known to have a disease that is caused by very tiny droplets that are suspended in the air (called aerosols) such as tuberculosis-causing bacillus, a HEPA (high-efficiency particulate air filter) mask must be worn. HEPA masks must be tightly fitted to the individual who will be wearing them. These masks readily filter the inhaled air to prevent aerosols from passing through. In some specific situations, a special mask, called a respirator mask or particulate mask, is used. This mask is used to filter out tiny particles.

The nurse assistant should follow the below measures for mask use:

- Mask should be put on before put on the gloves.
- Mask should not be touched until it is to be removed.
- Mask must be changed when soiled or moist.
- Hands should be washed and gloves should be removed before removing the mask.
- Masks should be handled by the strings or elastic only.
- Used mask should be disposed of immediately.
- Mask should not be left dangling around the neck.

Donning and removing a mask

1. Proper hand hygiene should be practiced.
2. Gown should be put on if required.
3. Mask should be picked up by its upper ties. It should not touch the part that will cover the face.
4. Mask should be placed over the nose and mouth.
5. Upper strings of the mask should be placed above the ears and should be tied them at the back in the middle of the head.
6. The lower strings should be tied at the back of the neck. The lower part of the mask should be under the chin.
7. The metal band should be pinched around the nose. The top of the mask must be snug over the nose. If there are eyeglasses, the mask must be snug under the bottom of the eyeglasses.
8. It should be ensured that the mask is snugged over the face and under the chin.
9. Goggles or a face shield should be put on if needed and if not part of the mask.
10. Gloves should be put on.
11. Sneezing, coughing, and unnecessary talking should be avoided.
12. The mask should be changed if it becomes wet or contaminated.
13. Gloves should be removed and discarded after their use. Goggles or face shield and gown should be then removed and discarded if worn.
14. Mask should be removed at the end. It should be removed as:
    - The lower strings of the mask should be untied first.
    - Then the top strings should be untied.
    - The top strings should be held and the mask should be removed.

- The mask should be discarded and proper hand hygiene should be practiced.

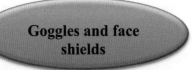

Goggles and face shields

Goggles and face shields protect mouth, eyes, and nose from spraying or splashing of body fluids, blood, secretions, and excretions. Sprays and splashes can occur during patient care, cleaning items, or disposing of fluids. The outside (front) of goggles or a face shield is considered as contaminated. The headband, ear-pieces, or ties used to secure the device are clean. They should be used to remove the device after hand hygiene. They are clean and safe to touch with bare hands. Disposable goggles or face shields should be discarded after use. Re-usable eyewear must be cleaned before re-use. It should be washed with water and soap.

Then a disinfectant should be used after their cleaning.

Encouraging safety and comfort
Eyeglasses and contact lenses usually cannot provide proper eye protection. If eyeglasses are worn, a face shield should be used that fits over glasses with minimal gaps. Goggles alone do not provide spray or splash protection to other parts of the face. Therefore, face shield should also be used along with goggles.

Transmission-based precautions

When a patient's primary care provider suspects or confirms that the patient has an infectious disease that can be spread to others, the nurse assistant must take additional precautionary measures to prevent the spread of the infection to other individuals. These precautionary measures are called as transmission-based precautions. The primary care provider takes decision about which transmission-based precautions should be followed. This decision is based on two factors: the pathogenic microorganism and how that pathogenic microorganism spreads. When transmission-based precautions are in effect, the nurse assistant will have to put on the proper PPE before entering the patient/resident's room, and remove it at the doorway right before leaving the patient/resident's room.

Standard Precautions should be used when caring for all patients/residents. Transmission-based precautions should be applied when caring for patients/residents with a suspected or known infectious disease, based on its route of transmission. Transmission-based precautions are designed to interrupt the transmission of pathogenic microorganisms in healthcare facilities. These precautions are used to break the "chain of infection", by providing a protective barrier for either the patient/resident or the healthcare worker. Transmission-based precautions are grouped into three types: airborne precautions, droplet precautions, and contact precautions. When caring patients/residents who need these precautions, healthcare workers should use them in addition to standard precautions.

■**Airborne precautions**
Airborne precautions are implemented when caring for a patient/resident who is known or thought to have a disease that is transmitted through the air. For example, rubeola virus (measles), varicella virus

(chickenpox), Mycobacterium tuberculosis (TB), and possibly SARS-CoV are spread in this manner. Airborne pathogens (pathogens which are expelled into the air when an infected individual coughs, breathes, or sneezes) may cover a long distance on air currents and through ventilation systems. Thus, airborne precautions should include placing the patient/resident in a private room and keeping the door closed. Other measures may include wearing a HEPA mask when providing care, and having the patient/resident wear a mask when he/she has to leave the room.

Airborne transmission occurs when tiny pathogenic microorganisms from evaporated droplets are carried on dust particles or remain suspended in the air. Air currents disperse these pathogenic microorganisms, which can be easily inhaled by a susceptible host. Special air handling and ventilation are needed to prevent this type of infection transmission. Tuberculosis (TB), chickenpox, measles, and COVID 19 are common examples of airborne-transmitted infections.

Patients/residents requiring airborne precautions are placed in a private room that has monitored negative airflow pressure. Many healthcare facilities have special portable air-filtering machines to maintain airborne precautions. Doors to rooms with patients/residents who need airborne precautions are kept closed. When caring for patients/residents requiring airborne precautions, respiratory protection is extremely necessary.

■ **Droplet precautions**
Droplet precautions are implemented when caring for a patient/resident who is known

or thought to have an infectious disease that is transmitted by large droplets in the air, such as a respiratory virus or meningitis. These droplets are spread by coughing, sneezing, singing, laughing, and talking. The droplets cannot travel too far. Droplet precautions are almost similar to airborne precautions, except the use of surgical (face) mask instead of a necessary HEPA mask.

Droplet transmission occurs when droplets with pathogenic microorganisms are propelled through the air from an infected individual and deposited on the host's nose, eyes or mouth. Transmission of infection can occur through coughing, sneezing, talking, or during certain procedures such as suctioning. Examples of infectious diseases spread by droplets may include pertussis, influenza, meningococcal meningitis, streptococcal pharyngitis (in young children and infants), mumps, and rubella. Patients/residents requiring droplet precautions should be placed in a private room. However, if a private room is not available, he/she can share a room with another patient/resident with the same infectious disease. The door of the room may remain open. Healthcare workers should wear a face mask when caring within 3 feet of the patient/resident. The patient/resident should also wear a mask if he/she needs to transport to an area outside the room.

■ **Contact precautions**
Contact precautions are implemented when caring for a patient/resident who is known or thought to have an infection that can be spread by direct or indirect contact. Some types of skin infections and wound infections can be spread in this way.

Contact precautions may include wearing a gown or apron and gloves when providing care, and disposing of contaminated items properly. When there are transmission-based precautions in effect, a sign may be posted outside the patient/resident's room so that all visitors (if allowed) and health care workers are aware of the precautions that must be taken. It should be ensured that visitors and other health care workers must follow these precautions.

Contact transmission is the most common mode of disease transmission in healthcare facilities. Transmission of these infections can occur as a result of direct contact between a susceptible host's body surface and an infected patient/resident. Indirect contact may occur when a susceptible host comes into contact with dirty instrument, needle, or hands (intermediate contaminated objects). Examples of infections spread by contact transmission may include respiratory and gastrointestinal, skin, and wound infections. Impetigo, scabies, hepatitis A, herpes simplex virus, and pediculosis are other examples. Precautionary measures are significantly important in cases caused by drug-resistant organisms, such as MRSA (Methicillin-resistant Staphylococcus aureus) or VRE (vancomycin-resistant Enterococcus). Patients/residents requiring contact - precautions can be placed in a room with other patients/residents who are infected with the same microorganism if a private room is unavailable. The door of the room may remain open. Healthcare workers should wear gloves when entering the room and remove them before leaving the room. Gloves should be changed after contact with a patient/resident's infective material (fecal matter or wound drainage).

Proper hand hygiene with an antimicrobial agent should be practiced. A gown, gloves, and mask should be worn before entering into the room or in case of contact with the patient/resident. When possible, it should be tried to restrict the use of noncritical equipment to one patient/resident only. If equipment is necessary to be used for multiple patients/residents, it should be cleaned and disinfected carefully and thoroughly before using it for other patients/residents.

Isolation

Both standard precautions and transmission-based precautions are the currently recommended isolation guidelines. Historically, two primary types of isolation techniques were used in healthcare settings: disease-specific isolation and category-specific isolation. Although standard precautions and transmission-based precautions have replaced the routine use of these techniques, some healthcare facilities still use them in addition to standard and transmission-based precautions. Disease-specific isolation applies a single all-purpose sign. Nursing assistants choose the items on the card that are specific for the specific types of diseases that are causing isolation. In category-specific isolation, special types of isolation (contact, enteric, respiratory, strict, or wound) are identified, using specific color-coded cards. This form of isolation is based on the patient/resident's diagnosis. The cards are posted outside the patient/resident's room and depicts that visitors must check with nursing assistant and other relevant staff before entering.

Body fluids, blood, secretions, and excretions can transmit infectious diseases. Sometimes barriers are needed to keep pathogenic microorganisms within a certain area. Usually the area is the patient/resident's room. This needs isolation precautions. These isolation precautions prevent the spread of contagious diseases (communicable diseases). They are diseases caused by pathogenic microorganisms that spread easily. Isolation precautions are based on the principles of clean and dirty. Clean objects or areas have no pathogenic microorganisms. They are not dirty or contaminated. Dirty objects or areas are contaminated with pathogenic microorganisms. If a clean object or area has contact with something contaminated, the clean object or area is now contaminated. Contaminated and clean also depend on how the pathogenic microorganism is spread.

Rules for isolation precautions

- All needed items should be collected before entering the room.
- There should be no contamination of equipment and supplies. Floors are considered as contaminated. So any object on the floor or that falls to the floor is also considered as contaminated.
- Floors should be cleaned with mops wetted with any disinfectant solution as floor dust is contaminated.
- Paper towels should be used to handle contaminated items.
- Objects should be removed from the room in leak-proof plastic bags.

- The objects should be in double-bag if the outside of the bag is or can be contaminated.
- The nurse assistant should follow agency policy to remove and transport re-usable and disposable items.
- Re-usable dishes, eating utensils, trays, and drinking vessels should be returned to the food service (dietary) department. Disposable dishes, eating utensils, drinking vessels, and trays should be discarded in the waste container in the patient/resident's room.
- The nurse assistant should not touch his/her nose, hair, eyes, mouth, or other body parts.
- They should not touch any clean object or area if hands are contaminated.
- They should wash their hands if they are visibly dirty or contaminated with body fluids, blood, excretions, or secretions.
- Clean items should be placed on paper towels.
- Paper towels should be used to turn faucets on and off.
- A paper towel should be used to open the door to the patient/resident's room and it should be discarded after use.

Nursing measures in setting up a patient/resident's room for isolation

Patients/residents who require isolation are usually confined to their rooms. The major goal is to protect other patients/residents, keep the patient/resident's environment contaminated only to that patient/resident, and facilitate concurrent and terminal disinfection. All healthcare facilities have pre-defined procedures and policies for isolation and for the use of specific PPE. The nurse assistant should check the healthcare facility's procedures and policies for specific measures to follow if the patient/resident needs to be brought out of the room for a test or treatment.

> **Psychological effects of standard and transmission based precautions on patients/residents**

Having standard and transmission-based precautions in effect can be very hard for the patient/resident. How would anyone feel if the door to his/her room had to be closed all the time for isolation? Perhaps he/she would feel as if no one wanted to be near him/her or that no one liked him/her. The patient/resident might feel lonely, depressed, angry, afraid, embarrassed, or all of these things. What if the other people caring for a patient/resident could not come near him/her without wearing masks, gowns, and gloves? Even though healthcare workers must follow standard and transmission-based precautions as ordered, they can also be sensitive to the patient/resident's feelings. It should be ensured that the patient/resident knows why the standard and transmission-based precautions are being taken, and stress that these preventive measures will aid to speed his/her recovery and prevent other people from getting sick. Healthcare workers should explain the purpose of the wearing PPE. This can help the patient/resident get used to watching healthcare workers in protective clothing. Healthcare workers

should make a special effort to check in on the patient/resident often, and should take time to talk with him/her. Spending time with the patient/resident and offering reassurance can support the patient/resident feel better about the time spent in isolation and may fulfill the basic needs such as love, belonging, affiliation, self-esteem, and self-actualization.

Education and Preparation

When setting up the patient/resident's room, it should be thoroughly explained the isolation precautions to the patient/resident and family. Both patient/resident and family will need to understand the reasons for these isolation procedures. Healthcare workers should explain that children are usually not allowed to visit a patient/resident with an infection requiring special precautions, because children are more susceptible to infection. Use of barrier techniques and PPE may frighten patients/residents, who may fear their infectious disease and believe that others are afraid to come near them. These patients/residents may experience loneliness and miss the companionship of their loved ones. Healthcare workers should make every effort to visit and communicate with patients/residents in isolation as much as possible. They should properly organize their workload so they can remain in their room for longer periods.

Supplies

The patient/resident's room should be equipped with

- A urinal and bedpan
- Wash basin and soap dish
- Water pitcher and glass
- Emesis basin

- Toilet and facial tissues
- Toothbrush and dentifrice
- Personal items, such as comb, shaving equipment, hair pick, and/or brush, shampoo, deodorant, and cosmetics

The patient/resident should be provided a telephone and television, if possible. Additional items may include paper towels, paper or plastic bags to line the wastebasket for trash disposal, washable blankets, bedspreads, pillows, impervious laundry bags, and the usual linens. A sink with knee or foot control and a covered linen stand and bag are ideal. The patient/resident should have a private bathroom and shower. Items to be placed outside the patient/resident's room or in an anteroom may include a cabinet or bedside stand stocked with PPE as required for the patient/resident's condition. A sink should be available for handwashing. Hand sanitization materials must also be available. Other items include large trash bags, biohazard bags, clean laundry bags, and tape or tags and marking pens for marking contaminated bags. Healthcare facilities also need a sign for the door, which may vary depending on the specific precautions the patient/resident's condition requires.

Helpful Resources

Burch, J., & Tort, S. (2020). Does healthcare worker education improve adherence to standard precautions for controlling health care-associated infections? *Cochrane Clinical Answers*. https://doi.org/10.1002/cca.3395

Chi-Chung Cheng, V., Fuk-Woo Chan, J., FN Hung, I., & Yuen, K. (2016). Viral infections, an overview with a focus on prevention of transmission. *Reference Module in Biomedical Sciences*. https://doi.org/10.1016/b978-0-12-801238-3.90174-0

Clinical manifestations of invasive fungal infections. (2005). *Fungal Infections in the Immunocompromised Patient*, 221-236. https://doi.org/10.1201/b14156-11

Electron microscopy of viral infections. (2016). *Lennette's Laboratory Diagnosis of Viral Infections*, 189-212. https://doi.org/10.3109/9781420084962-13

Gallucci, S. (2016). An overview of the innate immune response to infectious and Noninfectious stressors. *The Innate Immune Response to Noninfectious Stressors*, 1-24. https://doi.org/10.1016/b978-0-12-801968-9.00001-5

Godfrey, C., & Schouten, J. T. (2014). Infection control best practices in clinical research in resource-limited settings. *JAIDS Journal of Acquired Immune Deficiency Syndromes*, *65*(Supplement 1), S15-S18. https://doi.org/10.1097/qai.0000000000000034

Günther, J., & Seyfert, H. (2018). The first line of defence: Insights into mechanisms and

relevance of phagocytosis in epithelial cells. *Seminars in Immunopathology*, *40*(6), 555-565.

https://doi.org/10.1007/s00281-018-0701-1

Hierholzer, W. J. (1982). Nosocomial bacterial infections. *Bacterial Infections of Humans*,

367-392. https://doi.org/10.1007/978-1-4757-1140-0_20

Sanchez, E., & Doron, S. (2017). Bacterial infections: Overview. *International Encyclopedia

of Public Health*, 196-205. https://doi.org/10.1016/b978-0-12-803678-5.00030-8

Standard precautions and transmission-based isolation precautions. (2016). *Fast Facts for the

Pediatric Nurse*. https://doi.org/10.1891/9780826119827.ap01

Tappero, J. W., Cassell, C. H., Bunnell, R. E., Angulo, F. J., Craig, A., Pesik, N., Dahl, B. A.,

Ijaz, K., Jafari, H., & Martin, R. (2017). US Centers for Disease Control and Prevention and

its partners' contributions to global health security. *Emerging Infectious Diseases*, *23*(13).

https://doi.org/10.3201/eid2313.170946

Viral infections of the Immunocompromised host. (2016). *Lennette's Laboratory Diagnosis

of Viral Infections*, 474-490. https://doi.org/10.3109/9781420084962-29

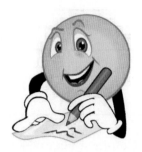

Chapter Seven:

Weights and Measures

Outline

I: Units of measurement used in the household and metric systems for weight, height, and volume

II: Equipment commonly used by the Nurse Assistant for measuring weight, length, and volume

III: Conversion of common measurements between the household and metric systems.

IV: Measurement of weight, length, and volume using metric and household systems.

V: Conversion between standard time and military time

Units of measurements used in the household and metric systems for weight, height, and volume

U.S. Customary weights and measurements (household)

The customary system of measurement, also known as U.S. Customary System, is based on the English system of measurement. The customary system may be defined as a set of weights and measures used for measuring weight, length, and volume.

Americans usually use customary units for commercial activities, as well as for social and personal use. In medicine, many sectors of industry, and some military and government areas, metric units are more commonly used.

Although customary units are seldom used in a medical setting, they may be sometimes used when providing patients instructions for administering medications at home.

U.S. Customary units for measuring length

The customary units to measure length in the customary system are inches, feet, miles, and yards.

Customary units for length			
Inch (in)	Feet (ft)	Mile (mi)	Yard (yd)

Common equivalents for conversion of one customary unit of length to another are:

Length
1 Foot = 12 inches
1 Yard = 3 feet = 36 inches
1 Mile = 5280 feet
1 Mile = 1760 yards

U.S. Customary units for measuring weight

The U.S. customary units for measuring weight are ounces, pounds, and tons.

Customary units for weight		
Ounce (oz)	Pound (lb)	Ton (tn)

Common equivalents for conversion of one customary unit of weight to another are:

Weight
1 Pound = 16 ounces
1 Ton = 2000 pounds

U.S. Customary units for measuring volume

The U.S. customary units for measuring volume are fluid ounces, pints, quarts, gallons, teaspoons, and tablespoons.

Customary units for volume					
Fluid ounce (fl oz)	Pint (pt)	Quart (qt)	Gallon (gal)	Teaspoon (tsp)	Tablespoon (Tbsp)

Common equivalents for conversion of one customary unit of volume to another are:

> **Volume**
> 16 Ounces = 1 pint
> 2 Pints = 1 quart
> 4 Quarts = 1 gallon

Metric system

It is a system of measurement that uses the meter, liter, and gram as base units of length, volume, and weight respectively.

The metric system is currently the most commonly used measurement system in the world. It is also the major primary measurement system that is used in the medical field. Healthcare professionals, including nursing assistants, must have the ability to understand and convert units of measurement within and between the metric and US customary systems. They should also be able to perform correct calculations with measurements and demonstrate the results with the accurate unit notations.

Metric units for measuring length

The metric units to measure length are millimeter (mm), centimeter (cm), meter (m).

Metric units for length		
Millimeter (mm)	Centimeter (cm)	Meter (m)

Common equivalents for conversion of one metric unit of length to another are:

> **Length**
> 1 cm = 1 centimeter = 1×10^{-2} meter = 0.01 meter

Metric units for measuring weight

The metric units for measuring weight are gram (gm) and kilogram (kg).

Metric units for weight	
Gram (gm)	Kilogram (kg)

Common equivalents for conversion of one metric unit of weight to another are:

> **Length**
> 1 kg = 1 kilogram = 1×10^{3} gram = 1000 gram

Metric units for measuring volume

The metric units for measuring weight are milliliter (ml), liter (L).

Metric units for volume	
Milliliter (ml)	Liter (L)

Common equivalents for conversion of one metric unit of volume to another are:

Equipment used for measuring weight, length, and volume

Volume measuring equipment

Liquid Volume Measuring Devices: The Graduated Cylinder

Like weighing, measuring volume is also a fundamental and frequently encountered task for nursing assistants. Graduated cylinder is commonly used for measuring liquid volume. As the name suggests, a graduated cylinder is a plastic tube or a cylindrical glass sealed at one end, with a calibrated scale marked on the outside wall. Graduated cylinders are available in a range of sizes, or volume capacities, and just like a measuring cup. The volume can be measured by adding liquid to the cylinder and comparing its level to the graduated scale. The measured volume correlates to the volume of liquid contained in the cylinder. Therefore, the graduated cylinder and equipment like it such as Erlenmeyer flasks, volumetric flasks, and beakers are classified as to-contain (TC) equipment. The volume of liquid in a graduated cylinder can be measured directly by reading the calibrated scale.

If the cylinder is made from glass, the liquid surface will be U-shaped (curved) rather than horizontal, due to the comparatively strong attractive force

between glass and water. The curved surface is named as meniscus. As a general rule, the bottom of the meniscus is considered as the level of liquid in a glass cylinder. If the cylinder is made from plastic, the liquid surface will be horizontal (flat). There will be no meniscus. The scale divisions on a graduated cylinder are usually determined by its size. The lines and numbers on graduated cylinder show the markings of milliliters and ounces. For example, the scale of a 10-mL graduated cylinder will be divided into 0.1 mL increments, and the scale of a 500-mL graduated cylinder is divided into 5 mL increments. The graduated cylinder scale is just like a ruled scale, which must be read like a ruler. The scale should be read to one digit beyond the smallest scale division by estimating between these divisions. The 10-mL graduated cylinder scale should be read to the nearest 0.01 mL and the 500-mL graduated cylinder scale must be read to the nearest 1 mL.

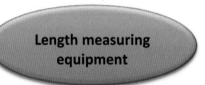

Length measuring equipment

The most common ways to measure length is by using a yard stick, measuring tape, or standing scale.

Yard stick

A yard stick measures the length by the yard. It only shows customary units of inches and feet. Since there are 3 feet in a yard, a yard stick can be used to measure the height of an infants and children. The height can also be measured with a tape measure; however, a yard stick is a rigid tool as compared to flexible tape measure.

Measuring tape

It is another tool to measure length. Since tape measure is a flexible tool, thus, it is often used to measure the heights of older patients/residents. Tape measures mostly show length in feet and inches, but sometimes, a tape measure may have both customary units and metric units marked.

Standing scale

When a patient/resident can stand independently for long time, an upright or standing scale can be used to measure the patient/resident's height. Standing scales show length in fractions of feet and inches, as well as centimeters. Therefore, they have both customary units and metric units to measure height.

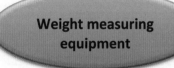

There are different types of scales for measurement of weight, for example standing, wheelchair, mechanical lift, bed scale, and chair scale. These scales are usually marked in ounces, pounds, grams, and kilograms. Both digital and mechanical scales can be used for measuring weight.

Digital scales

Digital scales make it extremely easy to determine the weight of a patient/resident on the scale. The numbers are usually bold and the screen is generally backlit, making it very difficult to mistake the numbers and almost impossible to make a mistake when reading the scale.

Mechanical scales

These scales are preferred by some individuals who want to be able to quickly gauge the weight, but aren't much worried about being exact.

Types of scales

There are different types of scales for measuring weight such as:

1. **Standing scales**

When a patient/resident can stand independently long enough to be weighed, an upright or standing scale can be used to measure the patient/resident's weight. Standing scales are usually marked in ounces, pounds, grams, and kilograms. Weight is measured through standing scales while a patient/resident must be steady on feet.

2. **Wheelchair scales**

Wheelchair scales are effective and reliable tools of weighing a patient/resident who cannot stand unassisted. The patient/resident is not required to move onto another chair, or any way discomforted by the process. For weighing through wheelchair scales, unoccupied wheelchair is weighed first, then the patient/resident in wheelchair is weighed, and finally wheelchair weight is subtracted from total weight.

3. **Mechanical lift**

If the patient/resident is unable to get out of bed at all, a sling scale can be used to weigh the patient/resident. The sling used depends on the patient/resident's size, condition, and other needs.

For weighing through mechanical lift, sling and any linen should be weighed first, then the patient/resident is weighed through the sling and hydraulic lift, and finally the sling's weight is subtracted from total weight.

5. Bed scale

A bed scale is a medical scale which enables a patient/resident to be weighed whilst still in bed. Depending on the patient/resident's size, condition, and other needs, these scales can be used in high-dependency areas.

6. Chair scale

When a patient/resident is able to get out of bed but is unable to stand long enough to be weighed using an upright scale, a chair scale can be used to weigh the patient/resident. Some chair scales contain a seat mounted on the scale and the nurse assistant simply helps the patient/resident to sit in the seat. When using this type of chair scale, the nurse assistant should first weigh the empty chair, and then should weigh the chair with the patient/resident in it. The patient/resident's weight would be the difference between the two measurements.

Conversion of common measurements between the household and metric systems

The metric system is the most commonly used measurement system in the worldwide. The household measures are those that usually use measuring tools found in most homes. Therefore, any medication orders written in metric systems should be converted to the household measurements for ease of drug administration.

Converting one system of measurement to another system of measurement requires that a nursing assistant should know and able to look up the equivalent unit of measurement for the different systems of measurement.

For weight:

Weight
1 Pound = 16 ounces
1 Ton = 2000 pounds

1 ton = 2000 pounds
1 pound = 16 ounces
1 ton = 2000 × 16 = 32000 ounces

Customary unit	Standard metric equivalent
1 ounce	28.35 grams
1 pound	453.6 grams
1 ton	907.2 kilograms

For length:

Length
1 Foot = 12 inches
1 Yard = 3 feet = 36 inches
1 Mile = 5280 feet
1 Mile = 1760 yards

Conversion of 3 foot to inches:
1 foot = 12 inches
3 foot = 12 × 3 = 36 inches

Customary unit	Standard metric equivalent
1 inch	2.54 centimeters
1 foot	0.3048 meters
1 yard	0.9144 meters
1 mile	1.6 kilometers

For volume:

Volume
16 Ounces = 1 pint
2 Pints = 1 quart
4 Quarts = 1 gallon

Conversion of 5 quarts to cups:
1 quart = 2 pint
5 quarts = 10 pints
1 pint = 2 cups
10 pints = 10 × 2 = 20 cups
So,
5 quarts = 20 cups

Customary unit	Standard metric equivalent
1 fluid ounce	30 ml (2 Tbsp)
1 cup	236.5 ml (8 fl oz)
1 pint	473 ml (2 cups)
1 quart	0.9 L (2 pints)
1 gallon	3.8 L (4 quarts)

Measurement of weight, length, and volume using metric and household systems

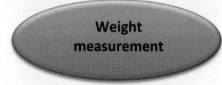

Weight measurement

Height and weight measurement on standing scale

The nurse assistant should assist in measuring height and weight on standing scales in following ways:

1. Hands should be washed properly.

2. The nurse assist should gather all supplies:
   - Upright scale
   - Paper towels
   - Pen and paper
3. The nurse assistant should knock, greet the patient/resident and should ensure his/her privacy.
4. The procedure should be explained thoroughly to the patient/resident.
5. Equipment should be adjusted for proper body mechanics and safety.
6. The balance of the scale should be checked by moving the weights all the way to the left (zero). The pointer should be evenly centered between the bottom and top bars. If the scale is not balanced, it should be notified to the nurse.
7. A paper towel should be put on the scale platform.
8. The patient/resident should be assisted to step onto the scale platform, facing the balance bar.
9. The bottom bar is marked in units of 50 pounds. The large weight should be moved on the bottom bar to the weight that is closest to the patient/resident's estimated weight in units of 50 pounds, without exceeding the patient/resident's estimated weight.
10. The top bar is marked in units of 1 pound and ¼ pound. The small weight should be moved on the top bar until the pointer is evenly centered between the bottom and top bars. 11. The weight on the top bar should be added to the weight on the bottom bar. This is the patient/resident's weight.
11. If the nurse assistant is measuring the patient/resident's height as well, the patient/resident should be assisted to turn around so that he/she is facing away from the balance bar.

12. The height scale should be slided all the way up and pulled out the height rod.

13. The height rod should be slided down until it touches the top of the patient/resident's head. The number on the height scale should be read. This is the patient/resident's height.

14. The patient/resident should be assisted to step off the scale.

15. It should be ensured the patient/resident's comfort and proper body alignment.

16. Hands should be properly washed, and observations should be reported and recorded at the end of the procedure.

Height measurement through measuring tape

Since measuring tape is a flexible tool, thus, it is often used to measure the heights of older patients/residents. Measuring tapes mostly show length in feet and inches, but sometimes a measuring tape may have both customary units and metric units marked.

If possible, the nurse assistance should ask someone for assistance while measuring the height with a measuring tape. Having assistance usually helps improve the accuracy of the measurement. To ensure the accurate measurement, shoes, hats, and other headwear should be removed before measuring. Keeping feet flat on the floor and standing straight with back flat against the wall, the nurse assistant should measure the distance from the floor to the spot on the wall to find out the height, keeping the patient/resident's chin parallel to the floor.

Safe care usually depends on accurate reporting and recording. Some agencies use kilograms (kg) for weight. Others use pounds (lb). For height, some agencies use

inches and feet. Others use inches only. If a nurse assistant does not know what measurements to use, he/she should ask the nurse. The nurse assistant should always follow agency policy to report and record weight and height.

Encouraging safety and comfort

The manufacturer's instructions should be followed when using wheelchair, chair, bed, or lift scales. The nurse assistant should also follow the agency's procedure and practice to prevent falls. The patient/resident should wear only pajamas or a gown for the weight measurement.

Volume measurement

Graduated cylinders are thin glass tubes used for measuring the volumes of liquids. The process of measuring volume through a graduated cylinder is straightforward, but following steps should be taken to make sure an accurate reading and maintain a safe working environment:

- An appropriate size cylinder that is large enough should be selected to hold the volume of liquid being measured.

- It should be ensured that the tube is dry and clean.

- The container should be placed on flat surface while pouring liquid into graduate container.

- The cylinder should be placed at eye level to take a reading. It should be ensure that cylinder is hanging straight down. The nurse assistant should avoid crouching to read the cylinder while it is resting on the flat surface.

- The liquid measurement should be taken at the very bottom of the dip in the surface of the liquid. This bottom of the dip is called the meniscus.

- The nurse assistant should look at the horizontal lines on the side of the cylinder and should note to which line the meniscus is closest.

- Measurement should be recorded using correct abbreviation for unit of measurement.

General guidelines when measuring volume, length, and weight

- Nurse assistants should always follow safety precautions for patient/resident and themselves. They should be familiar with how to use measuring equipment. Standing scales are used commonly to measure the height and weight. Wheelchair, chair, bed, and lift scales are used for patients/residents who cannot stand. The nurse assistant should follow the manufacturer's instructions and agency procedures.

- Proper hand hygiene should be practiced before, after, and as needed when doing any procedure.

- The nurse assistant should wear gloves when handling body fluids and should dispose of fluids appropriately.

- The scale should be balanced at zero (0) before weighing the patient/resident. For balance scales, the weights should be moved to zero. A digital scale should read at zero.

- The patient/resident should wear only pajamas or a gown. Clothes add more weight. No footwear should be worn as footwear also adds to the weight as well as height measurements.

- The patient/resident should void before being weighed. A full bladder adds more weight. A dry incontinence product should be worn as a wet product may add weight.

- Height and weight are generally measured on admission to the agency. Then the patient/resident is weighed daily, weekly, or monthly. This is done to measure weight loss or gain.

- The patient/resident should be weighed at the same time of day. Before breakfast is usually the best time as food and fluids may add weight.

- When a patient/resident can stand independently long enough to be weighed, an upright scale should be used. The upright scale is also used to measure the patient/resident's height.

- When a patient/resident is able to get out of bed but is unable to stand long enough to be weighed using an upright scale, a chair scale should be used to weigh the patient/resident.

- If the patient/resident is unable to get out of bed at all, a sling scale should be used to weigh the patient/resident. There should be at least one additional assistant, helping while using mechanical lifts.

- Equipment should be cleaned and placed to appropriate location. The nurse assistant should record findings and report any significant changes to the nurse.

- The nurse assistant should be well aware of how the patient/resident tolerates the procedure.

Standard time vs. Military time

There are two major systems for expressing time: the 12-hour clock (standard) and the 24-hour clock (military). In North America, civilians commonly use the 12-hour clock, in which the day is divided into two portions, the 12 hours from midnight to noon (a.m. — ante meridiem), and the 12 hours from noon to midnight (p.m. — post meridiem). In the 24-hour clock system, the hours of the day run 0-23, midnight to midnight. Midnight is considered as 00:00 and the last minute of the day is considered 23:59. Midnight may also sometimes render as 24:00 to depict the end of the day.

Nursing assistants in many healthcare settings record various documentation entries, including medications and treatments by using military time (the 24-hour clock). Military time uses 0000 for midnight, 0900 for 9 AM, 1200 for noon, and 2100 for 9 PM. This system eliminates errors in interpreting the exact time the entry is made (AM or PM).

The 12-hour clock (standard time) has many disadvantages. It may cause confusion over whether a time given is in the PM or AM, and whether 12:00 is midnight or noon. The 24-hour clock (military time) helps to prevent errors and misunderstandings. For example, 8 o'clock in the morning is 0800 and 8 o'clock in the evening is 2000. Therefore, these two will not be confused with each other when written in military time, and this enhances the accuracy of recording. The 24-hour clock (military time) contains four digits. The first two digits show the hours: 0200 = 2:00 AM; 1400 = 2:00 PM. The last two digits show minutes: 0220 = 2:20 AM; 1420 = 2:20 PM. Colons and AM and PM should not be used for documenting medications and treatments.

Standard time and military time

AM		PM	
Standard time	Military time	Standard time	Military time
12:00 Midnight	0000 or 2400	12:00 Noon	1200
1:00 AM	0100	1:00 PM	1300
2:00 AM	0200	2:00 PM	1400
3:00 AM	0300	3:00 PM	1500
4:00 AM	0400	4:00 PM	1600
5:00 AM	0500	5:00 PM	1700
6:00 AM	0600	6:00 PM	1800

7:00 AM	0700	7:00 PM	1900
8:00 AM	0800	8:00 PM	2000
9:00 AM	0900	9:00 PM	2100
10:00 AM	1000	10:00 PM	2200
11:00 AM	1100	11:00 PM	2300

Helpful Resources

Dolenska, S. Lung volumes and their measurement. *Basic Science for Anaesthetists*, 104-108. https://doi.org/10.1017/cbo9780511544545.030

Evans, S., Ashmore, C., Daly, A., & MacDonald, A. (2014). Accuracy of formula preparation equipment for liquid measurement. *Molecular Genetics and Metabolism Reports*, *1*, 141-147. https://doi.org/10.1016/j.ymgmr.2014.02.004

Fontanarosa, P. B., & Christiansen, S. (2009). Units of measure. *AMA Manual of Style*. https://doi.org/10.1093/jama/9780195176339.003.0018

Mari, L., Ehrlich, C., & Pendrill, L. (2018). undefined. *Metrologia*, *55*(5), 716-721. https://doi.org/10.1088/1681-7575/aad8d8

Pacchioni, G. (2018). Units of measurement. *Oxford Scholarship Online*. https://doi.org/10.1093/oso/9780198799887.003.0006

Swyt, D. (2001). Length and dimensional measurements at NIST. *Journal of Research of the National Institute of Standards and Technology*, *106*(1), 1. https://doi.org/10.6028/jres.106.002

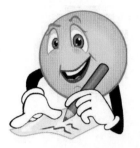

Chapter Eight:

Patient Care Skills

Outline

I: Assistance with daily routine care, promoting independence and dignity

II: Bathing and its benefits

III: Procedure for bathing patients/residents and safety guidelines

IV: The purposes and schedule for oral hygiene

V: Procedure of oral hygiene and denture care for a patient/resident needing assistance, and for the unconscious individual

VI: Nurse Assistant's role and responsibility for patient/resident nail care and foot care

VII: Nurse Assistant's role and responsibility for caring for hair of patients/residents

VIII: Procedure for shaving a patient/resident

IX: Ways to maintain healthy skin

X: Causes, signs and symptoms, and staging of pressure sores

XI: General nursing measures to prevent and treat pressure sores

XII: Guidelines for selecting and caring for patient's/resident's clothing

XIII: Guidelines for dressing or undressing a patient/resident

XIV: Usual frequency and pattern for urination

XV: Observations about urine

XVI: Urinary incontinence

XVII: The purpose and general rules of care for urinary catheters

XVIII: The goals and methods for bowel and bladder training

XIX: Normal pattern of bowel movements

XX: The purpose of an ostomy and the care of patients/residents with an ostomy

XXI: The procedures for weighing and measuring height of the patient/resident

XXII: Common prosthetic devices and their care

XXIII: The purpose of a hearing aid and the procedures for maintenance and care of the hearing aid

Personal care

Most people have hygiene habits and routines. For example, the face and hands are washed and teeth are brushed after sleep. These and other hygiene measures are usually taken before and after meals and at bedtime. The nurse assistant provides routine care during the day and evening. He/she also may assist with hygiene whenever it is needed. However, the right to privacy and to personal choice for the patients/residents should always be preferred.

The nurse assistant usually helps the patients/residents with the activities necessary for maintaining their personal cleanliness and a well-cleaned appearance. Personal hygiene (cleanliness), which can be achieved through regularly washing the hair and body and brushing the teeth, is vital for both physical and emotional well-being. These activities may help to keep the hair, skin, and mouth healthy by removing infectious agents. In addition, keeping the mouth and body clean prevents bad odors, which is an important factor for self-esteem. Grooming activities, such as shaving, dressing, and styling the hair, aid to maintain a neat appearance and are also vital for maintaining a patient/resident's emotional health. When the nurse assistant helps a patient/resident with personal hygiene and grooming activities, he/she actually helps the patient/resident feel attractive and confident. A patient/resident who feels attractive and confident is more likely to socialize with other people, and feels better about him/her in general. The way a person appears to others depicts a lot about who he/she is and how he/she lives. The decisions anyone makes may affect his/her outward appearance, such as how he/she choose to style his/her hair or what clothes he/she choose to wear, are deeply personal because they are so closely tied to the self-image and self-esteem. Religious and cultural beliefs can influence the decisions a patient/resident takes about his/her outward appearance. Many of the patients/residents need help to maintain personal cleanliness and a neat appearance. However, it does not mean that they have given up the desire to make their own decisions regarding grooming and hygiene. When a nurse assistant is assisting with personal care, he/she should always try to find out the patient/resident's preferences and honor them. In health care settings, activities related to personal grooming and hygiene usually take place at predictable times. Scheduling these activities is important because they must be accomplished in addition to other routine activities throughout the day, such as therapy sessions, meals, and social events. However, it is still possible to take a patient/resident's preferences into account when scheduling these activities. For example, some patients/residents may prefer to bathe in the night instead of in the morning. It is significant to try and accommodate the patient/resident's preferences as much as possible when scheduling care. Disability or Illness can make it difficult for a patient/resident to maintain his/her normal personal care routines. For many patients/residents, it can be embarrassing or difficult to accept help with activities of such a personal, private nature. The nurse assistant should be sensitive to the patient/resident's feelings, and remember to provide restorative care by encouraging the patient/resident to do as much for himself/herself as he/she is able. This is important for the patient/resident's self-esteem and sense of independence.

Daily care

Each healthcare facility has specific procedures and policies related to AM care, PM care and h.s. care. In general, daily care may include:

Early morning care (Before breakfast care or AM care)
- Preparation of patient/resident for breakfast or morning tests
- Assisting with elimination
- Cleaning incontinent patients/residents
- Changing soiled or wet linens and garments
- Assisting with face and hand washing along with oral hygiene
- Assisting with dressing and hair care
- Positioning patients/residents for breakfast—bedside chair, dining room, or in bed
- Making beds and straightening units

Morning care after breakfast
- Assisting with elimination
- Cleaning incontinent patients/residents
- Changing soiled or wet linens and garments
- Assisting with face and hand washing along with oral hygiene, bathing, back massage, and perineal care
- Assisting with shaving, hair care, dressing, and undressing
- Assisting with range-of-motion exercises and ambulation
- Making beds and straightening rooms

Afternoon care
- Preparing patients/residents for naps, visitors, or activity programs

- Assisting with elimination
- Cleaning incontinent patients/residents
- Changing soiled or wet linens and garments
- Assisting with face and hand washing along with oral hygiene and hair care
- Assisting with range-of-motion exercises and ambulation
- Straightening beds and units

Evening care (PM care, h.s. care)
- Preparing patients/residents for sleep
- Assisting with elimination
- Cleaning incontinent patients/residents
- Changing soiled or wet linens and garments
- Assisting with face and hand washing along with oral hygiene and back massages
- Helping patients/residents change into sleepwear
- Straightening beds and units

Scheduling og grooming and personal care

Care Type	Time of care	Activities
Early morning care	After waking up the patient/resident	Toileting Washing face and hands Mouth care Brushing the teeth Dressing
Morning care	After breakfast	• Toileting • Mouth care • Bathing • Washing and styling hair • Dressing • Shaving • Bedmaking
Afternoon care	Before and after lunch	• Toileting • Mouth care • Washing hands and face • Brushing the hair
Evening care	Before bed	• Toileting • Mouth care • Washing the hands and face • Changing into sleepwear • Back rub

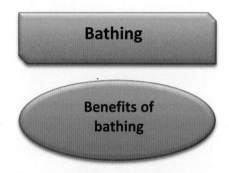

Bathing

Benefits of bathing

Bathing cleans the skin, and mucous membranes of the anal and genital areas. Microorganisms, perspiration, dead skin, and excess oils are removed through bathing. A bath is relaxing and refreshing. Body parts are exercised and circulation is stimulated through bathing. Certain useful observations can be made, and there may be more time to talk to the patient/resident. Complete or partial baths, showers, or tub baths are given. The method of bathing depends on the patient/resident's condition, personal choice, and self-care abilities. In hospital settings, bathing is common usually after breakfast. In nursing centers, bathing usually occurs after evening meal or breakfast. The patient/resident's choice of bath time should be preferred whenever possible. Bathing frequency is also a personal matter. Some patients/residents bathe daily. Others bathe one or two times a week. Personal choice, activity, weather, and illness affect bathing. Other illnesses and dry skin can limit bathing to every two or three days.

When a nurse assistant is assisting a patient/resident to bathe, he/she should be well aware that the patient/resident may be embarrassed about needing assistance. The patient/resident should be encouraged to complete as much of the bath as he/she can independently and appropriate measures should be taken to keep the patient/resident warm and protect his/her modesty. When a

nursing supervisor is scheduling bath times, he/she should take into account the patient/resident's preferences as well as employer's policies. It should be remembered that patients/residents in the care do have the right to refuse a bath. However, if this happens too frequently, the nurse assistant should talk to the nurse supervisor because regular bathing is necessary for good hygiene. Close attention should be needed to prevent accidents when bathing. Water on hard bathroom surfaces can be slippery. It should be ensured that tubs and showers have non-skid mats and the grab bars should be tightly fastened to the wall. To prevent burns, the temperature of shower or bath water should be checked by using a bath thermometer, which should be between 105° F and 115° F. If a thermometer is not available, the inside of wrist should be used to check the temperature of the water.

The nurse assistant should always follow the care plan for bathing method and skin care products:

- Patient/resident's personal choice should be preferred when possible.
- Standard Precautions and the Bloodborne Pathogen Standard should be followed while bathing patients/residents.
- All needed items should be collected before starting the procedure.
- Hearing aids should be removed before bathing because water may damage hearing aids.
- Proper privacy should be provided. Patient/resident should be screened. Doors and window coverings should be closed.

- Assistance should be provided for elimination as bathing usually stimulates the need to urinate. Relaxation and comfort increase if urination needs are met.
- Patient/resident should be covered for warmth and privacy.
- Drafts should be reduced. Doors and windows should be closed.
- Patient/resident should be protected from falling.
- Proper body mechanics should be practiced at all times.
- The rules to safely transfer and move the patient/resident should be followed.
- Appropriate water temperature should be ensured.
- Bar soap should be kept in the soap dish between latherings to prevent soapy water. It also prevents slipping and falls in tubs and showers.
- Washing should be from the cleanest areas to the dirtiest areas.
- Patient/resident should be encouraged to help as much as possible.
- The skin should be rinsed thoroughly and all soap should be removed.
- The skin should be dried to avoid irritation or skin breaks.
- It should be dried well under the breasts, in the perineal area, between skin folds, and between the toes.
- Skin should be bathed when urine or feces are present. This helps prevention of skin breakdown and bad odors.

Encouraging safety and comfort

Safety

Warm water can burn the skin. Thus, water temperature should be measured according to agency policy. If the nurse assistant is unsure whether the water is too hot, he/she should ask the nurse supervisor to check it. The patient/resident should be protected from falls and other injuries. Powders should not be used near patients/residents with respiratory disorders. Inhaling powder may irritate the lungs and airway. Before using powder, it should be checked with the nurse supervisor and the care plan.

For safe application of powder:
- A small amount of powder should be sprinkled onto the hand or a cloth. Powder should not be shaked or sprinkled directly onto the patient/resident.
- The powder should be applied in a thin layer.
- It should be ensured that powder does not get on the floor. Powder is usually slippery and may cause falls. The nurse assistant should make beds after baths. After making the bed, the bed should be lowered to a safe and comfortable level appropriate for the patient/resident. It should be ensured that the bed wheels are locked. Patient/resident should be protected from infection. During bedmaking and baths, contact with body fluids, blood, excretions, or secretions is more likely. Therefore, standard precautions and the bloodborne pathogen standard should always be followed.

Comfort: Before bathing, the nurse assistant should let the patient/resident meet elimination needs. Bathing may stimulate the need to urinate. Thus, comfort is greater when the bladder is empty. Also bathing should not be interrupted. Oral hygiene is usually common during bathing routines. Some patients/residents do so before bathing; others do so after. Personal choice should be preferred and the person's care plan should be followed. Warmth should be provided. The patient/resident should be covered with a bath blanket. It should be ensured that the water is warm enough for the patient/resident. Cool water usually causes chilling. If the patient/resident prefers, sleepwear should be removed after washing the face, eyes, ears, and neck. Removing sleepwear at this time can help the patient/resident feel less exposed and provides more mental comfort with the bath. If the patient/resident is able, the nurse assistant should let him/her wash the genital area. This promotes patient/resident's privacy and helps prevent embarrassment.

Assisting a patient/resident with bed bath

A complete bed bath involves bathing all parts of a patient/resident's body while he/she is in bed. A partial bed bath involves bathing only the hands, face, armpits (axillae), back, perineal area, and buttocks. A partial bath may be provided on days when a complete bath is not scheduled. A partial bath may also be a useful compromise when the patient/resident refuses a complete bath.

When assisting with a bed bath, the nurse assistant should help the patient/resident maintain his/her independence by discussing about how he/she can help. A patient/resident may be able to help only by washing his/her face, but any amount of self-care is good. If the patient/resident has more ability, the nurse assistant may suggest that he/she do his/her own perineal care.

Assisting a patient/resident with complete bed bath

The nurse assistant should assist the patient/resident with a complete bath in following ways:

1. Hands should be washed properly.
2. The nurse assist should gather all supplies:

- Washcloths
- Towels
- Bed protector
- Wash basin
- Bath blanket
- Paper towels
- Gloves
- Clean clothing
- Lotion (optional)
- Bath thermometer
- Soap

- Deodorant or antiperspirant (optional)
- Clean linens (if needed)

3. The nurse assistant should knock, greet the patient/resident and should ensure patient's privacy.
4. The procedure should be explained thoroughly to the patient/resident.
5. Equipment should be adjusted for proper body mechanics and safety: the bed should be raised to a comfortable working height. It should be ensured that the wheels on the bed are locked.
6. The over-bed table should be covered with the paper towels and the nurse assistant should arrange all supplies. The wash basin should be filled with warm water. The bath thermometer should be used to verify that the water temperature is between 105° F and 115° F. The wash basin should be placed on the over-bed table.
7. The head of the bed should be lowered as low as the patient/resident can tolerate.
8. The patient/resident should be helped to move closer to the side of the bed where the nurse assistant is working.
9. The bedspread and blanket should be removed or folded for reuse. Patient/resident and the top sheet should be covered with the bath blanket (to provide warmth and privacy).
10. The gloves should be put by the nurse assistant.
11. The patient/resident should be provided help to remove soiled clothing.

Washing the patient/resident's face, neck and ears
12. A towel should be placed on top of the bath blanket, across the patient/resident's chest. This helps to keep the bath blanket dry while the nurse assistant wash the patient/resident's face, neck and ears.
13. The washcloth should be wet and should be made a mitt.
14. Without using soap, the nurse assistant should use the washcloth to bathe the eye farther from him/her. The nurse assistant should begin at the inner corner of the eye, near the nose. Then he/she should move the washcloth across the eye to the outer corner. The towel should be used to dry the eye. The nurse assistant should rinse and dry the patient/resident's face, neck and ears.

Washing the patient/resident's arms and hands
15. The bath blanket should be folded back to expose the patient/resident's arm that is farther from the nurse assistant. The towel should be placed lengthwise under the arm.
16. A bed protector should be placed on the mattress near the patient/resident's hand, and the wash basin should be place on the bed protector. The nurse assistant should place the patient/resident's hand in the wash basin. He/she should wash, rinse and dry the patient/resident's hand.
17. After hands, the nurse assistant should rinse and dry the arm, shoulder, and axilla in the same way.
18. The towel should be removed from under the arm, and the arm should be covered with the bath blanket.

Washing the patient/resident's chest and abdomen

19. The towel on top of the bath blanket should be placed over the patient/resident's chest and abdomen (stomach).
20. The bath blanket should be folded down to the patient/resident's pubic area without exposing it and the towel should be left in place so that the patient/resident is not completely exposed.
21. The nurse assistant should wash, rinse, and dry the patient/resident's chest and abdomen.

Washing the patient/resident's legs and feet
22. The towel should be placed lengthwise under the patient/resident's leg and the nurse assistant should wash, rinse and dry the leg. The towel that was under the leg should be used to dry it.
23. A bed protector should be placed on the mattress near the patient/resident's foot, and the wash basin should be placed on the bed protector. The patient/resident's foot should be placed in the wash basin. The nurse assistant should wash, rinse and dry the patient/resident's foot.

Washing the patient/resident's back and buttocks
24. The nurse assistant should help the patient/resident turn onto one side so that his/her back is facing the nurse assistant.
25. The towel should be placed on the sheet behind the person's neck, back and buttocks. The bath blanket should be adjusted so that it covers the patient/resident's chest, shoulders, abdomen and legs.
26. The nurse assistant should wash, rinse and dry the patient/resident's neck, back and buttocks.

Washing the perineal area
27. The towel should be placed so that it should be under the patient/resident's hips. If the patient/resident is able to do his/her own perineal care, He/she should be provided a fresh washcloth, clean water, and soap. The patient/resident should be allowed a few minutes alone to complete perineal care. If the patient/resident is not able to do his/her own perineal care, the nurse assistant should provide him/her proper perineal care.

Helping the patient/resident to dress
28. The nurse assistant should help the patient/resident back into the supine position. They should help the patient/resident to apply deodorant or antiperspirant (optional).
29. They should also provide help the patient/resident to put on clean clothing.
30. If the linens are wet or soiled, these should be changed.
31. The top linens should be pulled up and the bath blanket should be removed.
32. It should be ensured the patient/resident's comfort and proper body alignment.
33. Hands should be properly washed, and observations should be reported and recorded at the end of the procedure.

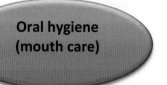

The partial bath

The partial bath involves bathing the hands, face, axillae (underarms), buttocks, back, and perineal area. Discomfort or bad odors may occur if these areas are not clean. Some patients/residents bathe themselves in bed or at the sink. The nurse assistant should only assist as needed. Most of the patients/residents only need help washing the back. The nurse assistant gives partial baths to patients/residents who cannot bathe themselves.

Assisting a patient/resident with a shower or tub bath

Patients/residents who are able to get out of bed may take a shower or a tub bath. Shower stalls in most of the health care facilities are usually large enough to accommodate a shower chair, so that the patient/resident can sit down while showering. A shower chair should be used if the patient/resident is not reliably steady on his/her feet. The nurse assistant may see several different types of bathtubs, used in a health care facility. Walk-in tubs usually have a door that swings open so that the patient/resident can easily enter the tub without stepping over a high edge. Some tubs may be equipped with a lift device that the patient/resident sits on it to be lowered into the tub. If using a standard bathtub, it should be ensured that the patient/resident can get in and out of the tub safely.

Oral hygiene (mouth care)

Purpose

It is a part of the nurse assistant's responsibility in assisting with personal care to help provide oral hygiene, also called as mouth care. Oral hygiene may include care of the gums, teeth, tongue, lips and soft parts of the inside of the mouth, such as the roof of the mouth and cheeks. Proper oral hygiene is important to keep the mouth and the body healthy. Regular brushing and flossing can remove plaque, a colorless, sticky layer of bacteria that is developed on the teeth. Starches and sugars in the food can cause the bacteria in plaque to grow. These bacteria may cause bad breath odors. In addition, they also produce acids, which may disrupt the outer surface of the tooth, leading to tooth decay. If plaque is not properly removed by brushing the teeth, it may harden into tartar. Tartar can cause gum infection and irritation, as well as tooth loss and decay. The same bacteria that cause gum infection and inflammation can also cause infection and inflammation in other parts of the body, putting the patient/resident at risk for stroke, heart disease, and other serious conditions. In addition to removing bacteria, regular oral hygiene also helps to keep the tissues of the oral cavity moist. A dry mouth may be extremely uncomfortable and can alter the taste of beverages and food, making them less appealing.

At minimum, the nurse assistant should assist those in his/her care with mouth care at:

- Every morning

- Every evening
- After each meal
- Every 2 hours, if the patient/resident is unconscious, on oxygen therapy, on "nothing by mouth" (NPO) status, or breathes through the mouth (all of these conditions may cause the mouth to become extremely dry and uncomfortable)
- After the patient/resident vomits.

When assisting with mouth care, the nurse assistant should follow standard precautions, and should take the opportunity to observe for changes that could indicate a health problem. These measures may include:

- Keeping the mouth and teeth clean.
- Preventing mouth odors and infections.
- Increasing comfort.
- Making food taste better.
- Reducing the risk for cavities (dental caries) and periodontal disease (pyorrhea, gum disease).

Encouraging safety and comfort

Safety
The nurse assistant should follow standard precautions and the bloodborne pathogen standard while providing oral hygiene. He/she may have contact with the patient/resident's mucous membranes. Gums may bleed during oral hygiene. Also, the mouth has many microorganisms.

Comfort
The nurse assistant should assist the patient/resident with oral hygiene after sleep, after meals, and at bedtime. Many individuals practice oral hygiene before meals. Some individuals need mouth care every 2 hours or more often. The nurse assistant should always follow the care plan.

Mouth care for a patient/resident with natural teeth

Natural teeth should be cared by using a soft-bristled toothbrush, toothpaste, and dental floss. The soft bristles of the toothbrush remove food particles and plaque from the tongue and teeth and stimulate circulation in the gums, which keeps them healthy. The toothbrush should be replaced after every 3 to 4 months, or when it starts to show wear. A toothbrush with frayed or worn bristles does not clean the teeth properly and may injure the gums. Unless instructed otherwise, the nurse assistant should use toothpaste that contains fluoride (a chemical that strengthens the tooth enamel and prevent tooth decay). In various regions of the United States where the water contains comparatively high levels of fluoride, dentists usually recommend using toothpaste without fluoride. After brushing, dental floss should be used to remove food particles and plaque between the teeth. Waxed dental floss slides more easily between the teeth than unwaxed dental floss does. Before flossing a patient/resident's teeth, the nurse assistant should check whether there are any special precautions or restrictions to be considered. For example, some patients/residents taking certain medications may bleed excessively if their teeth are flossed.

The nurse assistant should assist the patient/resident for brushing and flossing teeth in following ways:

1. Hands should be washed properly.
2. The nurse assist should gather all supplies:
   - Towel
   - Gloves
   - Protective eyewear and a gown (optional)
   - Paper towels
   - Toothbrush
   - Toothpaste
   - Emesis basin
   - Cup
   - Floss pick or dental floss
   - Mouthwash
   - Lip balm or petroleum jelly and cotton-tipped applicator
3. The nurse assistant should knock, greet the patient/resident and should ensure his/her privacy.
4. The procedure should be explained thoroughly to the patient/resident.
5. Equipment should be adjusted for proper body mechanics and safety: the bed should be raised to a comfortable working height. It should be ensured that the wheels on the bed are locked.
6. The over-bed table should be covered with the paper towels. In the cup, the nurse assistant should prepare a solution of half water and half mouthwash.
7. The patient/resident should be positioned in high Fowler's position.
8. The towel should be unfolded and should be placed across the patient/resident's chest.
9. The nurse assistant should put on the gloves and other relevant personal protective equipment.
10. The patient/resident should be given a mouthful of the mouthwash mixture to rinse his/her mouth. The emesis basin should be held under the patient/resident's chin to catch the liquid. The patient/resident's mouth and chin should be dried using the towel.
11. The toothbrush should be wet by pouring mouthwash solution over it.
12. Toothpaste should be put on the wet brush.
13. The upper teeth and gums should be brushed as:

- Starting at the back of the mouth, the toothbrush should be placed on the outer surface of the upper teeth at an angle of 45 degree. There should be gentle brushing the outer surface of each tooth by using short back-and-forth (tooth-wide) strokes.
- Next, the chewing surfaces of the upper teeth should be cleaned, moving from one part of the mouth to the other and using the same tooth-wide strokes.
- Finally, the brush should be put vertically against the inside surfaces of the front upper teeth and there should be gentle brushing with up-and-down motion. The lower gums and teeth should be brushed in the same way.

14. The tongue should be brushed after gum and teeth.
15. The patient/resident should be given a mouthful of the mouthwash mixture to rinse his/her mouth. The emesis basin should be held under the patient/resident's chin to catch the liquid. The patient/resident's mouth and chin should be dried using the towel.

16. Flossing the patient/resident's teeth

- **Floss pick**

Starting between the two front teeth, the nurse assistant should hold the handle of the floss pick and move the floss carefully between the teeth. The floss should be held against the tooth and scraping should be done at the side of the tooth by moving the floss away from the gum. It should be repeated with the next tooth, sliding from the front of the mouth to the back of the mouth on one side and then the other side. Then same process should be repeated for the lower teeth.

- **Dental floss**

The nurse assistant should break off about 18 inches of floss from the dispenser. The nurse assistant should wrap most of the floss around his/her middle fingers of both hands, leaving 1 inch of floss between his/her hands. The floss should be stretched tightly between the thumbs and index fingers. Starting between the two front teeth, the floss should be slid carefully between the teeth. The floss should be held against the tooth and scraping should be done at the side of the tooth, by moving the floss away from the gum. After flossing each tooth, a clean 1-inch section of floss should be unwrapped from the finger and the soiled floss should be wrapped around the other finger. Flossing should be done from the front of the mouth to the back of the mouth on one side and then the other side. Then the process should be repeated for the lower teeth.

17. The patient/resident should be given a mouthful of the mouthwash mixture to rinse his/her mouth. The emesis basin should be held under the patient/resident's chin to catch the liquid. The patient/resident's mouth and chin should be dried using the towel.
18. The patient/resident should be encouraged to apply lip balm or petroleum jelly to the lips.
19. It should be ensured the patient/resident's comfort and proper body alignment.
20. Hands should be properly washed, and observations should be reported and recorded at the end of the procedure.

A denture is an artificial tooth or a set of artificial teeth that are often called "false teeth". Full (complete) dentures replace all of the bottom teeth or all of the top teeth. Partial dentures replace only a few teeth. Mouth care should be given and dentures should be cleaned as often as natural teeth. Dentures can be slippery when wet. They may easily break or chip if dropped onto a hard surface such as sinks, floors, and counters. They should be held firmly when removing or inserting them.

Dentures are commonly removed at bedtime. Some patients/residents do not usually wear their dentures. Others wear dentures only during eating and remove them after meals. The nurse assistant should remind them not to wrap dentures in tissues or napkins. Otherwise, they can be easily discarded. Dentures should be cleaned by brushing them with a special kind of toothpaste made for dentures. Some patients/residents may also soak their dentures in a denture-cleansing solution as their routine denture-cleaning.

Dentures that have been soaking in a denture-cleansing solution should be properly brushed and thoroughly rinsed before placing them in the patient/resident's mouth. When the patient/resident is not wearing the dentures, they should be stored in a labeled denture-cleansing solution or denture cup in water to prevent warping. The nurse assistant should always handle a patient/resident's dentures carefully, so that they do not chip or break. Also, care should be taken about not to lose the patient/resident's dentures. Dentures are generally expensive and time-consuming to replace, because they are custom-made for the patient/resident.

The nurse assistant should assist in providing denture care in following ways:
1. Hands should be washed properly.
2. The nurse assist should gather all supplies:
- Washcloth
- Towel
- Gloves
- Paper towels
- Cup
- Emesis basin
- Denture cup
- Disposable mouth sponges
- Regular toothpaste, toothbrush and dental floss if the patient/resident has some natural teeth
- Denture brush or toothbrush
- Denture toothpaste
- Mouthwash
- Lip balm or petroleum jelly and cotton-tipped applicator

3. The nurse assistant should knock, greet the patient/resident and should ensure his/her privacy.
4. The procedure should be explained thoroughly to the patient/resident.
5. Equipment should be adjusted for proper body mechanics and safety: the bed should be raised to a comfortable working height. It should be ensured that the wheels on the bed are locked.
6. The over-bed table should be covered with the paper towels. In the cup, the nurse assistant should prepare a solution of half water and half mouthwash.
7. The patient/resident should be positioned in high Fowler's position.

Removing the denture
8. The towel should be unfolded and should be placed across the patient/resident's chest.
9. The nurse assistant should put on the gloves and placed the dentures, which were removed by the patient/resident, in the emesis basin. If the patient/resident needs assistance removing the denture, the nurse assistant should grasp the denture firmly with his/her thumb and index finger and should use a rocking motion to gently remove the denture a. A patient/resident may wear more than one denture (for example, one to replace the lower teeth and one to replace the upper teeth). If necessary, the same process should be repeated to remove the other denture.

Cleaning the denture
10. The nurse assistant should take the emesis basin, the washcloth, the denture cup, the denture brush or toothbrush, the denture toothpaste, and the denture-cleansing tablet (if used) to the sink.
11. The nurse assistant should line the sink with the washcloth or several paper towels.
12. Using a paper towel, it should be turned on the faucet and should adjust the water temperature so that it is cool.
13. The toothbrush should be wet and the denture toothpaste should be applied on it.
14. The sink should be allowed to fill halfway with cool water.
15. If the patient/resident has more than one denture, the nurse assistant should clean only one denture at a time. One denture should be removed from the emesis basin and should be held it in the palm of the hand over the sink. The toothbrush should be used to clean all surfaces of the denture, using circular movements.
16. The denture should be rinsed thoroughly under cool, running water and should be placed it in the denture cup. 18. The same process should be repeated to clean other denture. 19. If the patient/resident will not be putting the denture back in the mouth right away, sufficient cool water should be added to the denture cup to cover the denture.
17. The faucet should be turned off with a paper towel.

Providing care for the patient/resident's mouth
18. The nurse assistant should take the denture cup and the emesis basin back to the patient/resident's bedside.

19. The patient/resident should be given a mouthful of the mouthwash mixture to rinse his/her mouth. The emesis basin should be held under the patient/resident's chin to catch the liquid. The patient/resident's mouth and chin should be dried with the towel.
20. The patient/resident should be provided help to clean the roof of the mouth, the inside of the cheeks, under the tongue, the gums, and the lips with mouth sponges dipped in the mouthwash mixture. If the patient/resident has any natural teeth, the nurse assistant should help to brush and floss them.
21. Appropriate help should be provided to put the denture back in the patient/resident's mouth.
22. The patient/resident should be encouraged to apply lip balm or petroleum jelly to the lips.
23. It should be ensured the patient/resident's comfort and proper body alignment.
24. Hands should be properly washed, and observations should be reported and recorded at the end of the procedure.

Encouraging safety and comfort

Safety
Dentures are the patient/resident's personal property. They are generally costly. The nurse assistant should handle them very carefully. The denture should be labelled with the patient/resident's name and room and bed number. The nurse assistant should report lost or damaged dentures at once. Damaging or losing dentures is negligent conduct. Dentures should never be carried in hands. The nurse assistant should always use a denture cup or kidney basin.

Comfort
Many individuals do not like being seen without their dentures. Privacy is the most important thing. Privacy should be ensured when the patient/resident cleans dentures. If the nurse assistant cleans dentures, he/she should return them to the patient/resident as quickly as possible. Patients/residents with dentures may have some natural teeth. Therefore, they need to brush and floss the natural teeth.

Mouth care for a patient/resident who is unconscious

An unconscious patient/resident is not able to respond to his/her environment and will be totally dependent on the caregiver for mouth care. Patients/residents who are unconscious breathe through their mouths, which can cause extreme drying of the soft tissues of the mouth and may lead to the build-up of mucus and other secretions on the tongue and teeth. The nurse assistant should provide mouth care for an unconscious patient/resident every 2 hours throughout the day and night to remove these secretions for prevention of the mouth from becoming extremely dry.

When providing mouth care for a patient/resident who is unconscious, the nurse assistant should elevate the head of the bed (if allowed) and turn the patient/resident's head to the side to allow fluids to run out of the mouth instead of down the patient/resident's throat. It is important to prevent aspiration (inhalation of foreign materials or fluids into the lungs). Aspiration may lead to pneumonia. A mouth sponge should be used to clean the soft tissues of the patient/resident's mouth and a soft-bristled toothbrush should be moistened with water or a mixture of mouthwash and water to clean the patient/resident's teeth.

The nurse assistant should provide mouth care for a patient/resident who is unconscious in following ways:

1. Hands should be washed properly.
2. The nurse assist should gather all supplies:
   - Two towels
   - Gloves
   - Gauze squares
   - Tongue depressor
   - Tape
   - Paper towels
   - Cup
   - Disposable mouth sponges
   - Toothbrush
   - Mouthwash
   - Lip balm or petroleum jelly and cotton-tipped applicator
3. The nurse assistant should knock, greet the patient/resident and should ensure his/her privacy.
4. The procedure should be explained thoroughly to the patient/resident.
5. Equipment should be adjusted for proper body mechanics and safety: the bed should be raised to a comfortable working height. It should be ensured that the wheels on the bed are locked.
6. The over-bed table should be covered with the paper towels. In the cup, the nurse assistant should prepare a solution of half water and half mouthwash.
7. The patient/resident should be positioned in high Fowler's position and the patient/resident's head should be turned towards the nurse assistant.
8. The nurse assistant should unfold one towel and should place it across the patient/resident's chest. The other towel should be placed under the patient/resident's head.
9. The nurse assistant should put on the gloves and should place the emesis basin on the towel near the patient/resident's cheek.
10. The nurse assistant should pad the tongue depressor by wrapping the end in gauze and securing the gauze with tape.
11. Without applying force, the patient/resident's upper teeth should be gently separated from lower teeth.

12. The padded tongue depressor should be between the upper and lower teeth at the back of the mouth to hold the patient/resident's mouth open.
13. The nurse assistant should clean the roof of the mouth, the gums, under the tongue, the inside of the cheeks, and the lips with mouth sponges dipped in the mouthwash mixture. Gauze should be wrapped around the finger or a mouth sponge should be used to remove thick mucus or secretions.
14. Toothbrush moistened with diluted mouthwash should be used to clean the patient/resident's teeth.
15. Lip balm or petroleum jelly should be used to the patient/resident's lips.
16. It should be ensured the patient/resident's comfort and proper body alignment.
17. Hand should be properly washed, and observations should be reported and recorded at the end of the procedure.

Encouraging safety and comfort

Safety
Sponge swabs should be used with care. It should be ensured that the sponge pad is tight on the stick. The patient/resident may aspirate or choke on the sponge if it comes off the stick.

Comfort
Unconscious patients/residents should be re-positioned at least every 2 hours. To promote comfort, mouth care should be combined with skin care, re-positioning, and other comfort measures.

Hand, foot, and nail care

Hand, foot, and nail care prevents infection, odors, and injury. Ingrown nails (nails that grow in at the side), hangnails, and nails torn away from the skin may cause skin breaks. These skin breaks can be portals of entry for microorganisms. Broken or long nails can scratch the skin and may snag clothing. Dirty socks, feet, or stockings may nourish microorganisms and cause odors. Socks and shoes provide a moist, warm environment for microorganisms to grow. Injuries may occur from stepping on sharp objects, stubbing on toes, or being stepped on. Shoes that are poorly fit can cause blisters. Poor circulation further prolongs healing. Vascular diseases and diabetes are common causes of poor circulation. Foot injuries or infections are very serious problems for older individuals and persons with circulatory disorders. Clipping and trimming toenails can easily cause injuries. Nail clippers should be used to cut fingernails. Some agencies do not allow nursing assistants trim or cut toenails, therefore, nursing assistants should follow agency policy.

The nurse assistant should provide hand, foot, and nail care in following ways:

1. Hands should be washed properly.
2. The nurse assist should gather all supplies:

- Washcloth
- Towel
- Bed protector
- Emesis basin (hand care) or wash basin (foot care)
- Bath thermometer
- Nail clippers
- Orange stick
- Emery board (nail file)
- Soap
- Lotion
- Paper towels
- Gloves (optional)

3. The nurse assistant should knock, greet the patient/resident and should ensure his/her privacy.
4. The procedure should be explained thoroughly to the patient/resident.
5. Equipment should be adjusted for proper body mechanics and safety: the bed should be raised to a comfortable working height. It should be ensured that the wheels on the bed are locked.
6. The over-bed table should be covered with the paper towels. The emesis basin or wash basin should be filled with warm water. The bath thermometer should be used to verify that the water temperature is between 105 °F and 115 °F. The wash basin or emesis basin should be placed on the over-bed table.
7. The patient/resident should be provided help to transfer from the bed to a chair, or to sit on the edge of the bed. Alternatively, the patient/resident should be positioned in high Fowler's position.
8. The nurse assist should put on the gloves and should help the patient/resident to soak his/her hands or feet.

- Hand care: The emesis basin should be positioned within the patient/resident's reach. The nurse assistant should help the patient/resident put his/her fingertips in the basin. The fingertips should be soaked in the water for 5 minutes.

- Foot care: The nurse assistant should place the bed protector on the floor or the mattress near the patient/resident's feet. The wash basin should be placed on the bed protector, and should help the patient/resident put his/her feet in the basin. The feet should be soaked in the water for 5 minutes.

9. The washcloth should be wet with water and soap. The nurse assistant should lift the patient/resident's hand or foot from the water, one at a time. The hand or foot should be washed, then rinsed, and finally dried thoroughly, including the fingers and toes.
10. If the nurse is allowed to trim the fingernails, he/she should use nail clippers to trim the patient/resident's fingernails in a way that the nail extends slightly beyond the tip of the finger. The nurse assistant should trim the nails straight across, and then smooth and shape the edges with the emery board.

11. The nurse assistant should massage the patient/resident's hands or feet with lotion. He/she should begin with the fingers or toes and then move upward toward the ankles or wrists.

12. It should be ensured the patient/resident's comfort and proper body alignment.

13. Hands should be properly washed, and observations should be reported and recorded at the end of the procedure.

Encouraging safety and comfort

Safety

It should be remembered that some conditions and agencies do not let nursing assistants trim and cut toenails. The nurse or podiatrist usually cuts toenails and provides foot care for the patients/residents. The nurse assistant does not cut or trim the toenails for patients/residents who:

- Having diabetes
- Having poor circulation to the feet and legs
- Taking drugs that affect blood clotting.
- Having very thick nails or ingrown toenails.

The nurse assistant should check between the toes for sores and cracks. These areas are usually overlooked. If not properly managed, a serious infection may occur. The feet can be easily burned. Patients/residents with decreased sensation or circulatory problems may not feel warm temperatures. After soaking, the nurse assistant may apply lotion or petroleum jelly to the feet. This may cause slippery feet, thus help should be provided to the patient/resident to put on non-skid footwear before transferring the patient/resident or letting the patient/resident to walk. Bleeding and breaks in the skin can occur. Therefore, the nurse assistant should always follow standard precautions and the bloodborne pathogen standard.

Comfort

The nurse assistant sometimes just trims the fingernails. Sometimes he/she just gives foot care. When the nurse assistant does both, the patient/resident should be seated at the over-bed table to provide warmth and comfort. The nurse assistant should promote his/her own comfort during nail and foot care. The nurse assistant should be seated in front of the over-bed table to trim and clean fingernails. For foot care, the patient/resident's lower leg and foot should be placed on the nurse assistant's lap. A towel should be layed across the lap or a bath mat should be placed on the floor to protect the uniform. The patient/resident's foot and ankle should always be supported when giving foot care.

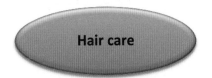

Hair care

Some individuals perform their own hair care. Most of the nursing centers have beauty and barber shops. The nurse assistant should assist patients/residents to comb, brush, and shampoo hair according to the care plan. Hair care usually includes washing, brushing, combing and styling the hair. It is important to keep the scalp and hair healthy, and to maintain a neat and clean appearance. Washing the hair and shampooing removes dirt, bacteria, and oil from the scalp and hair. Combing, brushing, and styling the hair provides a neat appearance and helps to prevent painful tangles. Many long-term care healthcare facilities have salons where patients/residents can go to have their hair professionally cut, styled, and washed. Many patients/residents can choose to take advantage of this service, but the nurse assistant is responsible for helping the patient/resident with hair care in between visits to the salon. Patients/residents often have strong preferences regarding what products should be used to care their hair. For example, some patients/residents may prefer a certain kind of shampoo, or may prefer to use a conditioning rinse in addition to shampoo.

Patients/residents of African descent, who often have curly hair and dry scalps, may prefer to use oils, creams or lotions to moisturize the scalp and to make the hair easier to comb. These products are generally applied to the scalp after shampooing and then massaged into the hair and scalp. When assisting a patient/resident with hair care, the nurse assistant should find out what products the patient/resident likes to use, and honor those preferences as much as possible.

The nurse assistant may observe the following skin and scalp conditions during hair care:

Alopecia: It means hair loss. Hair loss may be partial or complete.

Hirsutism: It is excessive body hair, which can occur in men, women, and children.

Dandruff: It is the excessive amount of dry, white flakes from the scalp.

Pediculosis (lice): It is the infestation with wingless insects (lice).

Scabies: It is a skin disorder caused by the female mite, which burrows into the skin and lays eggs.

Brushing, combing and styling the hair

Brushing and combing hair are components of early morning care, morning care, and afternoon care. Some patients/residents also do so at bedtime. Hair care should be provided when it is needed and before visitors arrive. Patients/residents should be encouraged to do their own hair care. The patient/resident chooses how to brush, comb, and style hair. Long hair may easily mat and tangle. Daily combing and brushing may prevent these problems. The nurse assistant needs the patient/resident's consent to braid hair. Special measures should be taken for curly, dry, and coarse hair. The patient/resident may have certain hair care practices and products. They are generally part of the care plan. Also, the nurse assistant should let the patient/resident to guide him/her when giving hair care.

The nurse assistant should provide assistance in brushing, combing and styling the hair in following ways:
1. Hands should be washed properly.

2. The nurse assist should gather all supplies:
- Comb and brush
- Towel
- Mirror
- Paper towels

3. The nurse assistant should knock, greet the patient/resident and should ensure his/her privacy.

4. The procedure should be explained thoroughly to the patient/resident.

5. Equipment should be adjusted for proper body mechanics and safety: the bed should be raised to a comfortable working height. It should be ensured that the wheels on the bed are locked.

6. The over-bed table should be covered with the paper towels and all supplies should be arranged.

7. The patient/resident should be positioned in high Fowler's position. If the patient/resident cannot tolerate having the head of the bed raised, the nurse assistant can comb his/her hair while he/she is lying in the supine position by turning his/her head to one side, and then to the other.

8. The towel should be placed over the patient/resident's shoulders (or under the shoulders if the patient/resident is in bed).

9. If the patient/resident wears glasses, they should be removed. Any hairpins or other styling aids should be removed from the hair.

10. The hair should be combed or brushed gently, beginning at the ends and working up in sections to the scalp. The patient/resident's hair should be styled the way he/she likes it.

11. The patient/resident should be provided a mirror so that he/she can see the way his/her hair is styled.

12. It should be ensured the patient/resident's comfort and proper body alignment.

13. Hands should be properly washed, and observations should be reported and recorded at the end of the procedure.

Encouraging safety and comfort

Safety
Sharp brush bristles may injure the scalp. Similarly, a comb with sharp or broken teeth may also injure the scalp. The nurse assistant should report any concerns about the patient/resident's brush or comb.

Comfort
A towel should be placed across the patient/resident's back and shoulders to protect garments from falling hair. If the patient/resident is in bed, hair care should be provided before changing linens and the pillowcase. If it is done after a linen change, a towel should be placed across the pillow to collect falling hair.

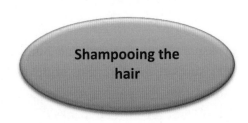

Shampooing the hair

Many individuals shampoo 1, 2, or 3 times a week. Others usually shampoo every day. In most of the nursing centers, shampooing is usually done on the patient/resident's bath or shower day. If it is done by a hairdresser or barber, the nurse assistant should not shampoo the patient/resident's hair. The nurse assistant should provide a shower cap for the bath or shower. The shampoo method generally depends on the patient/resident's condition, safety factors, and personal choice. The nurse supervisor guides one of the following methods to use:

Shampooing during the shower or tub bath

The patient/resident shampoos in the shower or tub bath. The nurse assistant uses a hand-held nozzle for those using shower chairs or taking tub baths and also directs a spray of water at the hair.

Shampooing at the sink

The patient/resident sits or lies facing away from the sink. A folded towel should be placed over the edge of sink to protect the neck. The patient/resident's head is tilted back over the edge of the sink. The nurse assistant uses a water pitcher or hand-held nozzle to wet and rinse the hair.

Shampooing in the bed

The patient/resident's head and shoulders are moved to the edge of the bed if possible. A shampoo tray should be placed under the head. The nurse assistant uses a water pitcher to wet and rinse the hair.

Hair should be dried and styled as quickly as possible after the shampoo. Women may want hair rolled up or curled before drying.

Encouraging safety and comfort

Safety

Shampoo should be kept away from and out of the eyes. To rinse, the nurse assistant should cup his/her hand at the patient/resident's forehead. This keeps soapy water from running down the patient/resident's forehead and into the eyes. Hearing aids should be removed before shampooing as water will damage hearing aids. Medicated products should be returned to the nurse supervisor. They should never be left at the bedside. The nurse assistant should wear gloves if the patient/resident has scalp sores. The nurse assistant should always follow standard precautions and the bloodborne pathogen standard. For a shampoo on a stretcher at a sink, the stretcher wheels should be locked and the safety straps and side rails should be used. Some patients/residents shampoo themselves during a tub bath or shower. A towel, shampoo, and hair conditioner should be placed within the patient/resident's reach.

Comfort

When shampooing during the tub bath or shower, the patient/resident usually tips his/her head back to keep shampoo and water out of the eyes. The nurse assistant should support the back of the patient/resident's head with one hand, and shampoo with his/her other hand.

Some patients/residents cannot tip their heads back. They usually lean forward and hold a folded washcloth over the eyes. The nurse assistant should support the forehead with one hand and hold shampoo with the other. It should be ensured that the patient/resident can breathe easily. Many patients/residents have limited range of motion in their necks. They should not be shampooed at the sink or on a stretcher.

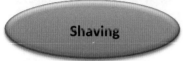

Shaving

Most of the males shave for comfort and well-being. Many women shave their underarms and legs. Some women also shave facial hair. Or they may use other hair removal procedures such as waxing, plucking, hair removal products, and threading. Safety razors or electric shavers are commonly used for shaving. Patients/residents usually have their own electric shavers. If the agency's shaver is used, it should be ensured that these are cleaned before and after use. To brush out whiskers, the nurse assistant should follow the manufacturer's instructions. Also the nurse assistant should follow agency policy for cleaning electric shavers. Safety razors have razor blades. They can cause cuts and nicks. Therefore, safety razors should not be used on patients/residents who have healing problems or for those taking anticoagulant medications. Electric shavers should be preferred over safety razors. The beard should be softened before shaving. To do so, a moist and warm washcloth or towel should be applied for a few minutes. For a safety razor, the face should be lathered with soap and water or shaving cream.

The nurse assistant should provide assistance for shaving a patient/resident in following ways:
1. Hands should be washed properly.
2. The nurse assist should gather all supplies:
   - Towel
   - Washcloths
   - Gloves
   - Paper towels
   - Wash basin
   - Bath thermometer
   - Soap (optional)
   - Aftershave lotion (optional)
   - Safety razor
   - Shaving cream, gel or soap Electric razor:
   - Electric razor
   - Pre-shave lotion
3. The nurse assistant should knock, greet the patient/resident and should ensure his/her privacy.
4. The procedure should be explained thoroughly to the patient/resident.

5. Equipment should be adjusted for proper body mechanics and safety: the bed should be raised to a comfortable working height. It should be ensured that the wheels on the bed are locked.

6. The over-bed table should be covered with the paper towels and all supplies should be arranged. The wash basin should be filled with warm water. The bath thermometer should be used to verify that the water temperature, which must be between 105° F and 115° F. The wash basin should be placed on the over-bed table.

7. The patient/resident should be positioned in high Fowler's position.

8. The towel should be unfolded and should be placed across the patient/resident's chest.

9. The nurse assistant should put on the gloves and should inspect the area to be shaved. The nurse assistant should also observe any moles, birthmarks, or sores during inspection.

10. The patient/resident should be assisted in washing his/her face with soap (optional) and warm water. Soap should be removed with a wet washcloth.

11. If the patient/resident is using a safety razor, the nurse assistant should assist him in applying shaving cream, soap, or gel to his face. If the patient/resident is using an electric razor, the nurse assistant should assist him to apply pre-shave lotion.

12. The nurse assistant should assist the patient/resident with shaving, if needed, as following:

- Safety razor: With the fingers of one hand, the nurse assistant should hold the patient/resident's skin on the cheek tight and the razor should be used to shave downward position, in the direction that the hair grows. Both cheeks should be shaved by rinsing the razor often in the washbasin. Shorter strokes should be used around the patient/resident's chin and lips. To shave the neck, the skin should be pulled tight and shave the neck, moving the razor up toward the chin.

- Electric razor: With the fingers of one hand, the nurse assistant should hold the patient/resident's skin tight and the razor should be used to shave in a circular motion. 14. The wet washcloth should be used to rinse the patient/resident's face.

13. The patient/resident's face should be dried with the towel, and the towel should be placed in the linen hamper.

14. The patient/resident should be provided a hand mirror so that he can inspect the shaved area.

15. The patient/resident should be assisted to apply aftershave lotion (optional).

16. It should be ensured the patient/resident's comfort and proper body alignment.

17. Hands should be properly washed, and observations should be reported and recorded at the end of the procedure.

Encouraging safety and comfort

Safety

Safety razors are really sharp. The patient/resident should be protected from nicks and cuts. The nurse assistant should prevent contact with blood. For an electric shaver, safety measures should be followed for electrical equipment. The safety razor should be rinsed often. Rinsing removes lather and whiskers. Then the razor should be wiped. To protect personal cuts and injuries:

- Several thicknesses of tissues or paper towels should be placed on the over-bed table.
- The razor should be wiped on the tissues or paper towels. The nurse assistant should always follow standard precautions and the bloodborne pathogen standard. Used razor blades should be discarded in the sharps container. The nurse assistant should not re-cap the razor.

Comfort

In some males, the neck area below the jaw is sensitive and tender. Some electric shavers may become very hot or warm while in use. The heat can further irritate the skin. Tender areas should be shaved first while the shaver is cool before moving other areas. Some patients/residents apply after-shave or lotion to the skin after shaving. Lotion generally softens the skin and after-shave closes skin pores.

Maintaining skin health

1. The patient/resident should be encouraged for well-balanced diet and plenty of fluids.
2. Appropriate skin care should be provided as:
- There should be bathing as necessary.
- There should be thorough rinsing off the skin with soap and water.
- Lotion and creams should be applied as necessary.
- There should be the massage for healthy skin.
- The skin should be kept clean and dry.
3. The nurse assistant should observe high-risk patients/residents for potential problems.

4. Special attention should be provided to bony prominences:
- The patient/resident should be turned and positioned correctly.
- Pressure should be kept off from reddened or irritated areas.
5. Massage should not be provided on red, purple, or irritated areas.
6. Bed should be kept free from small objects and linen should be free of wrinkles.
7. The patient/resident should be kept clean and dry.
8. There should be prevention for shearing and friction.
9. The observations should be reported and recorded.

Causes of Skin Breakdown

Disruption of skin integrity or non-intact skin is called as skin breakdown. It is a potential complication for any patient/resident confined to a bed or wheelchair. This may also include the patient/resident with a body cast, traction, or the patient/resident who is paralyzed or otherwise cannot move without assistance. In several other cases, skin breakdown may occur as a result of factors such as infection, moisture, external pressure, or rash, even in the ambulatory patient. A major cause is shearing force (friction) caused by bed linens, clothing, or patient safety devices.

The major conditions contributing to skin breakdown may include:

- Immobility, low level of activity (sitting/lying in one position for long periods of time as in paralysis)
- Inadequate nutrition (very thin person; insufficient protein, inadequate calories)
- Hydration levels (insufficient fluid intake, excess fluid retention as in edema)
- Presence of moisture (including urine, sweat, and feces); incontinence
- Altered mental status, alertness, or cooperation; heavy sedation or/and anesthesia
- Sensory loss
- Fever and low blood pressure
- Other causes may include CVA, COPD, and circulatory problems such as diabetes, poor circulation and healing, and neuropathy.

Pressure sores

Pressure sores are one of the major complications of immobility. A pressure sore is an ulcer that develops when part of a patient/resident's body presses against a hard surface (such as the seat of a chair or a mattress) for an extended period of time. Pressure sores usually develop over bony prominences. Examples of these areas may include the back of the head, elbows, shoulder blades, hips, knees, coccyx (tailbone), ankles and heels. When a patient/resident stays in one position for too long, the weight of his/her body squeezes the tissue between the surface and the bone, which slows down blood flow to the area. Because the tissue is not receiving sufficient oxygen and nutrients, it begins to die. This loss of healthy and intact skin is called skin breakdown, which can lead to a pressure sore.

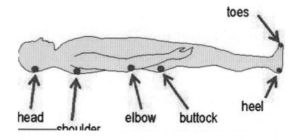

Patients/residents at risk

Patients/residents at risk for pressure sores are those who:

- Are confined to bed or wheelchair
- Need total or partial help moving
- Are agitated or having involuntary muscle movements
- Have fecal or urinary incontinence
- Are exposed to moisture—feces, urine, sweat, wound drainage, or saliva
- Have poor fluid balance or poor nutrition
- Have altered mental status
- Have problems sensing pressure or pain
- Have circulatory problems
- Are very thin or obese

- Have a healed pressure ulcer
- Taking medications that affect wound healing
- Refuse care and treatment measures
- Have health problems such as thyroid disease, kidney failure, or diabetes
- Smoke

Stages of pressure ulcer: Signs and symptoms

In patients/residents with light skin, a red or pink area is probably the first sign of a pressure sore. In patients/residents with dark skin, the skin may have no prominent color change or it may appear blue, red, or purple. Color does not fade on application of pressure. The area may feel cool or warm and firm or soft. The patient/resident may complain of burning, pain, tingling, or itching in the area. Some patients/residents do not feel anything unusual.

Stage I
An area is pale, red, or dark, and the normal color does not re-appear within a few minutes of relieving the pressure. The area may be softer, firmer, cooler, warmer, or more painful than the surrounding tissue. Detection may be more difficult in patients/residents with darker skin.

Stage II
The area may look like an open and shallow ulcer with red or pink exposed tissue at the bottom. Sometimes, instead of looking like a sore, the area may look like a blister.

Stage III
More tissue is damaged and lost. The fat that lies underneath the skin may be visible.

Stage IV
A deep crater is formed.

General nursing measures to prevent and treat pressure sores

Some pressure sores may be avoidable. That is, they are developed because of improper use of the nursing process. Some pressure sores unavoidable—they are developed despite efforts to prevent them. Nursing assistants should take following measures to prevent and manage them:

1. **Sensory/Mobility measures**
- The pressure should be controlled by special beds or pressure-reducing devices.
- The patient/resident should be re-positioned and turned every two hours at least.
- The patient/resident should be positioned with proper support of the body and limbs.
- Active range of motion exercises should be promoted or the nurse assistant should assist patient/resident with them.
- Assistance should be provided to the patient/resident using a wheel chair to change his/her position frequently.
- The nurse assistant should prevent friction and shearing during moving, lifting, transferring, and repositioning procedures.
- The bed linens should be kept crumb free, clean, and wrinkles-free.
- It should be ensured that tubing like foley catheter does not cause pressure.
- Patients/residents should be removed from toilets and bedpans promptly.

- Circulation should be encouraged by gentle massage around red or purple area. It should not be done over red area.
- The skin should be checked every eight hours.
- Head of bed (H.O.B.) should be kept at 30 degrees as much as possible to avoid sacral and coccygeal pressure.

2. Elimination measures

- Skin should be kept clean and dry; powder should be applied where skin touches skin. Diaphoretic patients/residents should be frequently watched and observed.
- Incontinent patient/resident should be checked every two hours and it should be ensured that skin is dried and clean (even when applying adult incontinence garment).
- Incontinence garment should be monitored because plastic edges near skin may cause skin irritation.
- Scrubbing or rubbing should be avoided when bathing and drying the patient/resident.
- Pillows and blankets should be used to prevent skin from being in contact with skin.

3. Fluid status

- Limbs should be elevated limb to prevent edema.
- Compression devices, such as anti-embolic stockings and ace bandages should be properly monitored. Skin should be checked and ensured that edges do not cut into skin.
- The patient/resident should be encouraged fluids intake from 1500-2000ml/day or as per care plan.

4. Nutrition status

- Patients/residents should be encouraged and assisted with proper balanced diet.
- The nurse assistant should check skin folds in obese patients/residents.
- The nurse assistant should monitor bony prominences on thin patients/residents.
- Braces, casts, and clothing items should be monitored and ensured that they are not causing pressure against skin.

5. Use of pressure-reducing devices

The physician may order wound care products, drugs, and special equipment to promote healing. Support surfaces are used to reduce or relieve pressure. Such surfaces usually include air, foam, gel, alternating air, or water mattresses. Protective devices are generally used to prevent and manage skin breakdown and pressure sores. These devices may include:

a) Bed cradle

It is a metal frame placed on the bed and over the patient/resident. Top linens are brought over the cradle to prevent pressure on the feet, legs, and toes.

b) Heel and elbow protectors

These devices are made of pressure-relieving gel, sheepskin, foam padding, and other cushion materials. They fit the shape of elbows and heels.

c) Heel and foot elevators

These devices raise the feet and heels off of the bed. They prevent pressure as well as footdrop.

d) Gel or fluid-filled pads and cushions

These devices involve a pressure-relieving gel or fluid-filled pads. They are used for wheelchairs and chairs to prevent pressure. The outer case is vinyl and the cushion or pad is placed in a fabric cover to protect the patient/resident's skin.

e) Special beds

Some special beds have air flowing through the mattresses. The patient/resident floats on the mattress. Body weight is evenly distributed. Therefore, there is very little pressure on body parts. Some special beds also allow re-positioning without moving the patient/resident. The patient/resident is turned to the supine or prone position or the bed is tilted various degrees. Alignment does not change; however, pressure points change as the position changes. Some special beds constantly rotate from one side to another. They are useful for patients/residents with spinal cord injuries.

f) Dressings

Sometimes dressings are also used to promote healing. If a pressure sore has drainage, a dressing that absorbs drainage is applied. The dressing absorbs slough, which is removed when the dressing is removed.

g) Other equipment

Foot boards, pillows, trochanter rolls, and other positioning devices can be used. They may help keep the patient/resident in good alignment.

General guidelines for selecting and caring for patient/resident's clothing

Most patients/residents wear street clothes during the day time and sleepwear at bedtime. Most patients/residents wear gowns that are mostly changed daily. Garments are usually changed:

- After bathing
- On admission and discharge
- When soiled or wet

Dressing and undressing

Some patients/residents may dress and undress themselves. Others may need assistance. Personal choice is a patient/resident right. Patients/residents should be allowed to choose what to wear.

When a nurse assistant assists with dressing and undressing, he/she should follow the below rules:

Rules for Dressing and Undressing

- The patient/resident should be provided proper privacy. The nurse should not expose the patient/resident.
- The patient/resident should be encouraged to do as much as possible.
- The patient/resident should be allowed to choose what to wear. The patient/resident should have the full right to choose undergarments.
- It should be ensured that garments and footwear are the correct size.
- Clothing from the strong or "good" side should be removed first. This is called the unaffected side.

- Clothing should be put on the weak side first. This is called the affected side.
- The arm or leg should be supported to remove or put on a garment.
- The body should be moved and handled gently. The nurse assistant should not force a joint beyond its range of motion or to the point of pain.
- When helping patients/residents select clothing, the nurse assistant should consider:
  - The patient/resident's preferences
  - The patient/resident's physical capabilities
  - What the patient/resident will be doing that day
  - The season and weather
- Clothing of the patient/resident should fit properly and be in good condition.
- If the nurse assistant notices that an article of clothing is ripped, stained, torn, missing buttons, or in need of alterations, the nurse assistant should talk to the nurse supervisor so that appropriate arrangements can be made to have the clothing altered, cleaned, replaced, or repaired.
- When helping a patient/resident with a weak, injured, or paralyzed leg or arm to dress, the garment should be put on the affected leg or arm first. Then, the opposite should be done when helping the patient/resident to undress i.e. the garment from the affected leg or arm should be removed last.
- Some patients/residents will be required to wear compression stockings, which are made of tightfitting elastic. They squeeze (compress) the veins in the legs. Squeezing the veins in the legs may help to return blood towards heart, preventing fatal complications such as blood clots. Because these stockings are so tight, these may be so difficult for a patient/resident to put on independently. These stockings must be put on before the patient/resident gets out of bed in the morning.

Encouraging comfort and safety

When assisting with dressing and undressing, the nurse assistant must turn the patient/resident from side to side. If the patient/resident uses bed rails, the nurse assistant should raise the far bed rail. If bed rails are not used, the nurse assistant should ask a co-worker to help turn and position the patient/resident. This protects the patient/resident from falling.

Characteristics of urine

Urine is observed for color, odor, clarity, and volume. The nurse supervisor makes these observations as part of routine data collection. Any deviations from the normal characteristics may indicate an abnormality.

- **Color**

Freshly voided urine is amber or light yellow in color. The degree of color in urine may vary with the body's level of hydration. Edema (too much fluid) or overhydration results in dilute urine that is nearly colorless. Dehydration (too little fluid) results in concentrated urine that may be orange-brown or dark amber. In addition, certain drugs and foods can alter the color of urine.

- **Clarity**

Freshly voided urine is transparent or clear. It may appear cloudy if it contains abnormal substances, such as blood, bacteria, mucous shreds, or pus, or if it has been standing for an extended period of time in a collection container.

- **Odor**

Freshly voided urine has a characteristic aromatic odor. Dilute urine has fewer odors than concentrated urine. When the urine has been exposed to the air for long time, it decomposes and emits a strong, ammonia-like odor. Sometimes drugs or foods may alter urine's usual odor. Usually a strongly offensive odor from freshly voided urine may suggest an abnormality like urinary tract infection.

- **Volume**

The normal average amount of urine that an adult voids at one time ranges between 250 and 400 mL. The exact urine output relates to each individual's size, hydration level, bladder condition, and other fluid losses or gains.

- **Specific Gravity**

Normal freshly voided urine has a specific gravity of 1.010 to 1.025. The specific gravity of urine is often measured by the laboratory as part of a routine urinalysis. It can be changed in various conditions.

- **Acidity**

The more acidic urine is, the greater the hydrogen ion concentration, and the lower the pH. Normal urine is slightly acidic, which helps to control bacterial growth in urine.

- **Abnormal Components**

Abnormal components such as microorganisms in urine suggest any disease somewhere in the body.

Color variations in urine

Clear, colorless (dilute)
- Large amount of liquids
- Diuretics (particularly if these are overused)
- Liver problems (acute viral hepatitis, cirrhosis)
- Conditions such as diabetes insipidus, diabetes mellitus

Bright, neon yellow
- Vitamin supplements

Cloudy
- Urine is left standing for an extended period of time
- Pyuria (pus in the urine)
- Epithelial cells
- Blood
- Leukocytes (white blood cells)
- Urinary tract infection
- Kidney stones

Green
- Pseudomonas infection
- Bile pigments

Dark yellow, gold
- Low fluid intake
- Dehydration (concentrated urine)
- Inability of kidneys to dilute urine

Bile Pink, red
- Hematuria—blood in urine
- Some foods (red berries, food dye, beets, red gelatin, some red juices)
- Some laxatives

Orange, red brown

- Some medications (rifampin, phenazopyridine, warfarin, doxorubicin)
- Some foods
- Some food coloring
- Dehydration

Blue, green
- Some medications (amitriptyline, indomethacin)
- Some food dyes
- Some foods (asparagus)

Smoky, hazy
- Prostatic fluid
- Yeast infection
- Hemoglobin (remnants of red blood cells)
- Chyle (product of digestion normally emptied into venous system)

Yellow brown
- Bile

Dark brown, black
- Methylene blue
- Typhus infection
- Some foods and food dyes
- Hematuria (blood in urine)
- Some medications (iron)
- Liver disorders (especially with light stools and jaundice)

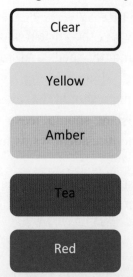

Patterns of urinary elimination

Although observation of the appearance of a patient/resident's urine may be an indication of renal or urinary problems, an alteration in the usual pattern of urinary elimination is also an important factor.

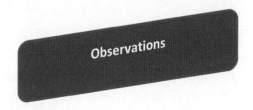

Normal urine is amber, pale yellow, or straw-colored, or amber. The nurse assistant should be familiar with these common signs and symptoms that may occur:

- **Urinary frequency**

It is voiding more often than usual without a significant increase in total urine volume, but often with a decrease in its volume per voiding.

- **Urgency**

It is the desire or sensation to urinate immediately. Often, the patient/resident is unable to delay voiding without some involuntary urine leakage.

- **Dysuria**

A painful or burning sensation when passing urine that is most commonly associated with an infection. The patient/resident may also experience shooting pain or cramping in the pelvis.

- **Nocturia**

It is the repeated or frequent voiding during the night. Sometimes, it may occur

223

when the patient/resident drinks a large amount of liquid before bedtime.

- **Enuresis**

Enuresis is the involuntary voiding in bed (bedwetting). It is a common problem in children, but may also occur in some adults. It may also be a side effect of certain medications.

- **Polyuria**

Polyuria is an increase in the expected amount of urine a patient/resident excretes over a period of time. It may occur when an individual drinks a larger than usual amount of liquids, but it can also be a symptom of various kidney diseases or diabetes mellitus. A daily urine output that is greater than almost 2,500 mL is considered as polyuria.

- **Incontinence**

Urinary incontinence is the inability to hold the urine or involuntary loss of urine from the bladder.

- **Urinary suppression**

The stopping or inhibition of urination is called as urinary suppression. It may involve suppression of secretion (urine is not formed) or suppression of excretion (urine is not expelled).

- **Oliguria**

Oliguria is a decrease in the expected amount of urine a patient/resident secretes and excretes. A less than 500 mL daily urine output is considered to be oliguria. It may be caused by kidney disorders or urinary tract obstruction.

- **Anuria**

It is the absence of urine secreted by the kidneys (100 mL/day). It is a very serious sign of kidney dysfunction.

- **Urinary retention**

It is inability to empty the bladder fully with attempts to void.

Assisting with urinary elimination

- Standard medical asepsis should be practiced.
- Standard precautions and the bloodborne pathogen standard should be followed.
- Sufficient fluids should be provided.
- The nurse assistant should follow the patient/resident's voiding routines and habits.
- The nurse assistant should help the patient/resident to the bathroom upon request. He/she should provide the commode, urinal, or bedpan.
- The patient/resident should be provided proper help to maintain a normal position for voiding if possible. Women usually squat or sit and males stand.
- The bedpan or urinal should be warmed.
- The patient/resident should be covered for warmth and privacy.
- To provide privacy, the curtain should be pulled around the bed, and room and bathroom doors along with window coverings should be closed. The nurse assistant should leave the room if the patient/resident wants to be alone.
- The nurse assistant should stay nearby if the patient/resident is weak or unsteady.

- The call light and toilet tissue should be placed within reach.
- The patient/resident should be allowed enough time. The nurse assistant should not rush the patient/resident.
- Water should be run in a sink if the patient/resident cannot start the stream. Or the patient/resident's fingers should be placed in warm water.
- Perineal care should be provided as needed.
- The nurse assistant should assist with hand washing after voiding. A wash basin, soap, washcloth, and towel should be provided.
- The nurse assistant should assist the patient/resident to the bathroom or should offer the urinal, bedpan, or commode at regular times.

Encouraging comfort and safety

Urinary elimination measures usually involve exposing and touching private areas—the rectum and perineum. Sexual abuse may occur in health care settings. The patient/resident may feel threatened or may be being abused. He/she needs to call for help. The call light should be placed within the patient/resident's reach at all times. The nurse assistant should always act in a professional manner. Urine may contain microorganisms and blood. Microorganisms can live and grow in dirty urinals, bedpans, commodes, and urinary drainage bags. The nurse assistant should always follow standard precautions and the bloodborne pathogen standards when handling urinary devices and their contents, including incontinence products. There should be thoroughly cleaning and disinfecting the urinals, bedpans, and commodes after use.

Urinary incontinence

Urinary incontinence is the involuntary leakage or loss of urine. It may be permanent or temporary. The basic types of incontinence may include:

- **Stress incontinence**
Urine leaks during certain movements and exercises that cause pressure on the bladder. Urine loss is usually less than 50 mL. It is also called as dribbling, and may occur with laughing, coughing, sneezing, lifting, or other activities.

- **Urge incontinence**
Urine is lost in response to a sudden, urgent need to urinate and the person cannot get to a toilet in time.

- **Overflow incontinence**
In overflow incontinence, a small amounts of urine leak from a full bladder. The person usually feels like the bladder is not empty.

- **Functional incontinence**
In this condition, the person has bladder control but cannot use the toilet in time. Immobility, unanswered call lights, restraints, no call light within reach, and not knowing where to find the bathroom are the major causes.

- **Reflex incontinence**
It is a condition in which urine is lost at predictable intervals when the bladder is full. The person usually does not feel the need to void in reflex incontinence.

- **Mixed incontinence**

In mixed incontinence, the patients have a combination of stress incontinence and urge incontinence.

- **Transient incontinence**

This refers to occasional or temporary incontinence that is reversed when the cause is treated.

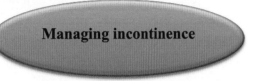

Managing incontinence

The main goals of incontinence management are to:

- Prevent urinary tract infections (UTIs)
- Restore normal bladder function as much as possible.

Incontinence is usually embarrassing. Garments are soiled or wet and odors develop. The patient/resident becomes uncomfortable. Skin irritation, pressure sores, and infection are risks. Falling is a major risk when trying to get to the bathroom quickly. Dignity, pride, and self-esteem are also affected. Loss of independence, social isolation, and depression are common. Overall the quality of life suffers. Appropriate skin care and dry garments and linens are essential. Encouraging normal urinary elimination prevents incontinence in some patients/residents, whereas others may need bladder training. Catheters are also required in some special cases.

Nursing measures for urinary incontinence

- Time and amount of voiding should be recorded. This also includes incontinent times as well as successful use of the toilet, bedpan, commode, or urinal.
- Call lights should be responded promptly because the need to void may be urgent.
- Normal urinary and bowel elimination should be promoted.
- The nurse assistant should assist the patient/resident with elimination after sleep, before and after meals, and at bedtime.
- The patient/resident's bladder training program should be followed.
- It should be ensured that the patient/resident has a clear pathway to the bathroom.
- The patient/resident should be encouraged to do pelvic muscle exercises as instructed by the nurse supervisor and care plan.
- The nurse assistant should frequently check the patient/resident to make sure he/she is clean and dry.
- Adequate fluid intake should be promoted as the nurse directs.
- The patient/resident should wear cotton underwear.
- The perineal area should be kept clean and dry.
- Fluid intake should be decreased at bedtime.
- Good skin care should be provided.

- A barrier cream or moisturizer (cream, lotion, and paste) should be applied as directed by the nurse.
- Dry garments and linens should be provided to the patient/resident.
- The patient/resident should be observed for signs of skin breakdown.
- Incontinence products should be used as the nurse directs.
- The nurse assistant should not leave urinals in place to catch urine in men who are incontinent.
- The nurse assistant should follow standard precautions and the bloodborne pathogen standard.
- The nurse assistant should protect the patient/resident, dry garments, and linen from the wet incontinence product.

Urinary catheters

A catheter is a tube used to inject or drain fluid through a body opening. It is inserted through the urethra into the bladder for urine drainage. An indwelling catheter (retention or Foley catheter) is generally left in the bladder. Urine constantly drains into a drainage bag. Catheter is connected to the drainage bag through tubing. The process of inserting a catheter is called as catheterization. It is done by a physician or nurse. With proper supervision and education, some agencies and states allow nursing assistants insert and remove catheters. Some patients/residents are too weak or disabled to use the urinal, bedpan, commode, or toilet. For them, catheters may provide comfort and prevent incontinence. Catheters may also protect wounds and pressure sores from contact with urine. Catheters also allow hourly

urinary output measurements. However, they are a last option for incontinence. It should be remembered that catheters do not treat the cause of incontinence.

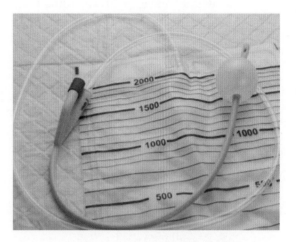

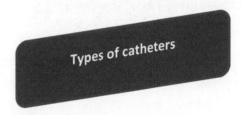

Types of catheters

A urinary catheter is a latex or vinyl tube that is used to drain urine. It is about 24 inches long and is inserted into the bladder through the urethra by using sterile technique. A straight catheter is inserted into the bladder through the urethra through which the urine is drained, and the catheter is removed and discarded. A retention catheter is inserted, remained in place, and continuously drains urine from the bladder. Retention catheter is also called an indwelling catheter because it is placed when a patient/resident is unable to void naturally or has had various types of surgery. There are multiple types of indwelling catheters, but the Foley catheter is most commonly used. This catheter usually has double tube-like cavities, called lumens, within it. One lumen is attached to a balloon that is inflated inside the bladder and plugged, to maintain the catheter in place. The other lumen drains the urine. The distal end of the catheter is usually attached to a drainage bag for collection of urine. There are some catheters which have a third lumen to provide a means for continuous bladder irrigation.

In some cases, a catheter is inserted via a very small incision through the lower abdominal wall above the pubis and into the urinary bladder. This is called a suprapubic catheter that is held in place by a balloon or by a hook-type apparatus, much like the Foley catheter.

Indwelling catheter care

- The rules of medical asepsis should be properly followed.
- The nurse assistant should always follow standard precautions and the bloodborne pathogen standard while caring an indwelling catheter.
- The nurse assistant should allow urine to flow freely through the catheter or tubing. Tubing should not contain kinks. The patient/resident should not lie on the tubing.
- The catheter should be connected to the drainage tubing.
- The drainage tube should be kept below the bladder to prevent urine from flowing backward into the bladder.
- The bag should be moved to the other side of the bed when the patient/resident is turned and re-positioned on his /her other side.
- The drainage bag should be attached to the back of the chair, bed frame, or lower part of the intravenous pole. The drainage bag should never be attached to the bed rail. Otherwise it may become higher than the bladder when the bed rail is raised.
- The drainage bag should not place on the floor. This may contaminate the system.
- The drainage tubing should be coiled on the bed. The nurse assistant should follow agency policy and may use a clip, tape, bed sheet clamp, pin with rubber band, or other device as the nurse directs. Tubing should not loop below the drainage bag.
- The catheter should be secured to the inner thigh or to the man's abdomen to prevent excess catheter movement and friction at the insertion site.
- The nurse assistant should check the site where the catheter connects to the drainage bag and should report any leaks to the nurse at once.
- Perineal care and catheter care should be provided according to the care plan—daily, twice a day, or when vaginal discharge is present.
- The drainage bag should be emptied at the end of the shift or as the nurse directs. Amount of urine should be measured and recorded. The nurse assistant should report an increase or decrease in the amount of urine.
- A separate measuring container should be used for each person to prevent the spread of infections from one person to another.
- The nurse assistant should report complaints at once—burning, pain, the need to void, or irritation. He/she should also report the color, clarity, and odor of urine and the presence of blood or particles.

- Signs and symptoms of a UTI (fever, chills, flank pain etc.) should be observed and reported immediately.

Encouraging safety and comfort

Safety
Special measures should be taken if using a safety pin and rubber band to secure the drainage tubing to the bottom linens.
- The safety pin and rubber band should be checked and ensured that they are working properly.
- The rubber band should be intact. It should not be over-stretched or frayed.
- The pin should not be inserted through the catheter.
- The pin should be pointed away from the patient/resident.

Comfort
The catheter should not be pulled at the insertion site. This may cause irritation and discomfort. The catheter should be held securely during catheter care. It should be ensured that the tubing is not under the patient/resident.

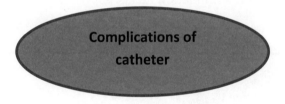

1. Urinary tract infections (UTIs). The symptoms of a UTI may include
   - Fever
   - Chills
   - Headache
   - Cloudy urine due to pus
   - Blood in the urine
   - Foul-smelling urine
   - Low back pain and achiness
   - Burning of the urethra or genital area
   - Leaking of urine out of the catheter
2. Other common complications from using a urinary catheter may include:
   - Allergic reaction to the material used in the catheter, such as latex or vinyl

- Bladder stones
- Injury to the urethra
- Kidney damage (with long-term indwelling catheters)
- Septicemia, or infection of the kidneys, urinary tract, or blood

Bladder or bowel training programs and scheduled toileting programs

A bowel or bladder training program is usually developed for a patient/resident who is incontinent of feces or urine and has the ability to recognize the urge to eliminate and to retrain the muscles used to control elimination. The bowel or bladder training program helps the patient/resident to regain control over elimination by promoting defecation or urination at predictable times. For example, as component of a bladder training program, the nurse assistant may be required to provide the patient/resident the opportunity to urinate at regular intervals according to the schedule recommended in the patient/resident's care plan. The nurse assistant should assist the patient/resident to the bathroom (or offer a urinal, bedpan, or portable commode) and should permit the patient/resident enough time to urinate each time. Supporting and assisting a bladder training program means proper following the schedule during the night as well (if the patient/resident typically gets up during the night to urinate), although the time intervals between using the toilet may be longer during the night time.

A bowel training program also works in much the same way as a bladder training program, except the patient/resident is only assisted to use the toilet (or bedside commode or bedpan) during the time when a bowel movement is expected, based on the patient/resident's usual bowel elimination routine and pattern. A patient/resident with dementia may become incontinent because he/she cannot remember how to control the muscles used for elimination or unable to recognize the urge to eliminate. In this special condition, a training program will not work. Instead of the training program, a scheduled toileting program should be set up for these patients/residents. The scheduled toileting program also involves providing the patient/resident the opportunity to eliminate at regular intervals based on the patient/resident's past elimination patterns. The scheduling toileting program helps to maintain the patient/resident's dignity by minimizing the likelihood of the occurrence of incontinence. Both toileting programs and training program are based on accurate assessment of the patient/resident's elimination patterns. It is a responsibility of a nurse assistant to gather data about when the patient/resident normally eliminates in preparation for placing the patient/resident on either type of program, thus, a nurse assistant may play a very important role in helping the patient/resident adhere to the plan by assisting the patient/resident with elimination at the scheduled times.

Bowel elimination

Bowel elimination is a basic physical need for every individual. Waste materials from the body are excreted from the gastro-intestinal (GI) system. The nurse assistant usually assists patients/residents in meeting elimination needs.

Normal patterns of bowel movements

Some individuals have a bowel movement (BM) every day. Most of the other people have one every 2 to 3 days. Some people may have 2 or 3 bowel movements a day. Many individuals have a bowel movement after breakfast. Others do so in the evening. To assist with bowel elimination, the nurse assistant should know these terms:

- **Defecation**

It is the process of excreting feces from the rectum through the anus (bowel movement).

- **Feces**

It is the semi-solid mass of waste products in the colon that is expelled out from the body through the anus. It is also known as stool.

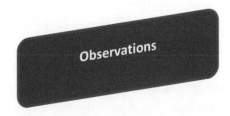

Stools are usually brown. Bleeding in the small intestine and stomach may cause black or tarry stools. Bleeding in the rectum and lower colon usually causes red-colored stools. Certain diseases and infection may cause white, clay-colored, pale, orange-colored, or green-colored stools. Stools are normally soft, moist, formed, and shaped like the rectum. They normally have a characteristic odor. Stools should be observed carefully. The nurse assistant should ask the nurse to observe abnormal stools. The nurse should observe and report the following:

- Color
- Amount
- Consistency
- Presence of mucus or blood
- Odor
- Size and shape
- Frequency of bowel movements
- Complaints of pain or discomfort

Encouraging comfort and safety
Assisting with bowel elimination usually involves exposing and touching the rectum. The nurse assistant may also have to provide perineal care. Sexual abuse may occur in health care settings. The patient/resident may feel threatened or may be being abused. He/she needs to call for help. The call light should be placed within the patient/resident's reach at all times. Healthcare workers should always act in a professional manner. Contact with feces is more likely while assisting with bowel elimination. Feces usually contain microorganisms and may contain blood. Therefore, the nurse assistant should always follow Standard Precautions and the Bloodborne Pathogen Standard.

Factors affecting on bowel movements

There are several factors that may affect stool frequency, color, consistency, and odor. They are component of the nursing process to meet the patient/resident's elimination needs. Normal, regular elimination is the major goal of normal bowel elimination.

1. Privacy

Lack of privacy may prevent a bowel movement despite the urge.

2. Habits
Many people have a bowel movement after breakfast. Change of bowel habits may prevent normal bowel movement.

3. Diet—high fiber foods
High-fiber foods produce a residue for needed bulk and prevent constipation. Vegetables, fruits, and whole-grain cereals and breads are high in fiber. Some older adults cannot chew these foods. They may

not have teeth. Lack of high fiber foods may cause constipation.

4. Fluids

Feces contain water and its consistency depends on the amount of water absorbed in the colon. Feces dry and harden when fluid intake is poor or when large amounts of water are absorbed. Hard feces move slowly through the colon and constipation may occur.

5. Activity

Lack of activity may prevent normal bowel elimination because exercise and activity usually maintain muscle tone and stimulate peristalsis.

6. Drugs

Several drugs can cause constipation and may prevent normal bowel movement.

7. Disability

Some people cannot control bowel movements. They have a bowel movement whenever feces enter the rectum.

8. Aging

Aging causes changes in the gastrointestinal tract, which may cause constipation.

The patient/resident with an ostomy

Sometimes a portion of the intestines is surgically removed due to bowel diseases, cancer, and trauma. An ostomy procedure is sometimes necessary in these conditions. An ostomy is a surgically created opening, which is seen through the abdominal wall (stoma). The patient/resident wears a pouch over the stoma to collect flatus and stools.

Colostomy

A colostomy is a surgically created opening between the abdominal wall and the colon. Portion of the colon is brought out onto the abdominal wall, and an opening (stoma) is made. Flatus and Feces pass through the stoma instead of the anus. The site for colostomy depends on the site of disease or injury. Stool consistency usually depends on the colostomy site. Appropriate skin care prevents skin breakdown around the stoma. The skin should be washed and dried. Then a skin barrier should be applied around the stoma, which prevents stools from having contact with the skin.

Ileostomy

An ileostomy is a surgically created opening between the abdominal wall and ileum. Part of the ileum is brought out onto the abdominal wall, and a surgical opening (stoma) is made. Liquid stools usually drain constantly from an ileostomy. Water is not properly absorbed because the colon was removed. Feces in the small intestine generally contain more digestive juices that can be very irritating to the skin. The ileostomy pouch should fit well and stools should not touch the skin. Appropriate skin care is required.

Ostomy pouches

The ostomy pouch has an adhesive backing that is usually applied to the skin. Some pouches may be secured to ostomy belts. The pouch should be changed every 3 to 7 days or when it leaks. Frequent pouch changes may cause damage in the skin.

Odors can be prevented by:
- Performing proper personal hygiene.
- Frequent emptying the pouch.

- Avoiding gas-forming foods.
- Putting deodorants into the pouch.

Caring for a patient/resident with an ostomy appliance

Changing an Ostomy Appliance
The nurse assistant should provide assistance for changing an ostomy appliance in following ways:
1. Hands should be washed properly.
2. The nurse assist should gather all supplies:
- Gloves
- Bed protector
- Toilet paper
- Washcloth
- Towel
- Clean ostomy appliance
- Ostomy appliance deodorant (if used)
- Skin adhesive (if used)
- Scissors
- Bedpan
- Bedpan cover
- Paper towels
- Soap or other cleansing agent
3. The nurse assistant should knock, greet the patient/resident and should ensure his/her privacy.
4. The procedure should be explained thoroughly to the patient/resident.
5. Equipment should be adjusted for proper body mechanics and safety: the bed should be raised to a comfortable working height. It should be ensured that the wheels on the bed are locked.
6. The over-bed table should be covered with the paper towels and all supplies should be arranged. The wash basin should be filled with warm water. The bath thermometer should be used to verify that the water temperature, which should be between 105° F and 115° F. The wash basin should be placed on the over-bed table.
7. The head of the bed should be lowered as low as the patient/resident can tolerate.
8. The top linens should be folded out of the way, keeping the patient/resident's legs covered. The patient/resident's clothing should be adjusted as needed to expose the stoma. The bed protector should be positioned alongside the patient/resident.
9. The nurse assistant should put on gloves and remove the soiled ostomy appliance by holding the skin and then peeling the appliance gently off, starting at the top. The soiled ostomy appliance should be placed in the bedpan.
10. The surroundings of the stoma should be wiped with toilet paper and the toilet paper should be placed in the bedpan. The bedpan should be covered properly.

11. The nurse assistant should wet the washcloth and make a mitt. Soap or other cleansing agent should be applied, if ordered. The area around the stoma should be washed, rinsed, and dried.
12. If the patient/resident uses as ostomy appliance deodorant, the deodorant should be placed in the new ostomy appliance. The new appliance should be applied over the stoma, making sure there are no wrinkles. The bedpan should be taken to the bathroom and should be disposed of the ostomy appliance by placing it in a labeled biohazard bag.
13. It should be ensured the patient/resident's comfort and proper body alignment.
14. Hand should be properly washed, and observations should be reported and recorded at the end of the procedure.

Weight and height

Although they are not purely considered as vital signs, weight and height measurements may provide important information about a patient/resident's health status. A patient/resident's height is usually measured only on admission to the health care facility, but weights may be obtained periodically. As with a patient/resident's vital signs, the frequency with which a patient/resident's weight is measured may vary from person to person. Also just like the vital signs, accuracy is very important. For patients/residents with certain medical conditions, such as heart failure and diabetes, changes in weight can be used to help monitor the patient/resident's condition, and even small changes may be extremely significant. Also, medication dosages are usually based on weight.

Height and weight are generally measured on admission to the agency. Then the patient/resident is weighed daily, weekly, or monthly. This is done to measure weight loss or gain. Standing scales are used commonly to measure the height and weight. Wheelchair, chair, bed, and lift scales are used for patients/residents who cannot stand. The nurse assistant should follow the manufacturer's instructions and agency procedures.

When measuring weight and height, these guidelines should be followed:

- The patient/resident should wear only pajamas or a gown. Clothes add more weight. There should be no footwear as footwear also adds to the weight as well as height measurements.
- The patient/resident should void before being weighed. A full bladder adds more weight.
- A dry incontinence product should be worn because a wet product may add weight.
- The patient/resident should be weighed at the same time of day. Before breakfast is usually the best time as food and fluids may add weight.
- The same scale should be used for daily, weekly, and monthly weights.
- The scale should be balanced at zero (0) before weighing the patient/resident. For balance scales, the weights should be moved to zero. A digital scale should read at zero.

Equipment used to measure weight and height

Depending on the situation, a patient/resident's weight and height can be measured in different ways:

- When a patient/resident can stand independently long enough to be weighed, an upright scale should be used. The upright scale is also used to measure the patient/resident's height.

- When a patient/resident is able to get out of bed but is unable to stand long enough to be weighed using an upright scale, a chair scale should be used to weigh the patient/resident. Some chair scales contain a seat mounted on the scale and the nurse assistant simply helps the patient/resident to sit in the seat. Several other chair scales are designed to be used with a wheelchair. When using this type of chair scale, the nurse assistant should first weigh the empty wheelchair, and then should weigh the wheelchair with the patient/resident in it. The patient/resident's weight is the difference between the two measurements.

- If the patient/resident is unable to get out of bed at all, a sling scale should be used to weigh the patient/resident. The patient/resident's height can be measured while he/she lies in bed, using a tape measure.

Encouraging comfort and safety
The patient/resident should wear only a gown or pajamas for the weight measurement. The nurse assistant should follow the manufacturer's instructions when using wheelchair, chair, bed, or lift scales. He/she should also follow the agency's procedures. Proper safety measures should be practiced to prevent falls.

Common prosthetic devices and their care

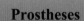

Prostheses

Prosthesis is an artificial device to replace part or all of a missing extremity. Over the years, the design of prostheses has significantly improved, and they have now become more reliable and lightweight. The use of modern computer technology has resulted in better-fitting prosthetic devices that are more natural looking. Patients/residents are fitted with prostheses as soon as possible after their surgery. Leg prostheses are more common and most successful. Trousers and skirts can conceal leg prostheses, which may be equipped with shoes that match. Physical therapists and specially trained nurses may assist the patients/residents in learning to walk with the new prostheses. Arm prostheses are usually more complicated because the hand is an exquisite sensory and motor organ. Thus, functional artificial hands generally do not look real. Above-the-elbow amputees may be used either as cosmetic or functional prostheses.

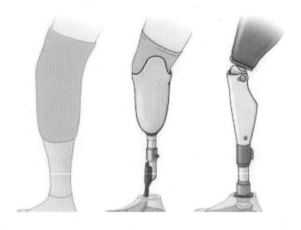

Nursing considerations

After amputation surgery, a compression or rigid dressing is usually applied to the stump to protect the limb, control edema, permit healing, and reduce pain and trauma. Two sets of compression bandages are generally needed so that bandages can be changed at least twice a day or more often if a patient/resident perspires freely. The patients/residents and their family members should be trained how to apply bandages.

Preventing complications

Potential complications following amputation may include infection, hemorrhage, failure of the stump incisions to heal, and deformity of proximal structures. The following nursing actions should be taken to prevent these complications:

- A tourniquet should be kept within reach at all times to be applied if severe and life-threatening bleeding occurs.
- The dressing should be observed for bleeding.
- The dressing should be changed using aseptic technique.
- If the surgeon has inserted drains, they should be monitored and documented the amount, color, consistency, and odor of drainage.
- Dislodging of drains should be avoided when turning the patient/resident.
- When changing dressings, the incision should be checked closely for signs of healing. Any signs of dark-red to black tissue or unusual drainage should be reported.
- The patient/resident who has had a leg amputation should be encouraged to lie in a prone position, rather than on the back. To prevent hip contractures, pillows should not be placed under the stump when the patient/resident is on the back.
- If ordered, skin traction should be applied to the stump as soon as the patient/resident returns from surgery.
- If no cast is in place, the nurse assistant should cleanse, dry, and carefully inspect the stump according to the agency policies.

Patient education

The patient/resident should be trained and encouraged for self-care of prosthesis. Patients/residents should be shown how to wash, rinse, and dry the stump. They should also be taught how to inspect the stump for signs of complications and how to use prosthesis. Patients/residents who are wearing limb socks should be taught to avoid skin problems by keeping the socks free of wrinkles.

Providing emotional support

Patients/residents who have amputations naturally react with grief because of the change in body image and their limb loss. They may exhibit anger, depression, irritability, and other emotions. They should be allowed time to express such feelings. Their concerns should be listened carefully and appropriate emotional support should be provided to them.

Contact lenses

These are placed directly on the eye to correct the vision. Some contact lenses are for single use that are worn once and discarded, while others need to be cleaned daily. The cleansing solutions used to clean and store contact lenses may vary, depending on the type of lens. If the nurse assistant is required to help a patient/resident maintain his/her contact lenses, it should be ensured that the nurse assistant knows what products to use. Because contact lenses are directly placed on the eye, it is very important to maintain the lenses properly. A dirty or damaged contact lens may scratch the eye or cause an infection. The nurse assistant should always wash his/her hands before handling a patient/resident's contact lenses. Contact lenses should be properly fit on the eye. They should be cleaned, removed, and stored according to the manufacturer's instructions.

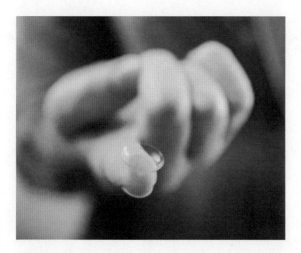

Contact lenses are costly. They should be properly protected from loss or damage. When not worn, they should be placed in

their case. The case should be placed in the top drawer of the bedside stand. Some agencies permit nursing assistants remove and insert contact lenses. Many others do not. The nurse assistant should know the agency's policy. If allowed to insert and remove contact lenses, the nurse assistant should always follow agency procedures.

Eyeglasses

These are worn to correct vision problems. The patients/residents who have glasses should be encouraged to wear them, especially when they are out of bed. This is very important for safety aspects. Eyeglasses are usually expensive and it can be inconvenient to replace them if they become lost or broken, so the nurse assistant should always handle them carefully. When the patient/resident is not wearing them, they should be placed in their case. The patient/resident may need help keeping the glasses clean. The nurse assistant should clean the glasses with water and soap or eyeglass-cleaning wipes, which should be moistened with a cleansing agent meant specifically for cleaning eyeglasses. If only water and soap used to clean the glasses, the nurse assistant should dry them with a soft cloth to avoid scratching the lenses.

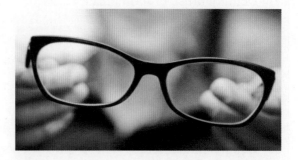

Eyeglasses are usually prescribed to correct the refractive errors of hyperopia, astigmatism, myopia, and presbyopia and for some low-vision individuals. Bifocals (two lenses in one) may be prescribed to correct the problem of presbyopia. Trifocals are also available to provide an extra option for vision correction.

Denture care

A denture is an artificial tooth or a set of artificial teeth that are often called "false teeth". Full (complete) dentures replace all of the bottom teeth or all of the top teeth. Partial dentures replace only a few teeth. Dentures are commonly removed at bedtime. Some patients/residents do not usually wear their dentures. Others wear dentures only during eating and remove them after meals. The nurse assistant should remind them not to wrap dentures in tissues or napkins. Otherwise, they can be easily discarded. Dentures should be cleaned by brushing them with a special kind of toothpaste made for dentures. Some patients/residents may also soak their dentures in a denture cleansing solution as their routine denture-cleaning. Dentures that have been soaking in a denture-cleansing solution should be properly brushed and thoroughly rinsed before placing them in the patient/resident's mouth. When the patient/resident is not wearing the dentures, they should be stored in a labeled denture-cleansing solution to prevent warping

The nurse assistant should assist in providing denture care in following ways:
1. Hands should be washed properly.
2. The nurse assist should gather all supplies:
- Washcloth
- Towel
- Gloves
- Paper towels
- Cup
- Emesis basin
- Denture cup
- Disposable mouth sponges
- Regular toothpaste, toothbrush and dental floss if the patient/resident has some natural teeth
- Denture brush or toothbrush
- Denture toothpaste
- Mouthwash
- Lip balm or petroleum jelly and cotton-tipped applicator
3. The nurse assistant should knock, greet the patient/resident and should ensure his/her privacy.
4. The procedure should be explained thoroughly to the patient/resident.
5. Equipment should be adjusted for proper body mechanics and safety: the bed should be raised to a comfortable working height. It should be ensured that the wheels on the bed are locked.
6. The over-bed table should be covered with the paper towels. In the cup, the nurse assistant should prepare a solution of half water and half mouthwash.

7. The patient/resident should be positioned in high Fowler's position.

Removing the denture

8. The towel should be unfolded and should be placed across the patient/resident's chest.
9. The nurse assistant should put on the gloves and placed the dentures, which were removed by the patient/resident, in the emesis basin. If the patient/resident needs assistance removing the denture, the nurse assistant should grasp the denture firmly with his/her thumb and index finger and should use a rocking motion to gently remove the denture. A patient/resident may wear more than one denture (for example, one to replace the lower teeth and one to replace the upper teeth). If necessary, the same process should be repeated to remove the other denture.

Cleaning the denture

10. The nurse assistant should take the emesis basin, the washcloth, the denture cup, the denture brush or toothbrush, the denture toothpaste, and the denture-cleansing tablet (if used) to the sink.
11. The nurse assistant should line the sink with the washcloth or several paper towels.
12. Using a paper towel, it should be turned on the faucet and should adjust the water temperature so that it is cool.
13. The toothbrush should be wet and the denture toothpaste should be applied on it.
14. The sink should be allowed to fill halfway with cool water.
15. If the patient/resident has more than one denture, the nurse assistant should clean only one denture at a time. One denture should be removed from the emesis basin and should be held it in the palm of the hand over the sink. The toothbrush should be used to clean all surfaces of the denture, using circular movements.
16. The denture should be rinsed thoroughly under cool, running water and should be placed in the denture cup.
17. The same process should be repeated to clean other denture.
18. If the patient/resident will not be putting the denture back in the mouth right away, sufficient cool water should be added to the denture cup to cover the denture.
19. The faucet should be turned off with a paper towel.

Providing care for the patient/resident's mouth

20. The nurse assistant should take the denture cup and the emesis basin back to the patient/resident's bedside.
21. The patient/resident should be given a mouthful of the mouthwash mixture to rinse his/her mouth. The emesis basin should be held under the patient/resident's chin to catch the liquid. The patient/resident's mouth and chin should be dried with the towel.
22. The patient/resident should be provided help to clean the roof of the mouth, the inside of the cheeks, under the tongue, the gums, and the lips with mouth sponges dipped in the mouthwash mixture. If the patient/resident has any natural teeth, the nurse assistant should help brush and floss them.
23. Appropriate help should be provided to put the denture back in the patient/resident's mouth.

24. The patient/resident should be encouraged to apply lip balm or petroleum jelly to the lips.
25. It should be ensured the patient/resident's comfort and proper body alignment.
26. Hand should be properly washed, and observations should be reported and recorded at the end of the procedure.

Encouraging comfort and safety

Dentures are the patient/resident's personal property. They are generally costly. The nurse assistant should handle them very carefully. The denture should be labelled with the patient/resident's name and room and bed number. The nurse assistant should report lost or damaged dentures at once. Damaging or losing dentures is negligent conduct.

Many individuals do not like being seen without their dentures. Privacy is the most important thing. Privacy should be ensured when the patient/resident cleans dentures. If the nurse assistant cleans dentures, he/she should return them to the patient/resident as quickly as possible.

Hearing aids

Hearing aids fit behind or inside the ear. They make sounds louder. They do not restore, correct, or cure hearing problems. Hearing aids are usually battery-operated. If the device does not work properly:

- It should be checked if the hearing aid is on. It has an off and on switch.
- The battery position should be checked.
- A new battery should be inserted if needed.
- The hearing aid should be cleaned. The nurse assistant should follow the nurse's directions and the manufacturer's instructions. Hearing aids should be turned off when not in use. And the battery should be removed. Hearing aids are usually costly. It should be handled properly. When not in the ear, it should be stored in its case. The case should be placed in the top drawer of the bedside stand.

An individual with impaired hearing usually uses a hearing aid. Some of the patients/residents may need help inserting or removing their hearing aids, and keeping them clean. The nurse assistant may also need to help the patient/resident to keep the hearing aid clean. It should be ensured that the patient/resident keeps an extra battery on hand, so that the battery may be replaced promptly when needed.

The nurse assistant should assist in inserting and removing a hearing aid in following ways:
1. Hands should be washed properly.
2. The nurse assist should gather all supplies.
3. The nurse assistant should knock, greet the patient/resident and should ensure his/her privacy.
4. The procedure should be explained thoroughly to the patient/resident.
5. Equipment should be adjusted for proper body mechanics and safety: the bed should be raised to a comfortable working height. It should be ensured that the wheels on the bed are locked.

6. Help should be provided to the patient/resident for a comfortable position that allows the nurse assistant to easily access his/her ear.

Inserting the hearing aid

7. It should be ensured that the hearing aid is turned off and the volume is turned down.
8. The nurse assistant should inspect the patient/resident's ear canal for excessive ear wax. If necessary, the ear canal should be gently wiped with a warm, wet washcloth, and then dried.
9. The narrow end of the hearing aid should be gently placed in the patient/resident's ear canal, and then the hearing aid should be rotated so that it follows the curve of the ear. While using one hand to gently pull down on the patient/resident's earlobe, the nurse assistant should use his/her other hand to gently push up and in to seat the hearing aid properly in place.
10. The hearing aid should be turned on and the volume should be adjusted until the patient/resident can hear.

Removing the hearing aid

11. The hearing aid should be turned off.
12. While using one hand to gently pull the top of the patient/resident's ear up, the nurse assistant should use his/her other hand to gently lift the hearing aid up and out of the ear canal.
13. The hearing aid should be placed in its case.
14. It should be ensured the patient/resident's comfort and proper body alignment.
15. Hands should be properly washed, and observations should be reported and recorded at the end of the procedure.

Caring for hearing aid

- The earpiece should be cleaned regularly with saline or the prescribed solution. It should not clean with alcohol.
- Batteries should be checked and replaced regularly. The patient/resident should be taught to have spare batteries on hand at all times.
- The volume should be adjusted to meet the individual's needs.
- The aid should be turned off when the patient/resident is not using it, to preserve the life of the battery.
- Batteries should be removed if the patient/resident will not use the aid for an extended period.
- If a hearing aid is removed from the patient/resident's ear, it should be placed in a plastic bag or other receptacle. The nurse assistant should carefully label it with the patient/resident's name and other pertinent information. The device should be stored in a safe place. It should be ensured that it is specified on the patient/resident's property list.
- The nurse assistant should avoid exposing the aid to moisture and heat.

- The volume should be turned down completely before inserting the aid into the patient/resident's ear.

Helpful Resources

Agrawal, K., & Chauhan, N. (2012). Pressure ulcers: Back to the basics. *Indian Journal of Plastic Surgery, 45*(02), 244-254. https://doi.org/10.4103/0970-0358.101287

Andrade, V. L., & Fernandes, F. A. (2016). Prevention of catheter-associated urinary tract infection: Implementation strategies of international guidelines. *Revista Latino-Americana de Enfermagem, 24*(0). https://doi.org/10.1590/1518-8345.0963.2678

Assadi, F. (2018). Strategies for preventing catheter-associated urinary tract infections. *International Journal of Preventive Medicine, 9*(1), 50. https://doi.org/10.4103/ijpvm.ijpvm_299_17

Baiju, R. (2017). Oral health and quality of life: Current concepts. *JOURNAL OF CLINICAL AND DIAGNOSTIC RESEARCH.* https://doi.org/10.7860/jcdr/2017/25866.10110

Bhattacharya, S., & Mishra, R. K. (2015). Pressure ulcers: Current understanding and newer modalities of treatment. *Indian Journal of Plastic Surgery, 48*(01), 004-016. https://doi.org/10.4103/0970-0358.155260

Cowley, K., & Vanoosthuyze, K. (2012). Insights into shaving and its impact on skin. *British Journal of Dermatology, 166*, 6-12. https://doi.org/10.1111/j.1365-2133.2011.10783.x

Goto, Y., Hayasaka, S., Kurihara, S., & Nakamura, Y. (2018). Physical and mental effects of bathing: A randomized intervention study. *Evidence-Based Complementary and Alternative Medicine, 2018*, 1-5. https://doi.org/10.1155/2018/9521086

Grant, M., McCorkle, R., Hornbrook, M. C., Wendel, C. S., & Krouse, R. (2012). Development of a chronic care ostomy self-management program. *Journal of Cancer Education*, *28*(1), 70-78. https://doi.org/10.1007/s13187-012-0433-1

Kane, D. P. (2013). Surgical management of pressure ulcers. *Pressure Ulcers in the Aging Population*, 99-126. https://doi.org/10.1007/978-1-62703-700-6_7

McNally, M. E., Martin-Misener, R., Wyatt, C. C., McNeil, K. P., Crowell, S. J., Matthews, D. C., & Clovis, J. B. (2012). Action planning for daily mouth care in long-term care: The brushing up on mouth care project. *Nursing Research and Practice*, *2012*, 1-11. https://doi.org/10.1155/2012/368356

Patel, A. (2014). Medical management of urinary incontinence. *Understanding Female Urinary Incontinence and Master Management*, 50-50. https://doi.org/10.5005/jp/books/12104_6

Richards, D. A., Hilli, A., Pentecost, C., Goodwin, V. A., & Frost, J. (2018). Fundamental nursing care: A systematic review of the evidence on the effect of nursing care interventions for nutrition, elimination, mobility and hygiene. *Journal of Clinical Nursing*, *27*(11-12), 2179-2188. https://doi.org/10.1111/jocn.14150

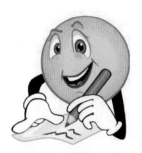

Chapter Nine:

Patient Care Procedures

Outline

I: The Nurse Assistant's role in specimen collection

II: Procedures for bedmaking and maintaining proper body mechanics

III: Types of hospital beds and bed positions

IV: General rules for maintaining the patient/resident's environment

V: The Nurse Assistant's role in administering an enema

VI: The Nurse Assistant's role in giving a suppository

VII: Enteral Nutrition or Tube Feeding

VIII: Nursing care for patients/residents with tube feeding

IX: Nursing care for a patient/resident receiving intravenous (IV) or parenteral therapy

X: The Nursing Assistant's role in maintaining fluid balance

XI: Measuring and recording fluid intake and output

XII: The Nursing Assistant role in applying bandages, binders, and dressings

XIII: The Nursing Assistant role in applying anti-embolic hose/elastic stockings

XIV: The Nurse Assistant's role in the patient/resident's skin care

XV: The Nurse Assistant's role in a patient/resident's admissions

XVI: The Nurse Assistant's role in a patient/resident's transfers

XVII: The Nurse Assistant's role in a patient/resident's discharge

The Nurse Assistant's Role in Specimen Collection

Specimens

Specimens are the samples that are collected and tested to diagnose, prevent, and treat disease. Specimens are usually tested in the laboratory. All specimens sent to the laboratory generally require requisition slips. The slip contains the patient/resident's identifying details and the test ordered. The specimen container should be labeled according to agency policy.

There are some tests that can be done at the bedside. While collecting specimens, these rules should be followed:

- The rules for medical asepsis along with Standard Precautions and the Bloodborne Pathogen Standard should always be followed.
- A clean container must be used for each specimen.
- The correct container should be used for each specimen and the inside of the container or the inside of the lid should not be touched.
- There should be proper identification of the patient/resident by check his/her ID (identification) bracelet against the laboratory requisition slip or assignment sheet.
- The specimen should be collected at the correct time.
- The patient/resident should be asked to void before collecting a stool specimen. The specimen must not contain urine.
- The lid on the specimen container must be secured tightly.
- The specimen container should be placed in a labeled BIOHAZARD plastic bag.
- The specimen and requisition slip should be taken to the laboratory or storage area as per agency policy.

Encouraging comfort and safety

Body fluids, blood, excretions, and secretions may contain pathogenic microorganisms. This includes stool, urine, and sputum specimens. Standard Precautions and the Bloodborne Pathogen Standard should always be followed when collecting, handling, and testing specimens.

Sputum specimens

Sputum specimens are studied for blood, microbes, and abnormal cells. For patients/residents with respiratory disorders, a sputum specimen may be sent to the laboratory for culture or other examination. It is often used to test the presence of the tubercle bacillus, the causative agent for tuberculosis. Often, sputum specimens are collected 3 days in a row. The ideal time to collect a sputum specimen is soon after the patient/resident awakens in the morning (sputum builds up during the night in the airways and expels more easily by coughing in the early morning). The first morning specimen is considered to be the most accurate. The sputum specimen should be collected before the patient/resident eats, brushes the teeth, or uses mouthwash. The inside of the specimen container should be kept sterile to ensure that organisms cultured from the sputum specimen are contained in the specimen and not be an outcome of a contaminated container. The cover on the container should be kept tight as much as possible to prevent contamination by particles in the air and to prevent the spread of organisms outward from the sputum specimen. When the cover is removed, the cover should be placed on the counter or table with the inside up. The inside of the container is considered to be sterile, and the outside is considered as contaminated. The physician may write an order to measure sputum. If so, it can be done in one of two ways:

1. If enough sputum is obtained in a graduated specimen container, the amount of the specimen should be read directly. OR

2. An equal amount of water should be poured into an identical container to measure the water.

In addition, the following points should also be kept in mind:

- The specimen should be weighed, if ordered. It should be weighed on a balance scale, subtracting the initial weight of the container.

- The specimen should be taken to the laboratory immediately after collection. A delay may change the result of a culture.

- The container should be labeled appropriately and the laboratory personnel should be notified about sputum specimen. It should be ensured that the proper requests are in place.

- The sputum's amount (copious, moderate, and small), color, and consistency should be documented appropriately.

Assisting with collecting a sputum specimen

The nurse assistant should provide assistance for collecting a sputum specimen in following ways:

1. Hands should be washed properly.
2. The nurse assist should gather all supplies:
- gloves and tissues
- Laboratory requisition slip
- Sputum specimen container and lid
- Specimen label
- Plastic bag
- BIOHAZARD label (if needed)
3. The nurse assistant should knock, greet the patient/resident and should ensure his/her privacy.
4. The procedure should be explained thoroughly to the patient/resident.
5. Equipment should be adjusted for proper body mechanics and safety: the bed should be raised to a comfortable working height. It should be ensured that the wheels on the bed are locked.
6. The nurse assistant should put on gloves.
7. The patient/resident should be asked to rinse the mouth out with clear water.

8. The patient/resident should hold the container. Only the outside of the container should be touched.
9. The patient/resident should be asked to cover the mouth and nose with tissues when coughing. Agency policy should be followed for used tissues.
10. The patient/resident should be asked to take 2 or 3 breaths and cough up the sputum.
11. The patient/resident should expectorate directly into the container. It should be remembered that sputum should not touch the outside of the container.
12. 1 to 2 teaspoons of sputum should be collected unless told to collect more.
13. The lid should be put on the container.
14. The container should be placed in the plastic bag. A BIOHAZARD label should be applied according to agency policy.
15. The specimen and the requisition slip should be delivered to laboratory or storage area according to agency policy.
16. It should be ensured the patient/resident's comfort and proper body alignment.
17. Hand should be properly washed, and observations should be reported and recorded at the end of the procedure.

Encouraging comfort and safety

The physician may order isolation precautions if the patient/resident has or may have tuberculosis (TB). The nurse assistant should protect himself/herself by wearing a TB respirator.

Urine specimens

Urine is the body's liquid waste product. It has typical physical and microscopic characteristics that are excellent indicators of an individual's state of health. Collecting and examining urine may provide significant information about an individual's health. The urine specimen ate tested for diagnosis of diseases and monitoring of the patient/resident's recovery or decline, assessment of liver or/and kidney status, presence of legal and illegal drugs, pregnancy, and identification of specific disease-causing agents.

A routine urine specimen is collected by having the patient/resident void directly into the specimen container, or by pouring urine from a bedpan, urinal, or urine drainage bag into a specimen container.

Promoting safety and comfort

Urine specimens may embarrass some patients/residents. They usually don't like clear specimen containers that show urine. It can be helpful to place the clear specimen container in a paper bag. A paper towel or washcloth may be used to wrap around the container.

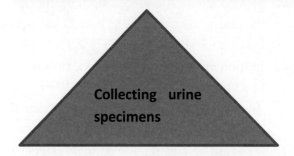

Collecting urine specimens

There are three methods of collecting a urine specimen i.e. random urine collection, clean catch (midstream) urine collection, and 24-hour urine collection.

Each method is ordered for a specific purpose, so only the ordered method should be used for collecting urine specimens.

Random urine specimen

The random urine specimen is collected for routine urinalysis. There are no special measures needed for collecting a random urine specimen. It may be collected any time during a 24-hour period. Many patients/residents can collect the specimen themselves. Weak and very ill patients/residents may need help.

Assisting with collecting a random urine specimen

The nurse assistant should provide assistance for collecting a random urine specimen in following ways:

1. Hands should be washed properly.
2. The nurse assist should gather all supplies:
   - Laboratory requisition slip
   - Specimen container and lid
   - Voiding device—bedpan and cover, urinal, commode, or specimen pan
   - Specimen label
   - Plastic bag
   - BIOHAZARD label (if needed)
   - Gloves
   - Graduated cylinder
3. The nurse assistant should knock, greet the patient/resident and should ensure his/her privacy.
4. The procedure should be explained thoroughly to the patient/resident.
5. The collected items should be arranged in the patient/resident's bathroom.
6. The patient/resident should be asked to void into the device. The nurse assistant should remind him/her to put toilet tissue into the wastebasket or toilet. Toilet tissue should not be put in the bedpan or specimen pan.
7. The voiding device should be taken to the bathroom.
8. About 120 mL (4 oz) should be poured into the specimen container.
9. The lid should be placed tight on the specimen container. The container should be put in the plastic bag. A BIOHAZARD label should be applied according to agency policy.
10. Urine should be measured if I&O are ordered.
11. Equipment should be emptied, rinsed, cleaned, disinfected, dried, and should be returned to its proper place.
12. The specimen and the requisition slip should be delivered to laboratory or storage area according to agency policy.
13. It should be ensured the patient/resident's comfort and proper body alignment.
14. Hand should be properly washed, and observations should be reported and recorded at the end of the procedure.

Clean catch (midstream) urine specimen

A midstream (clean catch) urine specimen is collected when the patient/resident is thought to have an infection e.g. urinary tract infection. A midstream or clean catch specimen can be collected while the patient/resident is using the toilet, portable commode, urinal, or bedpan. Before the patient/resident starts to void, the opening of the urethra should be cleaned to remove any microbes in the area. The patient/resident then starts to void (not in the container), then stops, and then voids into the container. The initial flow of urine washes away microorganisms that might be around the urethral opening. These steps may help to avoid contamination of the urine sample with microorganisms other than the ones causing the infection, providing more accurate test results.

Assisting with collecting a midstream specimen

The nurse assistant should provide assistance for collecting a midstream urine specimen in following ways:

1. Hands should be washed properly.
2. The nurse assist should gather all supplies:
-   Laboratory requisition slip
-   Midstream specimen kit—specimen container, label, towelettes, sterile gloves
-   Plastic bag
-   Sterile gloves if not part of the kit
-   Disposable gloves
-   BIOHAZARD label (if needed)
-   Graduated cylinder
-   Voiding device—bedpan and cover, urinal, commode, or specimen pan if needed
-   Supplies for perineal care
-   Paper towels
3. The nurse assistant should knock, greet the patient/resident and should ensure his/her privacy.
4. The procedure should be explained thoroughly to the patient/resident.
5. The collected items should be arranged in the patient/resident's bathroom.
6. The nurse assistant should wear gloves and provide perineal care:
-   **For a female**
a) The perineal area should be cleaned with towelettes.
b) The nurse assistant should spread the labia with thumb and index finger and clean down the urethral area from front to back.
c) A clean towelette should be used for each stroke.
d) The labia should be kept separated to collect the urine specimen.
-   **For a male**
a) The penis should be cleaned with towelettes.
b) The nurse assistant should hold the penis with non-dominant hand and clean the penis starting at the meatus.
c) It should be cleaned in a circular motion, starting at the center and working outward.
d) The nurse assistant should keep holding the penis until the specimen is collected.

7. The sterile specimen container should be opened and the lid should be set down so the inside is up.
8. The patient/resident should be asked to void into a device.
9. The specimen container should be passed into the urine stream. The labia should be kept separated and about 30 to 60 mL (1 to 2 oz) of urine should be collected.
10. The specimen container should be removed before the patient/resident stops voiding.
11. The labia or penis should be released and the patient/resident should be allowed to finish voiding into the device.
12. The lid should be put on the specimen container. The outside of the container should be wiped.
13. The nurse assistant should provide toilet tissue to the patient/resident when he/she is done voiding.
14. The voiding device should be taken to the bathroom.
15. The container should be put in the plastic bag. A BIOHAZARD label should be applied according to agency policy.
16. Urine should be measured if I&O are ordered.
17. Equipment should be emptied, rinsed, cleaned, disinfected, dried, and should be returned to its proper place.
18. The specimen and the requisition slip should be delivered to laboratory or storage area according to agency policy.
19. It should be ensured the patient/resident's comfort and proper body alignment.
20. Hand should be properly washed, and observations should be reported and recorded at the end of the procedure.

24-hour urine specimen

A 24-hour urine specimen is collected and obtained over 24 consecutive hours. To collect a 24-hour urine specimen, the patient/resident should empty his/her bladder. The urine should be discarded, and the time should be noted. For the next 24 hours, each time the patient/resident voids, the nurse assistant should collect the urine and transfer it to the specimen container. At the end of the 24-hour time period, the patient/resident should void one last time and add this urine to the specimen container. During the 24-hour urine collection period, the nurse assistant should make sure to label and store the specimen container according to his/her employer's policy.

For the 24-hour urine specimen, all urine voided during a 24-hour period is collected. Urine should be chilled on ice or refrigerated during this time to prevent the growth of microbes. For various tests, a preservative may be added to the collection container. The patient/resident voids to begin the test with an empty bladder. The nurse assistant should discard this voiding. All voidings should be saved for the next 24 hours. The test should be restarted if:

- A voiding was not saved.

- The specimen contains stools.
- Toilet tissue was discarded into the specimen.

Testing urine: Observations

The physician orders for the frequency and type of urine tests. The nurse may ask a nurse assistant to do these simple tests.

- **Testing for pH**: Urine pH is measured to test whether urine is acidic or alkaline. Changes in normal pH (4.6 to 8.0) may be resulted from food, illness, and medications.

- **Testing for blood**: Disease and Injury can cause hematuria i.e. blood (hemat) in the urine (uria). Sometimes blood is clearly observed in the urine. At other times it is not observed (occult).

- **Testing for glucose and ketones**: In diabetes patients, the pancreas does not release enough insulin. The body requires insulin to utilize sugar for energy. If not used, sugar may build up in the blood and may appear in the urine.

.

Glucosuria and ketonuria

Glucosuria (glycosuria) means sugar (glucos, glycos) in the urine (uria).The diabetic patients may also have ketones in the urine. Ketones (ketone bodies, acetone) are substances that often appear in urine from the breakdown of fat for energy. The body uses fat for energy utilization if it cannot use sugar. Tests for ketones and glucose are usually done 4 times a day (30 minutes before each meal and at bedtime). The physician uses the test to make drug and diet decisions.

Using urine dipsticks (Reagent Strips)

Dipsticks (Reagent strips) have sections that can change color on their reaction with urine. To use a reagent strip:

- The nurse assistant should not touch the test area on the strip.
- The strip should be dipped into urine.
- The strip should be compared with the color chart on the bottle.

Encouraging comfort and safety

The nurse assistant must be accurate when testing urine and should promptly report the results to the nurse. Ordered medications may depend on the results. When using reagent strips:

- The color of the reagent strips should be checked carefully. Discolored strips should not be used.
- The expiration date should be checked on the bottle. The strips should not be used if the date has passed.
- The nurse assistant should follow the manufacturer's instructions. Otherwise he/she could get the wrong results. The physician uses the test results in diagnosing and managing the patient/resident. A wrong result may cause serious harm.

Stool specimens

Stools are studied for microorganisms, worms, fat, blood, and other abnormal contents. Extreme care must be taken to make sure that urine must not contaminate the stool specimen. The patient/resident should use one device for voiding and another for bowel movements. Some tests need a warm stool. The specimen should be taken at once to the laboratory or storage area as per agency policy.

Promoting safety and comfort

Stools normally have a characteristic odor. A patient/resident may be embarrassed that someone needs to collect his/her stool specimen. The nurse assistant should complete the task quickly and carefully. Also he/she should act in a professional manner.

Assisting with collecting a stool specimen

The nurse assistant should provide assistance for collecting a stool specimen in following ways:

1. Hands should be washed properly.
2. The nurse assist should gather all supplies:

- Laboratory requisition slip
- Specimen pan for the toilet
- Specimen container and lid
- Specimen label
- Tongue blades
- Disposable bag
- Plastic bag
- BIOHAZARD label (if needed)
- Device for voiding—bedpan and cover, urinal, commode, or specimen pan
- Toilet tissue
- Paper towels

3. The nurse assistant should knock, greet the patient/resident and should ensure his/her privacy.
4. The procedure should be explained thoroughly to the patient/resident.
5. The collected items should be arranged in the patient/resident's bathroom.
6. The patient/resident should be asked to void. The nurse assistant should provide the voiding device if the patient/resident does not use the bathroom.
7. The specimen pan should be put on the toilet if the patient/resident needs to use the bathroom. It should be placed at the back of the toilet.
8. The patient/resident should be asked not to put toilet tissue into the commode, bedpan, or specimen pan. A bag should be provided for toilet tissue if the patient/resident uses the bedpan or commode.
9. The call light and toilet tissue should be placed within patients/resident's reach. Bed rails should be raised or lowered and the care plan should be followed.
10. The nurse assistant should note the amount, color, consistency, and odor of stools.
11. The specimen should be collected as:

- A tongue blade should be used to take about 2 tablespoons of stool to the specimen container. The sample should be taken from the middle of a formed stool.
- The nurse assistant should include mucus, pus, or blood present in the stool.
- The stool must be taken from two different places in the BM if required by agency policy.
- The lid should be put on the specimen container.

254

12. The container should be put in the plastic bag. A BIOHAZARD label should be applied according to agency policy.
13. Equipment should be emptied, rinsed, cleaned, disinfected, dried, and should be returned to its proper place.
14. The specimen and the requisition slip should be delivered to laboratory or storage area according to agency policy.
15. It should be ensured the patient/resident's comfort and proper body alignment.
16. Hand should be properly washed, and observations should be reported and recorded at the end of the procedure.

Bedmaking Procedures

A fresh and clean bed is important to almost everyone. It is especially important to residents who spend most of their time in bed. Nursing assistants are responsible for ensuring that the patient/resident in their care have dry and clean linens at all times. The frequency with which a nurse assistant changes bed linens depends on how much time the patient/resident spends in bed, and it also depends on employer's policies. In most healthcare settings, linens are routinely changed in the morning, after bathing, dressing, and when grooming are completed. But the time of day for changing linens may also vary according to the needs of the patient/resident.

One universal rule to follow is that "All linens must be changed immediately if they are wet or soiled" because soiled and wet linens may cause skin irritation that can lead to pressure sores.

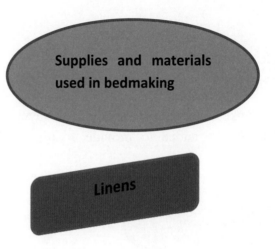

Supplies and materials used in bedmaking

Linens

There are the following types of linens that can be used to make a bed:

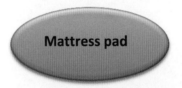

Mattress pad

The mattress pad is an absorbent and thick pad that is used to cushion the mattress. Because the mattress pad is thick and absorbent, it also protects the mattress from becoming wet and soiled. The mattress pad may be fitted or flat. Fitted mattress pads contain elastic edges that fit over the mattress to hold the mattress pad in proper place.

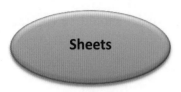

Sheets

A top sheet and a bottom sheet are used to make the bed. Often, in most of healthcare settings, both sheets are flat, although the bottom sheet may be fitted. When a flat sheet is used as a bottom sheet, the nurse assistant must miter the corners to hold the sheet in place.

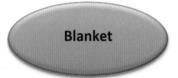

Blanket

A blanket is a heavier and thicker layer that can be added to provide additional warmth.

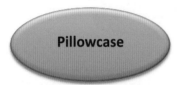

Pillowcase

A pillowcase may be used to cover the pillow and protect it from becoming wet and soiled.

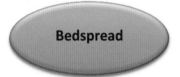

Bedspread

A bedspread is the finishing layer that covers and protects the linens underneath when the bed is not being used. It provides another layer for warmth when the patient/resident is in the bed.

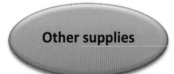

Other supplies

Depending on the procedure and the needs of the patient/resident, the nurse assistant may need additional supplies for bedmaking as well, such as:

Bath blanket

It is a lightweight flannel sheet that is used to provide warmth and privacy when performing personal care procedures (such as a linen change or bed bath with the patient/resident still in the bed). The bath blanket is draped over the patient/resident to minimize exposure during the procedure.

Draw (lift) sheet

It is a half-sized sheet that is placed over the middle of the bottom sheet and can be used to assist with repositioning the patient/resident in bed. The draw sheet extends from the patient/resident's shoulders to his/her thighs.

Bed protector

It is an absorbent pad that wicks moisture away from the patient/resident's body. A bed protector can be placed on top of the bottom sheet when a patient/resident has incontinent of urine, and has a heavily draining wound or is perspiring heavily.

Foam pads

Eggcrate foam pads or solid foam pads may be placed over the mattress for comfort. These pads may be dangerous, because they tend to slip. When making the bed of a patient/resident who uses a foam pad, it should make sure to cover the pad with a sheet and tuck the edges of the sheet tightly to minimize the risk of slipping. Extra caution should be taken when moving the patient/resident around in the bed or assisting the patient/resident to get out of the bed when one of these pads is in place, because of the tendency of the pad to slip. When the pad becomes wet and soiled, it must be replaced or cleaned according to facility policy.

Alternating-pressure pads

These pads work in much the same way as an alternating-pressure bed. An alternating-pressure pad may be used when a patient/resident is at high risk for developing pressure sores. Just as with a foam pad, there is an increased risk of slipping when an alternating-pressure pad is in place.

Foot board

It is a padded board that can be placed against the patient/resident's feet when he/she is in bed to keep his/her feet at right angles to the legs, with the toes pointed upward. The foot board can be used to maintain a position that will prevent foot drop.

Bed cradle

It is a frame that keeps the top bed linens from rubbing against and putting pressure on the tops of the patient/resident's feet, legs, and toes. The top linens are usually placed on the bed over the bed cradle.

Role of the nurse assistant to make a bed

The nurse assistant must take infection control measures when making beds in a healthcare setting. When making beds in a healthcare setting, the nurse assistant can save time and energy by:

- Stacking and gathering bed linens in the order, so that the mattress pad is on the top.
- Folding reusable linens, such as spreads and blankets, and putting them in a clean place, such as over the back of a chair, until the nurse assistant is ready to put them back on the bed.
- Checking the bed for personal objects, such as dentures and eyeglasses, before removing the linens from the bed.
- Making one side of the bed at a time. Working on one side of the bed at a time may help to prevent a nurse assistant from reaching across the bed, which is significant for good body mechanics. The bed should be raised to a comfortable working height so that a nurse assistant does not have to stoop and bend.

To practice infection control when making a bed, the nurse assistant should make sure to follow these precautions:

- The linens should be taken into the patient/resident's room. In a healthcare setting, once linens have been taken into a patient/resident's room, they cannot be used for another patient/resident, and they have to be laundered, even if they were not used.
- Clean linens should be placed on a clean surface, such as the over-bed table or a chair. Clean linens should not be placed on the floor.
- Soiled linens should be put directly in the linen hamper. Soiled linens should never be placed on the floor.
- Linens should be removed and replaced carefully, without shaking them. Shaking linens may cause air currents that can spread dust and microorganisms around the room.

- Linens (clean and soiled) should be kept away from the uniform.
- Glove should be worn when removing soiled linens from the bed.

After removing the gloves, the nurse assistant should wash his/her hands before touching the clean linens. If the bed has side rails, the nurse assistant can raise the side rail on the opposite side of the bed. Bedmaking is an opportunity for a nurse assistant to spend some time in conversation with the patient/resident in his/her care.

Preparing the bed for the patient/resident

After making the bed, the nurse assistant may need to prepare it for the patient/resident who will be using it. If the patient/resident will not be getting back into the bed right away, the nurse assistant may prepare a closed bed. A closed bed is generally a bed that is made, but not occupied. The bedspread should be pulled up to cover the linens, protecting them from becoming wet and soiled, and providing the bed a neat appearance. When a nurse assistant knows a patient/resident will be getting into the bed soon, he/she should "open" the bed. An open bed is one where the blanket, bedspread, and top sheet have been folded back toward the bottom of the bed, making it easier for the patient/resident to get into the bed. A surgical bed is a specific type of open bed that is prepared for a patient/resident who will be arriving on a stretcher. To prepare a surgical bed, the blanket, bedspread, and top sheet are fanfolded to the side of the bed, instead of to the bottom.

Beds should be made every day. Dry, clean, and wrinkle-free linens are used to:
- Promote comfort
- Prevent skin breakdown
- Prevent pressure sores

Beds are generally made in the morning after baths. They can be made while the patient/resident is in the shower, up in the chair, or out of the room. For keeping beds neat and clean:
- Linens should be changed when they are soiled, wet, or damp.
- Linens should be straightened when loose or wrinkled and at bedtime.
- Foods and crumbs should be checked and removed after meals and snacks.
- Linens should be checked for eyeglasses, dentures, sharp objects, hearing aids, and other items.
- Standard Precautions and the Bloodborne Pathogen Standard should be followed.

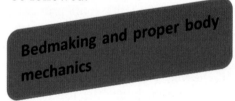

Bedmaking and proper body mechanics

Nursing assistants should require proper body mechanics to make a bed, in order to prevent fatigue and injury. They should know their limitations and should not attempt to turn, lift, or move a patient/resident alone if they have any doubts about their ability to turn, lift, or move a patient/resident alone.

Below guideline should be followed while making beds for body mechanics:
- The nurse assistant should not lean over a patient/resident to provide care. The nurse assistant should get close to sides of bed and should not make beds from the head of bed or foot positions.

- The bed should be elevated so that a nurse assistant can work at a safe and comfortable height.
- Wheels of the bed, stretcher, or wheelchair should be locked so that they do not slide while moving the patient/resident.
- The principles of proper body mechanics should be followed to prevent personal injury while working.
- The patient/resident's body should be supported well. The nurse assistant should avoid holding and grabbing an extremity by its muscles.
- The nurse assistant should keep his/her back straight and knees bent. The feet should be kept apart to provide a broader support base. The nurse assistant should keep his/her body in good alignment with a wide base of support.
- An upright posture should be used, which involve bending the legs. The back should not be bended to maintain an upright posture.
- Widening the base of support to pull or push is an important component of proper body mechanics. A person should move his/her front leg forward when pushing and he/she should move his/her rear leg back when pulling.
- The nurse assistant should face in the direction he/she is working at the side of the bed and should raise bed to comfortable height.

Types of Hospital Beds and Bed Positions

Hospital beds are especially constructed and designed to provide comfort, safety, and mobility for a wide range of patients/residents with varying conditions and treatment plans. The versatility and adaptability of hospital beds and related safety devices permit nursing assistants including caregivers to meet the diverse requirements of their patients/residents. Hospital beds can be operated manually or electrically:

Manual hospital beds

The height and positions of the manual bed is controlled manually, using a crank. Therefore, anytime if someone wants to change the position of the bed, there is manual effort required. Manual bed is the best for patients/residents who do not require constant position changing. It should be remembered that there are several manual beds that don't have the same range of positions as an electrical bed, so if the patient/resident needs to be put in many different positions, an electrical hospital would be a better option. The manual bed is generally a lot cheaper, so it is definitely the most economical way to go.

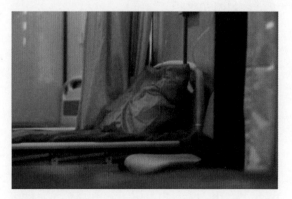

Manual hospital beds are usually operated by hand cranks situated at the bottom of the bed.

Manual beds may contain one, two or three gatches and will have one crank for each gatch.

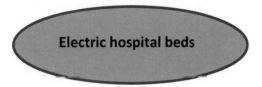
Electric hospital beds

It is a special bed that is plugged into an outlet and controlled with a remote that is usually attached to the side of the bed. In electric bed, all the different positions can be changed very easily. Therefore, it eliminates the need for any manual effort. In addition to the control over the head and feet, the height of a full electric bed can be easily adjusted with the push of a button. It may be important if the patient/resident needs the bed to be lowered to make it safer to get out and in the bed, and then raised again to permit caregivers to reach the patient easily.

Electric beds are the best options for patients/residents who spend most of their time in bed and benefit from regular changes in position for therapeutic or comfort purposes.

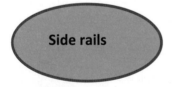
Side rails

Hospital beds often have side rails that can be lowered or raised. These side rails, which serve as protection for the patient/resident and can make the patient/resident feel more secure, may also include the buttons used for their operation to move the bed, to call the nurse, or even to control the television.

There are several types of side rails to serve multiple different purposes. While some side rails are simply used to prevent patient falls; however, many others have equipment that can support the patients/residents themselves without physically confining the patient/resident to bed.

Beds can be made in these ways.
1. A closed bed is not in use; therefore, top linens should not be folded back. The bed should be ready for a new patient or resident. In nursing centers, closed beds are usually made for residents who are up during the day.
2. An open bed is a type of bed that is in use. Top linens should be fan-folded back. A closed bed becomes an open bed by fan-folding back the top linens.
3. An occupied bed is a type of the bed that is made with the patient/resident in it.
4. A surgical bed is made to transfer a patient/resident from a stretcher to bed. This may include an ambulance stretcher.

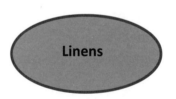
Linens

Linens should be collected in the order the nurse assistant will use them, such as:
- Mattress pad (if needed)
- Bottom sheet (fitted or flat)
- Waterproof pad or waterproof drawsheet (if needed)
- Cotton drawsheet (if needed)
- Top sheet
- Blanket
- Bedspread
- Pillowcases
- Bath towels
- Hand towel

- Washcloth
- Gown or pajamas
- Bath blanket

One arm should be used to hold the linens. The nurse assistant should use his/her other hand to pick them up. The first item should be at the bottom of the stack i.e. the mattress pad should be at the bottom and the bath blanket should be on top. To get the mattress pad on top, the nurse assistant should place his/her arm over the bath blanket and then turn the stack over onto the arm on the bath blanket. The arm that held the linens is now free. The clean linen should be placed on a clean surface. Dirty linen should be removed as one piece at a time.

Each piece should be rolled away from the nurse assistant. The side that touched the patient/resident should be inside the roll and away from the nurse assistant. Each piece should be discarded into a laundry bag. In healthcare settings, top and bottom sheets, the cotton drawsheet, and pillowcases are usually changed daily. If still clean, the mattress pad, waterproof drawsheet, blanket, and bedspread should only be re-used for the same patient/resident. In nursing centers, linens are generally not changed every day. A complete linen change is usually done on the patient/resident's shower day. This can be once or twice a week. Pillowcases, top and bottom sheets and drawsheets (if used) can be changed twice a week. Linens should not be re-used if wet, soiled, or wrinkled. Damp, wet, or soiled linens should be changed right away. Gloves should be worn and the nurse assistant should always follow Standard Precautions and the Bloodborne Pathogen Standard.

Waterproof pads and drawsheets

Waterproof Pads and Drawsheets absorb moisture and protect the skin. A drawsheet is a smaller sheet that is usually placed over the middle of the bottom sheet.

- A cotton drawsheet is made of cotton, which keeps the mattress and bottom linens clean.
- A waterproof drawsheet is a drawsheet made of rubber, plastic, or absorbent material. It protects the bottom linens and mattress from dampness and soiling.

Some linens have rubber or plastic on one side—the waterproof side. The waterproof side is placed down, away from the patient/resident. The other side is cotton, which is placed up, toward the patient/resident. Most waterproof drawsheets are disposable. They should be discarded when soiled, wet, or wrinkled. The cotton drawsheet protects the patient/resident from contact with plastic or rubber and absorbs moisture. Rubber and plastic retain heat.

Waterproof drawsheets are generally hard to keep tight and wrinkle-free. Discomfort and skin breakdown may occur. Many agencies also use incontinence products to keep the patient/resident and linens dry. Plastic-covered mattresses may cause some patients/residents to perspire, which may cause more discomfort. A cotton drawsheet minimizes heat retention and absorbs moisture. Cotton drawsheets are often used as assist devices to transfer and move the patient/resident in bed. If used as an assist device, the nurse assistant should leave the sides untucked if allowed by agency policy.

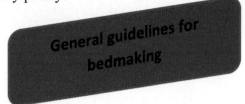

General guidelines for bedmaking

- Proper body mechanics should be used at all times.
- The nurse assistant should follow the rules to safely move and transfer the patient/resident.
- The nurse assistant should also follow the rules of medical asepsis.
- Standard Precautions and the Bloodborne Pathogen Standard should always be followed.
- Proper hand hygiene should be practiced before handling clean linen.
- Enough linen should be brought to the patient/resident's room. Clean linen should be placed on a clean surface. The nurse assistant should use the bedside chair, over-bed table, or bedside stand. A barrier (towel, paper towel) should be placed between the clean surface and the linen if required by agency policy.
- Extra linen should not be used in the patient/resident's room for another resident. Extra linen is generally considered contaminated and should be put with the dirty laundry.
- Torn or frayed linen should not be used.
- Linen should not be shaked. Shaking may spread microbes.
- Linens should be held away from the body and uniform.
- The nurse assistant should wear gloves to remove linen. Linens may contain body fluids, blood, secretions, or excretions. Proper hand hygiene should be practiced after removing the gloves.
- Dirty linens should never be put on the floor or on clean linens. The nurse assistant should always follow agency policy for dirty linen.
- The nurse assistant should keep bottom linens tucked in and wrinkle-free.
- A waterproof drawsheet should be covered with a cotton drawsheet. Rubber or plastic must not touch the patient/resident's body.
- Loose sheets, blankets, and bedspreads should be straightened and tightened as needed.
- Wet, damp, or soiled linens should be changed right away.

Encouraging safety and comfort

Safety

The nurse assistant needs to raise the bed for proper body mechanics. The bed must also be flat. If the bed is locked, the nurse assistant should unlock it and return it to the proper position. The nurse assistant should wear gloves to remove linen. He/she must also follow other aspects of Standard Precautions and the Bloodborne Pathogen Standard. Linens may contain body fluids, blood, secretions, or excretions. After making a bed, the bed should be lowered to the correct level for the patient/resident. For an occupied bed, bed rails should be raised or lowered according to the care plan.

Comfort

For an occupied bed, the patient/resident should be covered with a bath blanket before removing the top sheet. The patient/resident should not be left uncovered. The bath blanket provides privacy and warmth. The nurse assistant should adjust the patient/resident's pillow as needed during the procedure. After the procedure, the patient/resident should be positioned as directed by the nurse and the care plan. The nurse assistant should always make sure that linens are straight and wrinkle-free.

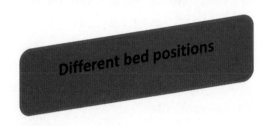
Different bed positions

Fowler's position

It is a semi-sitting position. The head of the bed is generally raised between 45 and 60 degrees. The knees can be elevated slightly. For good alignment:

- The spine should be straight.
- The head should be supported with a small pillow.
- The arms should be supported with pillows.

The nurse assistant may place small pillows under the thighs, lower back, and ankles of the patient/resident. Patients/residents with respiratory and heart disorders usually breathe much easier in Fowler's position.

Semi-Fowler's position

It is position is a position in which patients/residents are lying on their back with the head and torso raised between 15 and 45 degrees. The most common and frequently used bed angle for this position is 30 degrees.

The Semi-Fowler's position is commonly used for purposes same to those of the Fowler's position, including lung expansion, feeding, cardiac or respiratory conditions, and for patients/residents with a nasogastric tube.

Trendelenburg's position

In the Trendelenburg's position or head-down position, the body is laid flat or supine on the back with the feet elevated above the head. The Trendelenburg position is often used in surgery, especially of the genitourinary system and abdomen. It permits better access to the pelvic organs due to gravitational pull of the intra-abdominal organs away from the pelvis.

Reverse Trendelenburg's position (head elevated)

In Reverse Trendelenburg's or head elevated position, head is kept higher than feet. Pillow should be placed between the patient/resident's feet and footboard of bed. This position is used to facilitate tube feedings, and emergency treatment in head injury and severe bleeding

High position

High position promotes and encourages the health care workers to apply proper body mechanics when providing care to patients/residents, when making beds, or moving patients/residents to stretchers.

Low position

It is the position that is used to encourage the ambulatory patient/resident to get out and in the bed with safely and easily.

General Rules for Maintaining the Patient/Resident's Environment

- The nurse assistant should make sure that the patient/resident can reach

- bedside stand and overbed table comfortably.
- Personal belongings should be arranged in the way that patient/resident prefers. The patient/resident safety should be kept in mind and within easy reach for him/her.
- Environment should be kept clean.
- The call light should be placed within the patient/resident's reach at all times.
- The nurse assistant should meet the needs of patients/residents who cannot use the call system.
- It should be ensured that the patient/resident can reach the over-bed table and the bedside stand.
- Personal items should be arranged as the patient/resident prefers. They should be within easy reach.
- The nurse assistant should place the phone, TV, bed, and light controls within the patient/resident's reach.
- Enough tissues and toilet paper should be provided to the patient/resident.
- The nurse assistant should adjust lighting, temperature, and ventilation for the patient/resident's comfort.
- Equipment should be handled carefully to prevent noise.
- The causes of strange noises should be explained to patients/residents.
- Room deodorizers should be used according to agency policy.
- Wastebaskets should be emptied at least once a day. In some agencies, they are usually emptied every shift. They should always be emptied when full.

- The nurse assistant should respect the patient/resident's belongings. An item may not seem important to a nurse assistant. But even a scrap of paper may mean a great deal to the patient/resident.
- The nurse assistant should not throw away any items that belong to the patient/resident.
- The nurse should not move furniture or the patient/resident's items. Patients/residents with poor vision rely on memory or feel to find items.
- Bed linens and towels should be straightened as often as needed.
- A safety check should be completed before leaving the room.

The Nurse Assistant's Role in Administering an Enema

Assisting with enemas

Enema is the introduction of fluid into the rectum and lower colon through the anus to remove feces from the bowel.

Physicians order enemas to:
- Remove feces.
- Relieve constipation, flatulence, or fecal impaction.
- Clean the bowel of feces before diagnostic procedures and certain surgeries.

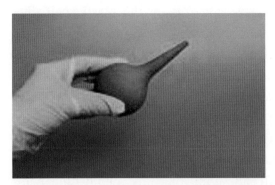

Licensed nurses are usually responsible for administering enemas; however, nurse assistants with the proper training may be allowed to administer enemas in some facilities. The nurse assistant should always act within his/her scope of practice.

If a nurse assistant responsible for administering an enema, he/she should follow the written orders exactly and should know what type of enema was ordered, and how many times the patient/resident is allowed to receive enema within a provided period of time. If the patient/resident complains of pain while administering an enema, the procedure should be stopped and waited until the pain goes away. If the pain continues, the nurse assistant should stop and report the situation to the nurse.

Encouraging safety and comfort

Safety
Enema is generally a safe procedure. Many individuals an administer enemas themselves at home. However, enemas are dangerous for older people and those with certain kidney and heart diseases.

Comfort
Before starting the procedure, the nurse assistant should make sure the bathroom is ready for the patient/resident's use. If the patient/resident will use the commode or bedpan, the nurse assistant should ready the device. A bedpan should always be kept nearby in case the patient/resident starts to expel the enema solution and stools. Mental comfort should be promoted when the patient/resident knows the bathroom, commode, or bedpan is ready for use. The patient/resident needs to retain the solution as long as possible. The nurse assistant should make sure that the patient/resident is comfortable in the Sims' or left side-lying position. When comfortable, it is easier to tolerate the procedure. To prevent abdominal cramping:

- The correct water temperature should be used as cool water may cause cramping.
- The solution should be administered slowly.

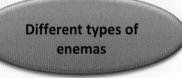

Different types of enemas

There are different types of enemas. Commercially prepared enemas are available in pre-filled plastic bottles with a tip that is designed to be inserted into the anus. Alternatively, an enema may also be administered using an enema bag and tubing. An enema bag and tubing are generally used to administer soap solution or tap water enemas. The bag is filled with tap water and a small amount of a castile soap (for a soap solution enema) or warm tap water (for a tap water enema). The nurse assistant should always follow the written orders exactly regarding the amount of water to be used while preparing the enema solution. He/she should also make sure that the enema solution has the proper temperature of around105° F. If the solution is too cold, the patient/resident may experience pain and cramping. A solution that is too hot may cause more serious injury.

1. The Cleansing Enema

Cleansing enemas clean the bowel of flatus and feces. They can relieve constipation and fecal impaction. They are needed before certain diagnostic procedures and surgeries. Cleansing enemas may effect in 10 to 20 minutes. The physician orders a tap water, saline, or soapsuds enema. The physician may order enemas until the return solution is clear and free of stools. The nurse assistant may allow repeating enemas 2 or 3 times according to agency policy.

2. The Small Volume Enema

Small-volume enemas distend and irritate the rectum to stimulate a bowel movement. They are generally ordered for relieving constipation or when the bowel does not need complete cleansing. These enemas are ready to administer. The solution is generally administered at room temperature. To administer the small-volume enema, the nurse assistant should squeeze and roll up the plastic container from the bottom. Pressure should not be released on the bottle. Otherwise, solution can be drawn from the rectum back into the bottle. The patient/resident should be urged to retain the solution until he or she needs to have a bowel movement. It may take about 5 to 10 minutes. Staying in the left side-lying or Sims' or position helps retain the enema.

3. The Oil-Retention Enema

Oil-retention enemas are administered to relieve constipation and fecal impaction. The oil should be retained for 30 to 60 minutes or longer (1 to 3 hours). Retaining oil may soften feces and lubricate the rectum. This lets feces to pass with more ease. Most oil retention enemas are prepared commercially. Administering an oil-retention enema is just like administering a small volume enema. After administering an oil-retention enema:

- The patient/resident should be left in the Sims' or left side-lying position and should be covered for warmth.
- The patient/resident should be urged to retain the enema for the time ordered.
- Extra waterproof pads should be placed on the bed if needed.
- The patient/resident should be checked as often while he or she retains the enema.

Administering an enema
The nurse assistant should administer an enema to a patient/resident in following ways:
34. Hands should be washed properly.
35. The nurse assist should gather all supplies:

Tap water or soap solution enema

- Enema unit (bag, tubing and clamp)
- Lubricating jelly
- Packet of castile soap (if giving a soap solution enema)
- Bath thermometer
- Gloves
- Bedpan or portable commode
- Bedpan or collection container cover
- Bed protector
- Bath blanket
- Washcloth
- Towel

Commercially prepared enema
- Commercially prepared enema
- Bath thermometer
- Gloves
- Bedpan or portable commode
- Bedpan or portable commode cover
- Bed protector
- Bath blanket
- Washcloth
- Towel

36. The nurse assistant should knock, greet the patient/resident and should ensure patient's privacy.
37. The procedure should be explained thoroughly to the patient/resident.
38. Equipment should be adjusted for proper body mechanics and safety: the bed should be raised to a comfortable working height. It should be ensured that the wheels on the bed are locked.
39. **Preparation of the enema**
■ **Tap water enema**
The tubing should be clamped and the enema bag should be filled with the amount of warm water (usually 500 to 1000 mL, 105° F on the bath thermometer), according to the written orders.

■ **Soap solution enema**
The tubing should be clamped and the enema bag should be filled with the amount of warm water (500 to 1000 mL, 105° F on the bath thermometer), according to the written orders. The packet of soap should be added and the nurse assistant should gently rotate the enema bag to mix the solution. Shaking the enema bag for mixing should be avoided.

■Commercially prepared enema
The nurse assistant should open the enema package and take off the protective cover.
40. The head of the bed should be lowered as low as the patient/resident can tolerate.

41. The patient/resident should be covered with top linens and the bath blanket. The patient/resident should be asked to hold the edge of the bath blanket while the nurse assistant folds the top linens down to the bottom of the bed.

42. The patient/resident should be assisted to turn onto his/her left side with back toward the nurse assistant and the right knee flexed (Sims' position).

43. The nurse assistant should adjust the bath blanket and the patient/resident's clothing as necessary to expose the buttocks. The bed protector should be positioned alongside the patient/resident.

44. If administering a tap water or soap solution enema, the tip of the tubing (2 to 4 inches) should be lubricated by placing a small amount of lubricating jelly on a tissue and dipping the tip of the tubing into it. Commercially prepared enemas generally have a pre-lubricated tip.

45. The nurse assistant should put on gloves.

46. The nurse assistant should lift the patient/resident's upper buttock and insert the tubing or the tip of the commercially prepared enema into the anus no more than 2 to 4 inches. If the nurse assistant has difficulty inserting the tubing or the tip of the commercially prepared enema bottle at least 2 inches into the patient/resident's rectum, he/she should stop the procedure and inform the nurse.

14. **Administration of the enema solution**

■ **Tap water or soap solution enema**

The clamp should be opened and the bag should be held no higher than 12 inches above the anus to allow the solution to flow slowly into the patient/resident's rectum. The tubing should be held in place so that it does not slip out of the rectum.

■**Commercially prepared enema**

The plastic bottle should be squeezed to administer commercially prepared enema.

15. When all of the enema solution has been administered, the nurse assistant should remove the tubing or the tip of the commercially prepared enema from the patient/resident's rectum and should encourage the patient/resident to hold the solution in a side-lying position for as long as possible.

16. The patient/resident should be provided proper help to eliminate the enema solution, using a bedpan, portable commode or the toilet.

17. The wash basin should be filled with warm water and help should be provided to the patient/resident to wash and dry his/her hands. The nurse assistant should assist the patient/resident with perineal care as needed.

18. The bed protector should be removed and the patient/resident's clothing should be adjusted to cover the buttocks.

19. If the patient/resident used a bedpan or portable commode, the bedpan or collection container should be covered and taken to the bathroom. The contents of the bedpan or collection container should be thoroughly observed before emptying it and cleaning it.

20. It should be ensured the patient/resident's comfort as well as proper body alignment.

21. Hands should be properly washed, and observations should be reported and recorded at the end of the procedure.

The Nurse Assistant's Role in Giving a Suppository

The nurse assistant should provide proper help to the patient/resident for a sidelying position and help him/her to unwrap the suppository, if necessary. The nurse assistant should place suppository 1 to 1-1/2 inches past anal sphincter using gloved hand and index finger. After insertion of the suppository, the nurse assistant should hold the patient/resident's buttocks together for a few minutes to help the patient/resident retain the suppository. Proper help should be provided to the patient/resident for coming back into a comfortable position. After the nurse assistant assists a patient/resident with taking a medication, he/she should make sure to document the medication that was taken, the amount, the time and the route.

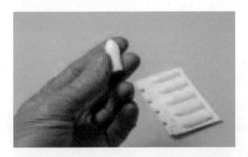

Enteral Nutrition or Tube Feeding

Enteral nutrition is generally called tube feeding because the patient/resident receives nutrition (in the form of a nutrient-rich formula) and fluids through a tube that is placed directly into the stomach or intestines. If the patient/resident will only need enteral nutrition for a few days, a nasogastric or nasointestinal tube may be placed. These types of tubes are inserted through the patient/resident's nose and passed down the patient/resident's throat to the stomach or the intestines. If the patient/resident is expected to require enteral nutrition for more than a few days, a gastrostomy tube may be placed. The gastrostomy tube is inserted directly into the stomach through an incision made in the abdomen. The tube is clamped and held in place by stitches and covered with a dressing.

Enteral nutrition may be necessary in certain conditions that prohibit the patient/resident from taking adequate oral nourishment. Examples may include inability to swallow, loss of consciousness, oral trauma, mouth surgery, esophageal or gastric cancer or trauma, or anorexia. Those suffering from conditions with increased nutritional needs, such as infection, burns, surgery, or fractures, may also need enteral nutrition.

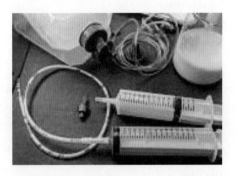

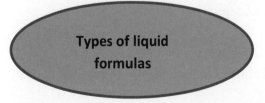

Types of liquid formulas

The liquid formulas for enteral nutrition contain adequate amounts of fat, protein, carbohydrate, minerals, and vitamins to maintain good nutrition. Routine formulas often provide about 1 calorie per milliliter.

They are low in fiber, lactose free, and contain 14% to 16% protein. Routine formulas are also available in high-protein, high-fiber, and high-calorie varieties. Specialized formulas marketed specifically for renal failure, liver failure, stress, diabetes, acquired immunodeficiency syndrome (AIDS), and other disorders are also available. A dietitian may help the physician to choose the right formula for a patient.

Different types of tubes

The name that is given to an enteral tube may be derived from a particular device, the type of procedure used, or the insertion of the tube.

There are following common types of tubes:

Nasogastric
It is inserted through the nose into the stomach.

Percutaneous endoscopic gastrostomy (PEG)
It is placed through the skin.

Endoscopic
It is placed with an instrument called an endoscope.

Gastrostomy
It is inserted directly into the stomach.

Button feeding device
It is a small silicone device used in place of a gastrostomy tube.

Nursing Care for Patients/Residents with Tube Feeding

General observations with tube feeding

Constipation, diarrhea, delayed stomach emptying, and aspiration are major risks of tube feeding. The nurse assistant should report the following at once:

- Nausea
- Discomfort during the feeding
- Distended (enlarged and swollen) abdomen
- Coughing
- Complaints of indigestion or heartburn
- Vomiting
- Redness, swelling, drainage, odor, or pain at the ostomy site
- Fever
- Signs and symptoms of respiratory distress
- Increased pulse rate
- Complaints of flatulence
- Diarrhea

Preventing aspiration

Aspiration is a main risk from tube feedings. It may cause pneumonia and death. Aspiration may occur:

- **During insertion**

A nasogastric tube can slip into the airway. An X-ray should be taken after insertion to check tube placement.

- **From tube movement out of place**
Sneezing, coughing, suctioning, vomiting, and poor positioning are common causes. A tube can move from the intestine or stomach into the esophagus and then into the airway. The registered nurse checks tube placement before a tube feeding. The nurse assistant should never check feeding tube placement.

- **From regurgitation**
Regurgitation is the backward flow of gastric contents into the mouth. Over-feeding and delayed stomach emptying are common causes.

To help prevent regurgitation and aspiration:

- The patient/resident should be positioned in Fowler's or semi-Fowler's position before the feeding. The nurse assistant should follow the care plan and the nurse's directions.
- Fowler's or semi-Fowler's position should be maintained after the feeding. This allows formula to move through the GI tract. The position is needed for 1 to 2 hours after the feeding or at all times.
- The left side-lying position should be avoided. It prevents the stomach contents from emptying into the small intestine.

Comfort measures

Patients/residents with feeding tubes usually are NPO. Dry lips, dry mouth, and sore throat may cause discomfort. Sometimes gum or hard candy is allowed. These measures are common every 2 hours while the patient/resident is awake.

a) Oral hygiene
b) Lubricant for the lips
c) Mouth rinsing
d) Cleaning the nose and nostrils every 4 to 8 hours.
e) Securing the tube to the nose.
f) Securing the tube to the patient/resident's garment at the shoulder area.

Nursing Care for a Patient/Resident Receiving Intravenous (IV) or Parenteral Therapy

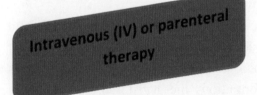
Intravenous (IV) or parenteral therapy

Although a patient/resident's nutritional needs cannot be met using IV therapy, IV therapy is important for administering fluids. It involves injecting into a vein any number of sterile solutions that the body needs, including electrolytes and drugs. IV solutions are used on a short-term basis to maintain or restore fluid and electrolyte balance. Because it is nutritionally inadequate, simple IV therapy is generally not used for more than a few days without addition of some sort of supplementation.

Intravenous or parenteral therapy is used when the patient/resident cannot take adequate amounts of nutrients via the enteral route. These patients/residents include those with severe burns or a disorder of the GI tract that may inhibit absorption of nutrients. A small catheter (tube) is inserted and placed in a vein on the back of the patient/resident's hand or in the patient/resident's arm. Fluid slowly drips from the IV bag, through the IV tubing and into the catheter. Sometimes drugs may be administered through the IV tubing as well. Although nursing assistants will not be responsible for administering IV therapy, they may care for patients/residents who are receiving IV therapy.

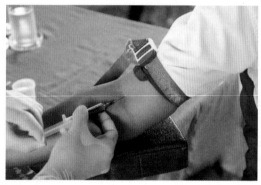

Flow rate

The physician orders the amount of fluid to administer (infuse) and the amount of time to administer it. With this information, the registered nurse figures the flow rate. The flow rate is the milliliters per hour (mL/hr) or number of drops per minute (gtt/min). The registered nurse sets the clamp for the flow rate or an electric pump can be used to control the flow rate. The flow rate is generally displayed in mL/hr. An alarm sounds if something shows wrong. The nurse assistant should tell the nurse at once if he/she hears an alarm. The nurse assistant can check the flow rate if a pump is not used. The RN tells the nurse assistant the

number of drops per minute (gtt/min). To check the flow rate, the number of drops in 1 minute should be counted. The nurse assistant should tell the RN at once if:

- No fluid is dripping.
- The rate is too rapid.
- The rate is too slow.
- The bag is close to being empty or empty.

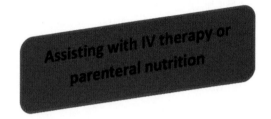

Assisting with IV therapy or parenteral nutrition

- Nurse assistants should always follow Standard Precautions and the Bloodborne Pathogen Standard.
- They should not move the needle or catheter. Needle or catheter position must be maintained. If the catheter or needle is moved, it may come out of the vein. Then fluid may flow into tissues or the flow may stop.
- They should follow the safety measures for restraints. The nurse may splint or restrain the extremity to prevent movement, or may apply a protective device. This helps prevent the catheter or needle from moving.
- The IV bag, tubing, and needle or catheter should be protected when the patient/resident walks. Portable IV stands should be rolled along next to the patient/resident.
- Proper assistance should be provided to the patient/resident with turning and re-positioning. The IV bag should be moved to the side of the bed on which the patient/resident is lying. There should always be allowed enough slack in the tubing. The needle or catheter may move from pressure on the tube.

- The nurse assistant should tell the nurse at once if bleeding occurs from the insertion site.
- The nurse assistant should report signs and symptoms of IV therapy complications. These signs and symptoms may include:

- **Local—at the IV site**: Bleeding, puffiness or swelling, pale or reddened skin, hot or cold skin near the site, blood backing up into the IV tube, and complaints of pain at or above the IV site.

- **Systemic—involving the whole body**: Fever, itching, pulse rate greater than 100 beats per minute, drop in blood pressure, cyanosis, confusion or changes in mental function, loss of consciousness, irregular pulse, decreasing or no urine output, chest pain, nausea, difficulty breathing, and shortness of breath.

Encouraging comfort and safety

The patient/resident can suffer serious harm if the flow rate is too slow or fast. The flow rate may change from:
- Position changes
- Kinked tubes
- Lying on the tube

The nurse assistant should never change the position of the clamp or adjust any controls on IV pumps. He/she should inform the nurse at once if there is a problem with the flow rate.

The Nursing Assistant's Role in Maintaining Fluid Balance

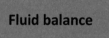

Fluid balance takes place when the amount of fluids an individual takes in equals the amount of fluids the individual loses. When sufficient fluid balance is not maintained, the patient/resident develops either edema (too much fluid in the body) or dehydration (too little fluid in the body).

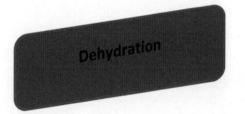

Dehydration may result from conditions such as diarrhea, vomiting, fever, severe blood loss, or not drinking enough fluids. Many patients/residents have conditions that put them at risk for not taking enough fluids and becoming dehydrated. For example, a patient/resident who has problems with mobility or other disabilities may have a difficult time getting up to take a drink. The patient/resident may also cut back on fluids because he/she is trying to minimize the number of times he/she needs to get up and go to the bathroom. Some patients/residents who are incontinent of urine may also minimize their fluid intake because they believe this will reduce their risk for having an episode of incontinence. However, it is significant to know that reducing fluid intake does not decrease incontinence, nor does it minimize trips to the bathroom.

Nurse assistants can play an important role in helping to ensure that those in their care take enough fluids through following:

- Frequently offering fluids that the patient/resident likes at the temperature he/she prefers.
- Encouraging the patient/resident to drink plenty of fluids with each meal.
- Frequently providing the patient/resident with a pitcher of clean, fresh water.
- It should be ensured that the patient/resident has a clean drinking glass or cup of water within easy reach. The glass should be refilled if the patient/resident cannot do it. A drinking straw may make it easier for some patients/residents to drink independently.
- If the patient/resident frequently refuses beverages, the nurse assistant should check with the nurse to see if he/she can offer fluid-rich foods instead, such as popsicles, gelatin, ice cream, or fruit.

If a patient/resident becomes dehydrated, the patient/resident's primary care provider may give an order to "push fluids" or "encourage fluids". This means that the patient/resident should be urged to drink as much fluid as possible. The nurse assistant

should keep a record of the amount of fluid the patient/resident does drink.

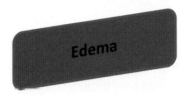

Edema

Edema is the state of retaining too much water, which can result from medical conditions (such as chronic kidney disease or heart failure) that makes it difficult for the body to rid itself of excess water. The individual's primary care provider may place restrictions on the amount of fluid the individual is allowed to have each day. When a nurse assistant is caring for a patient/resident and fluid restrictions are in place, the nurse will tell him/her how much fluid the patient/resident is allowed to have over the course of the shift. The nurse assistant should offer small amounts of fluid at regular intervals. This will help to prevent the patient/resident from becoming too thirsty.

Measuring and Recording Fluid Intake and Output

When the orders to restrict or encourage fluids are in place, the nurse assistant will need to measure and record the patient/resident's fluid intake. A patient/resident's fluid intake may include all of the liquids the patient/resident drinks, as well as foods that are liquid at body temperature (such as ice cream or popsicles)or that are primarily liquid (such as soups). Although in everyday life fluids are generally measured in ounces (oz); however, in healthcare settings, fluids are usually measured in milliliters (mL) or cubic centimeters. The nurse assistant should follow his/her employer's policy regarding which abbreviation (cc or mL) to use when documenting fluid intake. With pre-packaged items, printed information on the container shows how much it holds. For example, a small pre-packaged milk container contains 240 mL or 8 ounces. In other cases, the nurse assistant will need to determine how much fluid the container holds. Most healthcare facilities have a list that can be checked to determine the amount of fluid the glasses, cups, and bowls in use in the facility hold.

Intake and output

The physician or nurse may order intake and output (I&O) measurements.

1. Intake is the amount of fluid taken in. All oral fluids are recorded and measured—milk, water, tea, coffee, soups, juices, soft drinks, ice cream, custard, sherbet, gelatin, pudding, and Popsicles. The nurse assistant often measures intravenous fluids and tube feedings.
2. Output is the amount of fluid that is lost. Output includes vomitus, urine, diarrhea, and wound drainage.

I&O records should be kept safe and used to evaluate fluid balance as well as kidney function. They are also used when the patient/resident has special fluid orders.

Encouraging safety and comfort
Safety
Urine may contain blood and microorganisms. Microorganisms can grow in commodes, urinals, specimen pans, bedpans, and drainage systems. The nurse assistant should always follow Standard Precautions and the Bloodborne Pathogen Standard when handling such equipment. The item should be thoroughly cleaned with a disinfectant after it is used.

Comfort
The contents of urinals, bedpans, commodes, and specimen pans should be measured promptly. This helps reduce or prevent odors. Odors can disturb the patient/resident.

The Nursing Assistant Role in Applying Bandages, Binders, and Dressings

Some agencies permit nursing assistants to apply simple, dry, non-sterile dressings to simple wounds. The nurse assistant should apply dressings (if allowed) in following ways:
- The nurse assistant should let pain-relief drugs take effect, which may usually take 30 minutes. The dressing change may cause discomfort. The nurse administers the drug and tells the nurse assistant how long to wait.
- Fluid and elimination needs should be met before dressing change.
- Equipment and supplies should be collected before dressing change.
- The nurse assistant should control nonverbal communication. Wound odors, drainage, and appearance may be unpleasant. The nurse assistant should not communicate his/her thoughts or reactions to the patient/resident.
- Soiled dressings should be removed so the patient/resident cannot see the

soiled side. The drainage and its color may upset the patient/resident.

- A wound may affect body image and self-esteem. The nurse assistant should help the patient/resident to deal with the wound.
- Tape should be removed by pulling it toward the wound.
- Dressings should be removed gently. They may stick to the drain, wound, or surrounding skin. If the dressing sticks, the dressing can be wet with a saline solution. A wet dressing is easier to remove.
- Only the outer edges should be touched of new and old dressings.
- The nurse assistant should report and record his/her observations after dressing change.

Encouraging safety and comfort
Safety
Contact with body fluids, blood, secretions, or excretions are likely. Nurse assistants should always follow Standard Precautions and the Bloodborne Pathogen Standard. They should wear personal protective equipment (PPE) as needed. Tape should not be applied to injured, irritated, or non-intact skin. Tape may further damage the skin.

Comfort
Wounds and dressing changes may cause pain or discomfort. The nurse may administer a pain-relief drug before the dressing change. The nurse assistant should allow sufficient time for the drug to take effect. Tape and dressing should be applied and removed gently. The patient/resident may not report discomfort from a dressing. The nurse assistant should ask:
- "Is the dressing comfortable?"
- "Does the tape cause itching or pain?"

Binders and compression garments

Binders are wide and broad bands of elastic fabric. They are usually applied to the chest, abdomen, or perineal area. Binders promote healing by supporting wounds and keeping dressings in place. They also reduce or prevent swelling, promote comfort, and prevent injury. There are following binders that are commonly used:

Abdominal binders

These binders provides abdominal support and hold dressings in place. The top part should be at the waist. The lower part should be over the hips. Binders are secured with hook or Velcro and loop closures.

Breast binders

Breast binder supports the breasts after surgery. It may be secured with Velcro or padded zippers. Compression garments are made of a stretchy and tight fabric. Compression garments may help to:

- Reduce swelling
- Hold the skin against the body
- Achieve the desired shape
- Prevent fluid build-up at the surgical site

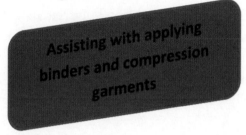

- The nurse assistant should follow the manufacturer's instructions.
- The device should be applied so it is snug. It must not interfere with circulation or breathing.

- The patient/resident should be positioned in good alignment.
- The device should be re-applied if it is out of position or causing discomfort.
- Safety pins should be secured, if used, pointing away from the wound.
- The device should be changed if it is moist or soiled. This prevents the growth of microorganisms.
- The nurse assistant should inform the nurse at once if there is a change in the patient/resident's breathing.
- The skin under and around the device should be checked. The nurse assistant should tell the nurse at once if there is irritation, redness, or other signs of a skin problem.

Promoting safety and comfort

Safety

Binders and compression garments should be applied properly. Otherwise, severe discomfort, skin irritation, respiratory and circulatory problems may occur. Correct application of binders and compression garments is needed for safety and for the device to work properly.

Comfort

A binder or compression garment usually promotes comfort. The nurse assistant should tell the nurse if the device causes discomfort or pain.

Elastic Bandages

They have the same purposes as elastic stockings. Elastic bandages provide support and reduce swelling from injuries. Sometimes they can be used to hold dressings in place. They are applied to legs and arms. To apply elastic bandages:

- These should be used in the correct size (length and width).
- The patient/resident should be positioned in good alignment.

- The nurse assistant should face the patient/resident during the procedure.
- The nurse assistant should start at the lower (distal) part of the extremity and then should work upward to the top (proximal) part.
- The fingers or toes should be exposed if possible. This permits circulation checks.
- The bandage should be applied with firm, even pressure.
- The color and temperature of the extremity should be checked every hour.
- A loose or wrinkled bandage should be re-applied.

- A moist or soiled bandage should be replaced immediately.

Promoting safety and comfort

Safety

Elastic bandages must be snug and firm, but not tight. A tight bandage may affect circulation. Bandages should be secured in place with tape, clips, or Velcro. Clips can injure the skin if they are loose or cause pressure. The nurse assistant should use clips only if the nurse orders to do so. The bandage should be checked often to make sure the clips are correctly in place. Some agencies do not allow nursing assistants to apply elastic bandages. The nurse assistant should know his/her agency's policy.

Comfort

A tight bandage may cause discomfort and pain. The nurse assistant should apply it with firm, even pressure. The bandage should be removed if the patient/resident complains of pain, numbness, or tingling.

Assisting with applying an elastic bandage

The nurse assistant should apply an elastic bandage to a patient/resident in following ways:

1. Hands should be washed properly.
2. The nurse assist should gather all supplies:
   - Elastic bandage as directed by the nurse
   - Tape or clips (unless the bandage has Velcro)
3. The nurse assistant should knock, greet the patient/resident and should ensure patient's privacy.
4. The procedure should be explained thoroughly to the patient/resident.
5. Equipment should be adjusted for proper body mechanics and safety: the bed should be raised to a comfortable working height. It should be ensured that the wheels on the bed are locked.
6. The bed rail should be lowered.
7. The nurse assistant should expose the part that will be bandaged.
8. It should be ensured that the area is clean and dry.
9. The nurse assistant should hold the bandage so the roll should be up. The loose end should be on the bottom.
10. The bandage should be applied to the smallest part of the foot, wrist, ankle, or knee.
11. The nurse assistant should make 2 circular turns around the part.
12. Over-lapping spiral turns should be made in an upward direction. Each over-lap should be equal.
13. The bandage should be applied smoothly with firm, even pressure. It should not be tight.
14. The bandage should be ended with 2 circular turns.
15. The bandage should be secured in place with Velcro, tape, or clips.

16. The fingers or toes should be checked for coldness or cyanosis (bluish color). The nurse assistant should ask the patient/resident about pain, itching, numbness, or tingling and should remove the bandage if any are noted.
17. It should be ensured the patient/resident's comfort as well as proper body alignment
18. Hands should be properly washed, and observations should be reported and recorded at the end of the procedure.

The Nursing Assistant's Role in Applying Anti-Embolic Hose/Elastic Stockings

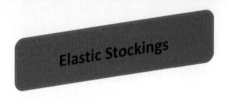

Elastic stockings exert pressure on the veins to promote venous blood return to the heart. The elastic stockings help prevent blood clots (thrombi) in leg veins. A blood clot is known a thrombus. If blood flow is stagnant, blood clots may develop in the deep veins in the lower leg or thigh. A thrombus can break loose and travel through the bloodstream to become an embolus (a blood clot that moves through the vascular system until it lodges in a blood vessel). An embolus from a vein may lodge in the lungs (pulmonary embolism). A pulmonary embolism is a serious condition that can cause severe respiratory problems and death. The nurse assistant should report chest pain or shortness of breath at once. Patients/residents at risk for thrombi may include those who:

- Have cardiovascular disorders
- Are on bedrest
- Have had surgery
- Are older
- Are pregnant

Elastic stockings also are known AE stockings (anti-embolic or anti-emboli stockings). They are also called TED hose (TED: thrombo-embolic disease). The patient/resident usually has 2 pairs of stockings. 1 pair should be washed while the other pair is worn. They should be washed by hand with a mild soap and should be hanged to dry.

Promoting safety and comfort
Safety
The stocking should be applied so the toe opening should be over the top of the toes or under the toes. The nurse assistant should follow the manufacturer's instructions. Stockings should not have creases, twists, or wrinkles after applying them. Twists may affect circulation. Similarly, stockings that roll or bunch up may also affect circulation. Wrinkles and creases can cause skin breakdown. Loose stockings may not promote venous blood return to the heart. Stockings that are too tight may affect circulation. The nurse assistant should tell the nurse if the stockings are too tight or too loose.
Comfort

Stockings should be applied before the patient/resident gets out of bed. Otherwise the patient/resident's legs can swell from sitting or standing. Stockings are difficult to put on when the legs are swollen. The patient/resident lies in bed while they are off. This prevents the legs from swelling. The patient/resident's foot and leg should be handled and moved gently. The nurse assistant should not force the joints (foot, toes, ankle, knee, and hip) beyond their range of motion or to the point of pain.

Assisting with applying elastic stockings

The nurse assistant should apply elastic stockings to patients/residents in following ways:

1. Hands should be washed properly.
2. The nurse assistant should obtain elastic stockings in the correct size and length. The location of the toe opening should be noted
3. The nurse assistant should knock, greet the patient/resident and should ensure patient's privacy.
4. The procedure should be explained thoroughly to the patient/resident.
5. Equipment should be adjusted for proper body mechanics and safety: the bed should be raised to a comfortable working height. It should be ensured that the wheels on the bed are locked.
6. The bed should be raised for proper body mechanics. Bed rails should be up if used.
7. The patient/resident should be in supine position. The legs should be exposed. Top linens should be fan-folded up toward the thighs.
8. The stocking should be turned inside out down to the heel.
9. The foot of the stocking should be slipped over the foot, toes, and heel. The nurse assistant should make sure that the heel pocket is properly positioned on the patient/resident's heel. The toe opening should be over or under the toes.
10. The stocking top should be grasped and the stocking should be pulled up the leg. The stocking should be even and snug.
11. Twists, creases, or wrinkles should be removed appropriately.
12. It should be ensured the patient/resident's comfort as well as proper body alignment.
13. Hands should be properly washed, and observations should be reported and recorded at the end of the procedure.

The Nursing Assistant's Role in Patient/Resident's Skin Care

The nurse assistant can provide foot care, and care for dry skin and dandruff to patients/residents.

Hand, foot, and nail care prevents infection, odors, and injury. Ingrown nails (nails that grow in at the side), hangnails, and nails torn away from the skin may cause skin breaks. These skin breaks can be portals of entry for microorganisms.

The nurse assistant should observe and report the following existing skin conditions and scalp to the licensed nurse:

- Alopecia

- Dandruff
- Pediculosis (lice)
- Acne
- Poison ivy or poison oak
- Insect bites or stings
- Minor burn
- Minor wounds
- Rash
- Excoriation, abrasions, skin tears
- Eczema or psoriasis

The patient/resident should be encouraged for well-balanced diet and plenty of fluids.

10. Appropriate skin care should be provided as:
    - There should be bathing as necessary.
    - There should be thorough rinsing off the skin with soap and water.
    - Lotion and creams should be applied as necessary.
    - There should be the massage for healthy skin.
    - The skin should be kept clean and dry.
11. The nurse assistant should observe high-risk patients/residents for potential problems.
12. Massage should not be provided on red, purple, or irritated areas.
13. Bed should be kept free from small objects and linen should be free of wrinkles.
14. The patient/resident should be kept clean and dry.
15. There should be prevention for shearing and friction.
16. The observations should be reported and recorded.

The nurse assistant should apply OTC ointment, lotion, or powder to the patient/resident in following ways:

1. Hands should be washed properly.
2. The nurse assistant should collect the OTC ointment, lotion, or powder ordered by the nurse and care plan.
3. The nurse assistant should knock, greet the patient/resident and should ensure patient's privacy.
4. The procedure should be explained thoroughly to the patient/resident.
5. Equipment should be adjusted for proper body mechanics and safety: the bed should be raised to a comfortable working height. It should be ensured that the wheels on the bed are locked.
6. The bed should be raised for proper body mechanics. Bed rails should be up if used.
7. The nurse assistant should cleanse the patient/resident's skin and protect the surrounding skin.
8. The nurse assistant should wear gloves.
9. Creams or liniments should be rubbed in by hand, lotions should be patted on with a cotton ball, and ointments should be applied with a wooden tongue blade or a cotton swab. The nurse assistant should sprinkle powder onto hand or cloth, and then apply it to patient/resident.
10. It should be ensured the patient/resident's comfort as well as proper body alignment.

11. Hands should be properly washed, and observations should be reported and recorded at the end of the procedure.

The Nursing Assistant's Role in Admission, Transfer, and Discharge

Nurse assistants can play an important role in assisting with admissions, transfers and discharges. Admission is the patient's formal entry into the healthcare facility. One of the tasks of the nurse assistant is to make the admission process as smooth as possible. How a nurse assistant performs his/her role in admitting a patient to a health care facility may influence the patient's attitude about the care he/she receives. Sometimes a patient must be moved from one portion of the facility to another during his/her stay. For example, as a patient/resident's medical condition improves, he/she may be required to move from the intensive care unit of a hospital to a general medical-surgical unit. This movement or change is called a transfer. The nurse assistant may assist with transfers by communicating significant information about the care that a patient/resident has received. The nurse assistant also ensures that the patient/resident and his/her belongings are moved safely. A discharge is the formal release of the patient/resident from the healthcare facility where he/she is receiving care. The care that a nurse assistant provides in helping to discharge a patient/resident when he/she leaves a health care situation may leave a long lasting impression about the care that he/she received.

Although specific procedures for admitting, transferring and discharging patients/residents may vary from one employer to another; however, the role of the nurse assistant is basically the same i.e. to look after and to ensure the safety and comfort of the patient/resident as he/she is admitted, transferred and discharged.

The Nursing Assistant's Role in a Patient/Resident's Admission

When a patient is admitted to a healthcare facility, the nurse assistant and other members of the staff usually follow a planned series of events. To get ready for a patient's arrival, the nurse assistant should follow the admission sheet and instructions from the nurse. He/she should find out whether the patient has any special requirements or needs. He/she should collect and bring the equipment and materials to the patient's room that are required for the admission process, such as a stethoscope, blood pressure cuff, thermometer, and a personal belongings inventory sheet. The nurse assistant should put a pitcher of water and a cup on the bedside table. He/she should provide a gown, a towel and washcloth, equipment for personal care (such as an emesis basin, wash basin, or a bedpan) and toiletry items (such as toothpaste and soap) to the patient. The bed should be opened by fan-folding the top linens down to the bottom of the bed. If the patient will be arriving on a stretcher, the nurse assistant may need to prepare a surgical bed instead.

Welcoming the patient/resident

A registered nurse along with nurse assistant and one member from the health care team (such as the social worker or admissions coordinator) manages the admission process, including any important paperwork. The nurse assistant may be asked to assist escort the patient to his/her room. However, if the nurse assistant is meeting the patient for the first time without a formal introduction, he/she should knock on the door, smile and greet the patient with a friendly "hello." The nurse assistant should make the patient feel welcome by introducing himself/herself. To support lessen feelings of anxiety about the health care experience, the nurse assistant should explain what is happening and what is going to happen. Next, he/she should wash his/her hands and check the patient's name band or photo identification. If someone has come from a hospital facility into a nursing home, the nurse assistant should remove the hospital name band if this has not been done already. The nurse assistant should explain that he/she is a nurse assistant and will be providing care to the patient. The patient should be asked what he/she would like to be called. The nurse assistant should not use the patient's first name unless he/she gives permission. The patient should be asked if he/she needs to use the bathroom before continuing the admission process. One way to learn more about the patients is to ask questions. Although the RN is responsible for completing the formal health history interview, the nurse assistant may encourage the patient to tell about anything that would make his/her stay more convenient. The nurse assistant should ask the patient about special preferences, habits or problems. The answers should be recorded and important information should be reported to the nurse. Admission to a healthcare facility can be very stressful for the patient and the family. The nurse assistant should be aware that the patient's first impressions of the healthcare facility may influence how he/she feels about being there. First impressions may also influence the feelings of family members about the care that their loved one will receive while in the facility. The nurse assistant's approach may go a long way toward making a great first impression and providing the patient and family confidence in the care that will be provided.

To support the patient and family for feeling more comfortable, the nurse assistant should take the following steps:

- Each time a nurse assistant greets the patient, he/she should smile and call the patient by his/her preferred name.
- The nurse assistant should ask the patient and his/her family members about the patient's preferences, and should take these preferences into account while providing care.
- The nurse assistant should always welcome information that the family provides and should use this information to guide the care.
- The nurse assistant should always include the patient in conversations that concern him/her.
- Before the nurse assistant leaves the patient's room, he/she should always ask if there is anything else that the patient needs.

Looking after the patient/resident's belongings

As part of the admission process, the nurse assistant may be responsible for filling out a personal belongings inventory sheet. When the nurse assistant describes belongings such as jewelery, he/she should use words that do not assign value to the object. For example, a ring should be described as "a yellow metal ring with one clear stone," and should be careful not using words such as silver, gold, or diamond. The patient should be encouraged to send as many valuables home as possible. If necessary, the nurse assistant can arrange for valuable items to be locked in the facility's safe. After completion of the inventory sheet, it should be given to the nurse. In a nursing home, the nurse assistant may need to label the patient's clothing with the patient's name. In some health facilities, other members of the health care team, such as the laundry aide or social worker, handle this responsibility. If the nurse assistant has this responsibility, he/she should follow the employer's policies and procedures for labelling the patient's clothing.

Measuring and recording vital signs, weight and height

When a patient is first admitted to a healthcare facility, the nurse assistant should measure and record the patient's vital signs, weight and height. These initial measurements may help the health care team to determine a point of reference, or baseline, for the patient. Subsequent measurements can be compared with the baseline measurements to trace changes in the patient's condition. The nurse assistant should perform the tasks in a warm, unhurried manner to help the patient relax and feel better about being in a health care situation.

Familiarizing the patient with the new surroundings

Another significant component of the admission process is familiarizing the patient with his/her new environment. The nurse assistant should explain the facility's policies, schedules and visiting hours to the patient and his/her family. The patient should be shown how the call signal works. The nurse assistant should demonstrate how to adjust the bed and lower and raise the over-bed table. If any other equipment is in the room, such as a phone or a TV, the nurse assistant should also ensure that the patient knows how to use it. When a patient is being admitted to a nursing home, the nurse assistant should offer to take him/her and his/her family on a tour of the unit or facility. If the patient wishes to go, the nurse assistant should introduce him/her to other members of the staff and other residents. After the tour, the nurse assistant should help the patient get comfortable in his/her room and should put the call signal within his/her reach. The nurse assistant should ask him/her whether he/she needs anything. When the nurse assistant has finished duties related to admitting the patient to the facility, he/she should report to the nurse. The nurse assistant should make sure to include observations about the patient's physical condition, emotional status or both in his/her report to the nurse.

The Nursing Assistant's Role in a Patient/Resident's Transfers

Transfers generally take place because a patient/resident's condition gets worse or better and his/her health care needs change. Most transfers occur within a facility, to a different unit or room. A resident of a nursing home can also be transferred temporarily from the nursing home to a hospital for treatment of an acute condition, such as bronchitis. Any transfer may have an emotional impact on the patient/resident. When a nurse assistant assists with transfers, he/she should encourage the patient/resident to talk about his/her feelings and reassure him/her, if necessary.

Within facility transfers

When a nurse assistant assists with a transfer within the facility, he/she will need to help the patient/resident pack his/her belongings. After washing hands and greeting the patient/resident, the patient/resident should be explained about the transfer. The nurse assistant should help him/her to get ready for transfer. The nurse assistant should pack personal care equipment, such as the bedpan and wash basin, in addition to the personal belongings. After completion of these tasks, the nurse assistant should wash his/her hands. If applicable, the patient/resident should be given time to say good-bye to his/her roommate.

The nurse should be asked for the records and charts that must go with the patient/resident, and should be asked if the receiving unit has been notified that the transfer is in process. The nurse will notify the receiving unit and provide the receiving nurse a report of the patient/resident's condition. The time of the patient/resident's arrival on the new unit may need to be adjusted so that the receiving staff should be available to receive the patient/resident. The nurse assistant should provide help to the patient/resident into a wheelchair (some healthcare facilities prefer that the nurse assistant should move the patient/resident in his/her bed from one room to another). The nurse assistant should ask a co-worker to help, if necessary. The patient/resident and his/her possessions should be moved to his/her new room, and the patient/resident should be introduced to his/her new nurse and nurse assistant. Important information should be recorded and reported, as necessary.

To help the patient/resident make a comfortable transition from one unit or room to another and as a courtesy to the new nurse assistant, the information about the patient/resident's preferences and care needs should be shared with the new nurse assistant who will take over. The nurse assistant may also stay and assist the new nurse assistant with some of the tasks regarding helping the patient/resident get settled in his/her new environment. After returning to his/her own unit, the nurse assistant should report to the nurse that the patient/resident's transfer has been completed. All relevant details such as the time of the transfer and the mode of transportation should be provided, and observations about the patient/resident's physical or emotional status should be shared with the nurse. The nurse assistant should follow employer's policy for preparing the room for use by another patient/resident. The nurse assistant should remove any equipment that the patient/resident did not take from his/her old room. If the patient/resident was not moved in his/her bed, the nurse assistant should remove dirty linens. After finishing these tasks, the nurse assistant should wash his/her hands.

Temporary transfers

A resident of a nursing home or a home health resident may need to be transferred to another type of healthcare setting to receive care for an acute medical condition. This type of transfer is known as a temporary transfer, because the patient/resident is expected to return to the nursing home or to his/her own home after receiving treatment for the acute medical condition. If the individual is a resident of a nursing home, a bed hold may be put into effect for the period that the resident is expected to be away. The bed hold reserves the resident's place at the nursing home. When a nurse assistant assists a patient/resident with a temporary transfer, he/she should pack only the belongings and clothing that the patient/resident will need for a hospital stay (for example, a robe, comb, slippers, brush, toothbrush, eyeglasses and dentures). If circumstances and time permit, the nurse assistant should help the patient/resident bathe. He/she should also help the patient/resident dress. Clothing that is easier to remove is usually the great choice. If the individual is a resident of a nursing home, valuable belongings can be placed in the facility's safe or any other safe area until the resident returns. The nurse assistant should follow his/her employer's policy for listing and storing the patient/resident's personal belongings while the patient/resident is away.

The Nursing Assistant's Role in a Patient/Resident's Facility Discharge

A patient/resident is released or discharged from the health care setting when the care provided by the current health care setting no longer meets the patient/resident's requirements. For example, a patient/resident may be discharged from a hospital to a nursing home, a sub-acute care facility, or his/her own home as his/her condition improves and he/she no longer needs hospital care. To ensure that the patient/resident's health care requirements continue to be met after the patient/resident leaves the healthcare facility where he/she is receiving care, the health care team including the nurse assistant should follow a process called discharge planning. Discharge planning involves identifying the patient/resident's ongoing care requirements and making arrangements to have those requirements met after he/she leaves the healthcare facility. Discharge planning initiates as soon as the patient/resident is admitted to the healthcare facility and continues throughout his/her stay. The discharge planner and nurse are primarily responsible for discharge planning, although the nurse assistant may help with discharge planning by communicating information about the patient/resident's requirements to the other members of the health care team.

On the day that a patient/resident is ready to be discharged from the healthcare facility, the nurse assistant should help him/her to gather all his/her belongings and pack his/her suitcase. Items should be checked against the personal belongings inventory list to ensure that he/she has everything that was brought with him/her. The nurse assistant should check with the nurse to ensure that the proper forms are filled out and ready to go with the patient/resident. If the patient/resident is being discharged to another healthcare facility, it is generally beneficial to send a detailed description of the patient/resident's personal habits and physical needs, as well as usual vital signs and medications, to the receiving facility. The nurse assistant should stay with the patient/resident and comfort him/her until the patient/resident is discharged because he/she may be very frightened. The nurse assistant should help the patient/resident into a wheelchair or onto a stretcher and should transport him/her to the exit.

The patient/resident should be told how much the nurse assistant has enjoyed helping him/her, and should wish him/her well in the recovery. If the patient/resident is being transported by ambulance, the patient/resident should be introduced to the ambulance crew. If necessary, the nurse assistant should help the ambulance attendants to transport the patient/resident into the ambulance. It should be ensured that the patient/resident's belongings and forms are placed in the vehicle with him/her. The nurse assistant should report to the nurse that the patient/resident's discharge has been completed. Important information such as the time of the discharge, mode of transportation, and how the patient/resident responded should be reported to the nurse.

Helpful Resources

Allen, L. V. (1997). Suppositories as drug delivery systems. *Journal of Pharmaceutical Care in Pain & Symptom Control, 5*(2), 17-26. https://doi.org/10.1300/j088v05n02_03

Blakeborough, L., & Watson, J. S. (2019). The importance of obtaining a sputum sample and how it can aid diagnosis and treatment. *British Journal of Nursing, 28*(5), 295-298. https://doi.org/10.12968/bjon.2019.28.5.295

Cadena, A. J., Habib, S., Rincon, F., & Dobak, S. (2019). The benefits of parenteral nutrition (PN) versus enteral nutrition (EN) among adult critically ill patients: What is the evidence? A literature review. *Journal of Intensive Care Medicine, 35*(7), 615-626. https://doi.org/10.1177/0885066619843782

Chinegwundoh, F. (2018). Urine sample collection: Issues and a solution. *Trends in Urology & Men's Health, 9*(1), 16-18. https://doi.org/10.1002/tre.615

Chowdary, K. V., & Reddy, P. (2010). Parenteral nutrition: Revisited. *Indian Journal of Anaesthesia, 54*(2), 95. https://doi.org/10.4103/0019-5049.63637

Doulla, B. (2018). Sputum specimen processing for culture procedure v1 (protocols.io.uvzew76). *protocols.io*. https://doi.org/10.17504/protocols.io.uvzew76

Gail, K. (2018). Monitoring the parenteral nutrition patient. *Total Parenteral Nutrition in the Hospital and at Home*, 57-59. https://doi.org/10.1201/9781351077330-7

Gowda, S. (2010). Monitoring intravenous therapy. *Intravenous Therapy for Nurses*, 20-20. https://doi.org/10.5005/jp/books/10401_4

Gowda, S. (2010). Initiating intravenous therapy. *Intravenous Therapy for Nurses*, 31-31. https://doi.org/10.5005/jp/books/10401_6

Hansen, D., Krude, J., Blahout, B., Leisebein, T., Dogru-Wiegand, S., Bartylla, T., Raffenberg, M., Benner, D., Biedler, A., & Popp, W. (2010). Bed-making in the hospital setting – Does it pose infectious risks? *Healthcare infection*, *15*(3), 85-87. https://doi.org/10.1071/hi10012

Lecky, D. M., Hawking, M. K., & McNulty, C. A. (2014). Patients' perspectives on providing a stool sample to their GP: A qualitative study. *British Journal of General Practice*, *64*(628), e684-e693. https://doi.org/10.3399/bjgp14x682261

Mitchell, A. (2019). Administering an enema: Indications, types, equipment and procedure. *British Journal of Nursing*, *28*(3), 154-156. https://doi.org/10.12968/bjon.2019.28.3.154

Peate, I. (2015). How to administer an enema. *Nursing Standard*, *30*(14), 34-36. https://doi.org/10.7748/ns.30.14.34.s43

Pellatt, G. C. (2007). Clinical skills: Bed making and patient positioning. *British Journal of Nursing*, *16*(5), 302-305. https://doi.org/10.12968/bjon.2007.16.5.23010

Rae, M., Macintyre, L., & Dahale, M. (2017). Anti-embolism stockings, the similarities and differences. *The Journal of The Textile Institute*, *108*(11), 1933-1939. https://doi.org/10.1080/00405000.2017.1301018

Specimen collection and transport. (2018). *Pocket Guide to Clinical Microbiology*, 81-126. https://doi.org/10.1128/9781683670070.ch3

Tzeng, H., Prakash, A., Brehob, M., Devecsery, D. A., Anderson, A., & Yin, C. (2012). Keeping patient beds in a low position: An exploratory descriptive study to continuously monitor the height of patient beds in an adult acute surgical inpatient care setting. *Contemporary Nurse*, 2695-2710. https://doi.org/10.5172/conu.2012.2695

Zhang, Q., McGuigan, C., Lew, K., & Chris Le, X. (2012). Urine sample collection and handling. *Comprehensive Sampling and Sample Preparation*, 123-142. https://doi.org/10.1016/b978-0-12-381373-2.00069-7

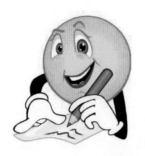

Chapter Ten:

Vital Signs

Outline

I: What are the Vital Signs?

II: Use of the body temperature as an indication of body functioning

III: Nursing measures to raise and lower the body temperature

IV: Pulse and identification of common pulse sites

V: Factors that increase and decrease the pulse rate

VI: Respiration and factors affecting respiratory rate

VII: Observations when measuring respirations

VIII: Altered respiratory function and abnormal breathing pattern

IX: Taking TPR as a combined procedure

X: Blood pressure

XI: Factors that raise and lower blood pressure

XII: Equipment for measuring blood pressure

XIII: Measuring blood pressure

XIV: Observation and recording of patient/resident's pain

XV: Recording vital signs on chart, graph and nursing assistant notes

What are the Vital Signs?

In health care, there are four basic measurements that may indicate a great deal about how an individual's body is functioning. These four measurements are:

1. Temperature
2. Pulse
3. Respiration
4. Blood pressure

These measurements are called vital signs because they depict functions that are essential for life. Nurse assistants are usually responsible for measuring and recording the vital signs of those in their care. These measurements are always taken when an individual is first admitted to a healthcare setting, at regular intervals throughout the patient/resident's stay at the facility, and before the patient/resident is discharged from the facility.

When a patient/resident first begins receiving care, the nurse assistant may be asked to take the patient/resident's vital signs frequently because these frequent readings may assist the health care team to determine what is baseline for that patient/resident. After the baseline measurements are established, the patient/resident's primary care provider may order the patient/resident's vital signs to be taken on a less frequent but regular basis. The frequency may vary from one individual to another. The nurse assistant may also take a patient/resident's vital signs on an "as-needed basis," such as when he/she notices a variation in the patient/resident's usual condition, or when the nurse asks him/her to do so.

Accuracy is extremely important while measuring vital signs. Vital sign measurements usually affect decisions that are made about the patient/resident's medical care. The significance of these measurements to the patient/resident's care makes it essential that a nurse assistant should measure these signs accurately, should record them correctly, and should report any variations in them promptly to the nurse. The other staff members of the health care team are dependent on vital signs measurements that should be provided in a timely manner.

Vital signs may reflect the functions of three basic body processes i.e. regulation of body temperature, breathing, and heart function. Vital signs are measured to detect variations in normal body function. They may show even minute changes in the patient/resident's condition. They may tell about treatment responses. Vital signs may indicate life-threatening events. Accuracy is essential while measuring, recording, and reporting vital signs. If the nurse assistant is unsure of measurements, he/she should promptly ask the nurse to take them again. Unless otherwise ordered, vital signs should be taken with the patient/resident at rest (sitting or lying). The nurse assistant should report the following at once:

- Any change of vital sign from a prior measurement
- Vital signs below or above the normal range.

Factors affecting vital signs

- Activity
- Anger
- Anxiety
- Drugs
- Eating
- Exercise
- Fear
- Illness
- Noise
- Pain
- Sleep
- Weather

Pain as a 5th vital sign

Pain or discomfort means to hurt, ache, or be sore. It is often called the fifth vital sign. Pain signals any tissue damage and is often causes the individual to seek health care. Pain is personal. It may differ for each individual. What hurts to one individual may ache to another. What one individual calls ache, another may call it sore.

Different types of pain

There are different types of pain, such as:

E. Acute Pain

It is a type of pain that is felt suddenly due to any disease, injury, trauma, or surgery. Acute pain usually indicates tissue damage. It may last for a short time. It reduces with healing.

F. Chronic Pain

It is a persistent pain that continues for a long time (months or years) or may occur off and on. Chronic pain generally persists long after healing. Arthritis is a common cause of chronic pain.

G. Radiating Pain

It is felt at the site of tissue damage and in surrounding areas. Pain from a heart attack is usually felt in the left jaw, left side of the chest, left arm, and left shoulder. Gallbladder disease may cause pain in the back, right upper abdomen, and the right shoulder.

H. Phantom Pain

It is a type of pain that is felt in a body part that is no longer there. An individual with an amputated leg may still sense leg pain.

Use of body temperature as an indication of body functioning

Body temperature represents the amount of heat produced by the body. Human body normally maintains a fairly constant temperature. A specific area in the brain regulates the body temperature and makes adjustments as required to maintain the body temperature within the normal range. An individual's temperature usually moves up and down within the normal range, depending on various factors like the time of day, the individual's level of activity, the individual's emotional status, and the temperature of the surrounding air. A temperature above the normal range is considered as fever and is a common response to an infection. A temperature below the normal range is called as hypothermia.

The normal range of body temperature may vary according to the body site as well as the age of the individual

Body site

Common sites to measure an individual's body temperature may include the mouth (an oral temperature), the rectum (a rectal temperature), armpit (an axillary temperature), ear (a tympanic temperature), and temporal artery (a forehead temperature). As the variation occurs from site to site, it is significant to note the site of the measuring temperature. The nurse assistant should always follow his/her employer's policy regarding how to note the site. A routine practice is to write an "O" after the measurement if the temperature was obtained orally, an "R" if the temperature was measured rectally, a "TY" if the temperature was obtained in the ear, and an "A" if the temperature was taken in the armpit.

Age

Body temperature is generally higher in infants or pediatric age groups and lower in older adults. Body temperature is often taken in degrees. Degrees may be measured on two different temperature scales i.e. Celsius (°C) or Fahrenheit (°F). In the United States, the commonly used scale is the Fahrenheit scale. Below table summarizes normal temperature ranges and average temperatures in degrees Celsius and degrees Fahrenheit and for each of the major sites where temperature can be obtained.

Site	°F		°C	
	Normal Range	Average	Normal Range	Average
Oral	97.6-99.6	98.6	36.4-37.5	36.9
Rectal	98.6-100.6	99	37-38.1	37.5
Axillary	95.3-98.4	96.8	35.2-36.9	36
Tympanic	96.6-99.7	98.1	35.9-37.6	36.7
Temporal artery	99.6	99.6	`37.5	37.5

Ensuring safety and accuracy while measuring a temperature

Measuring an accurate temperature measurement safely needs to use the right equipment in the right way. It also requires considering conditions the patient/resident may have that make one method of measuring a temperature preferable over another one.

Oral site

Oral temperatures should not be taken if the patient/resident:

- Is unconscious
- Is under 4 or 5 years of age
- Has had surgery or an injury to the neck, face, nose, or mouth
- Is receiving oxygen
- Has a nasogastric tube
- Breathes through the mouth
- Is delirious, confused, restless, or disoriented
- Has a sore mouth
- Is paralyzed on one side of the body
- Has a convulsive (seizure) disorder

Rectal site

The rectal site should be used for infants and children under 3 years old. Rectal temperatures are obtained when the oral site cannot be used. Rectal temperatures should not be taken if the patient/resident:

- Has a rectal disorder or injury
- Has diarrhea
- Has heart disease
- Had rectal surgery
- Is confused or agitated.

Tympanic membrane site

The site has fewer microorganisms than the mouth or rectum. Therefore, there is a minimum risk of spreading infection. This site should not be used if the patient/resident has:

- An ear disorder
- Ear drainage

Temporal artery site

It is used to measures body temperature at the temporal artery in the forehead. The site is non-invasive.

Axillary site

Axillary site is less reliable than the other sites. It is used when the other sites cannot be used.

Promoting safety and comfort

The rectal site is dangerous for patients/residents with cardiac problems. The thermometer may stimulate the vagus nerve that affects the heart. Vagus nerve stimulation slows down the heart rate and may cause serious complications.

Equipment consideration for measuring temperature

The nurse assistant should always follow the manufacturer's instructions and agency procedures to clean, use, and store thermometers.

Electronic thermometers

Electronic thermometers are battery operated thermometers, in which the temperature is shown on the front of the device. Standard electronic thermometers are used to take body temperature at the oral, rectal, and axillary sites.

Digital thermometers

Digital thermometers are used to take body temperature at the oral, rectal, and axillary sites. Depending on the type, the temperature can be measured in 6 to 60 seconds.

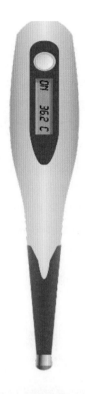

Glass thermometers

These are long- or slender-tip thermometers, which are used for taking oral and axillary temperatures. These thermometers may have stubby and pear-shaped tips. Rectal thermometers contain stubby tips.

Glass thermometers are generally color-coded.

- Blue for oral and axillary thermometers
- Red for rectal thermometers

Glass thermometers are re-usable; however, the following problems may occur while using glass thermometers:

- They may take a long time to measure the temperature (3 to 10 minutes) depending on the body site.
- They can be broken easily. Broken rectal thermometers may injure the rectum and colon.
- The patient/resident may bite down and break an oral thermometer. Cuts in the mouth are major risks. If the thermometer contains mercury, swallowed mercury may cause severe mercury poisoning.

Glass thermometers

Glass thermometers contain a hollow glass tube and a bulb tip. The device is filled with a substance that rises in the tube when heated, and moves down the tube when cooled. The nurse and care plan guides the nurse assistant about:

- When to take the patient/resident's temperature
- What site to use
- What thermometer to use

Before using a glass thermometer, the nurse assistant should always inspect the thermometer to make sure that it is not

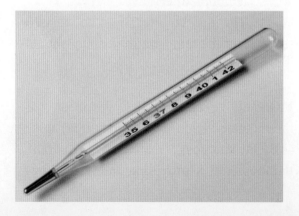

cracked, chipped, or broken. To prevent the spread of infection, thermometer should be washed with cool water and soap before and after using it (Hot water should not be used to wash a glass thermometer because this can cause the thermometer to break). Before using the thermometer, the mercury or mercury-like substance should be moved into the bulb by "shaking down" the thermometer with a rapid downward flick of the wrist. The mercury or mercury-like substance should start below the 34° C mark on a Celsius thermometer or the 94° F mark on a Fahrenheit thermometer, in order to provide an accurate temperature measurement. The nurse assistant should make sure to place the thermometer properly, and should leave it in place for the specified amount of time.

Encouraging safety and comfort

Mercury-glass thermometers are not commonly used currently. If a thermometer breaks, the nurse assistant should tell the nurse at once. Mercury is a dangerous substance. The nurse assistant should always follow agency special procedures for handling hazardous materials.

Electronic thermometers

Electronic thermometers contain probe covers or caps to prevent the spread of infection. Electronic thermometers are usually batteries operated. Some electronic thermometers are kept in chargers when not in use.

- Standard electronic thermometers may take temperature in a few seconds.

They usually have oral (blue) and rectal (red) probes. The oral (blue) probe is also used for taking axillary temperatures.

- Tympanic membrane thermometers take temperature in 1 to 3 seconds. They are comfortable and non-invasive. There are fewer microorganisms in the ear than in the rectum or mouth. There is the minimum risk of spreading infection. To use the tympanic membrane thermometers, the covered probe should be gently inserted into the ear.

- Temporal artery thermometers usually take temperature in 3 to 4 seconds. They are non-invasive and measure the temperature of the blood in the temporal artery. To use temporal artery thermometers:
  a) The side of the head that is exposed should be used. The nurse assistant should not use the side covered by hair, a hat, a dressing, or other covering. The side that was on a pillow should also not be used.
  b) A disposable cap or cover should be placed on the thermometer.
  c) The device should be placed in the center of the forehead.
  d) The scan button should be pressed.
  e) The device should be slid across the forehead and across the temporal artery.
  f) The scan button should be released and the temperature display should be read.

It should be ensured that the electronic thermometer is fully charged. If a nurse assistant notices that the electronic thermometer is providing faulty readings (for example, a temperature that is extremely low or extremely high, or the same temperature for every individual), he/she should report the problem to the nurse so that the device can be repaired or replaced. Electronic thermometers are often used for many individuals, so the nurse assistant should always practice proper infection control procedures. The thermometer should not be placed on dirty surfaces, and if the thermometer has a cord, the cord should be kept in the nurse assistant's hand. It should be ensured that the only part of the device that contacts the patient/resident or his/her surroundings has the probe cover. To ensure an accurate measurement, the nurse assistant must place the thermometer probe properly, and leave it in place for the recommended time.

Temperature Measurement Methods: Individual-Specific Considerations

The method used to measure an individual's temperature depends on various factors. Using the wrong method to take a patient/resident's temperature may affect the patient/resident's safety, the accuracy of the measurement, or both. Different methods to measure a patient/resident's body temperature along with individual-specific considerations may include:

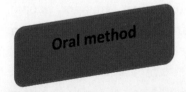

The oral method is generally the preferred way to measure a patient/resident's body temperature because it is easy, causes the minimum personal discomfort and embarrassment, and provides a measurement that accurately depicts the internal body temperature.

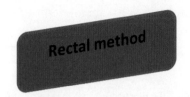

The rectal method for obtaining a patient/resident's body temperature also accurately depicts internal body temperature, but it may cause more personal discomfort and embarrassment. A rectal temperature is measured when measuring an oral temperature might cause injury or inaccurate results.

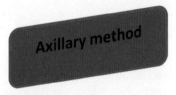

The axillary method is the least accurate method to take a patient/resident's body temperature. An axillary temperature should be taken only if the patient/resident cannot tolerate measuring an oral or a rectal temperature. To ensure that the measurements obtained are as accurate as possible, the armpit should be dried with a tissue before placing the thermometer (moisture may affect the measurement). The nurse assistant should make sure that the patient/resident stays seated or lies down while the temperature is being taken.

Encouraging comfort and safety

Thermometers should be placed into the mouth, rectum, axilla, and ear. Each area has infectious microorganisms. The area may also contain blood. Therefore, each patient/resident should have his/her own glass or digital thermometer. Disposable covers (sheaths) or caps should be used for other electronic thermometers to prevent the spread of microbes and infection. The nurse assistant should always follow Standard Precautions and the Bloodborne Pathogen Standard. With rectal temperatures, the nurse assistant's gloved hands may have contact with feces. If so, he/ should remove gloves and practice proper hand hygiene.

Nursing Measures to Lower and Raise Body Temperature

Measures to raise the body temperature

a) The temperature of the room should be increased.
b) Coverings should be added to the body.
c) Hot liquids should be provided to drink.
d) Warm baths or soaks should be provided to the patient/resident.

Measures to lower the body temperature

a) The temperature of the room should be decreased.
b) Coverings from the body should be removed.
c) The patient/resident should be offered plenty of liquids to drink.
d) Cool bath or sponging should be provided to patients/residents.

Temperature control

Body temperature represents the amount of heat produced by the body. Human body normally maintains a fairly constant temperature. A specific area in the brain regulates the body temperature and makes adjustments as required to maintain the body temperature within the normal range. An individual's temperature usually moves up and down within the normal range, depending on various factors like the time of day, the individual's level of activity, the individual's emotional status, and the temperature of the surrounding air. A temperature above the normal range is considered as fever and is a common response to an infection. A temperature below the normal range is called as hypothermia.

A person cannot be comfortable if there is too hot or too cold. Loss of body fat is a basic component of aging. As a result, older people are more likely to have lower body temperature than younger people. People who are ill may also feel more chilled. Many healthcare settings have individual room-temperature controls. The temperature should be set for the comfort of the patient/resident receiving care. The nurse assistant may still need to provide the patient/resident with an extra blanket for the bed, a sweater, or a lap blanket to help ensure that he/she is warm enough.

Pulse and Identification of Common Pulse Sites

Every time the heart beats, it forces blood through the arteries that carry blood away from the heart and throughout the body. The heartbeat produces a wave of blood, which can be felt passing through the artery if the fingers are put over certain body sites where the artery lies closer to the surface of the skin. Between heart beats, the heart gets a bit rest and then it beats again, causing another wave that can be felt. The wave that is felt is called the pulse.

Features of a pulse

The pulse provides significant information about how an individual's heart is working. When a patient/resident's pulse is being evaluated, there are several things should be noted, such as:

Pulse rate

The pulse rate is the number of pulses or heartbeats heard or felt in 1 minute. Pain, fever, activity, significant blood loss, and emotions such as fear, anger, agitation, or excitement may cause the increased pulse rate. Sleep, some drugs, and conditions such as depression may cause the decreased pulse rate. In adults, the normal pulse rate is usually between 60 and 100 beats/min. A pulse rate of more than 100 beats per minute is called as tachycardia and less than 60 beats per minute is known as bradycardia. Both these conditions are usually considered abnormal. The nurse assistant should report abnormal pulses to the nurse at once.

Pulse rhythm

When the pulse rhythm is described, it generally demonstrates how regular the pulse is. A pulse that comes at regular intervals is called as a regular rhythm. If the length of time is uneven between pulses, the rhythm is considered as irregular. The normal pulse rhythm should be regular (pulses should be felt in a pattern). The same interval occurs between heart beats. A pulse is described as irregular pulse when the beats are skipped or not evenly spaced.

Pulse force

If the pulse is easy to feel, it is demonstrated as a strong or full pulse. A bounding pulse is a pulse that looks like pushing up against the examiner's fingertips. A weak pulse that is very difficult to feel is described as thready pulse.

Age group	Normal resting pulse (beats/min)
Children and adults older than 10 years	60-100
Children between 1 and 10 years	70-130
Infants between 1 and 11 months	80-120
Newborns between 1 and 30 days	100-150

Different sites for evaluating a pulse

The carotid, temporal, radial, brachial, popliteal, femoral, posterior tibial, and dorsalis pedis pulses are felt on each side of the body. The most commonly used site for evaluating the pulse is radial pulse, which is easy to reach and find. The patient/resident is not exposed.

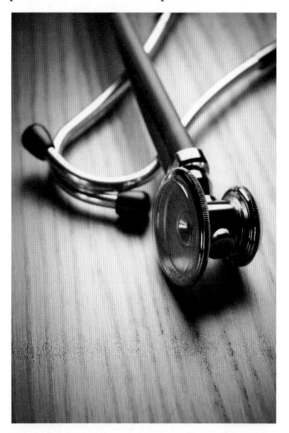

The apical pulse is evaluated over the heart. The apex (apical) of the heart lies at the tip of the heart, just beneath the left nipple. The apical pulse is taken with a stethoscope, which is an instrument used to listen the sounds produced by the lungs, heart, and other body organs. It can be used to evaluate apical pulses and blood pressures.

To use a stethoscope:

- The ear-pieces and diaphragm should be wiped with antiseptic before and after use.
- The ear-piece tips should be paced in the examiner's ears. The bend of the tips should be pointed forward. Ear-pieces should fit snugly to inhibit noises. They should not cause discomfort or pain.
- The diaphragm should be tapped gently. The examiner should hear the tapping. If not, the chest piece should be turned at the tubing. The diaphragm should be tapped gently again and should be proceeded after listening the tapping sound. The nurse assistant should check with the nurse if he/she does not hear the tapping.
- The diaphragm should be placed over the pulse site to evaluate i
-

Encouraging comfort and safety

Safety

Stethoscopes are in direct contact with many patients/residents and staff. The nurse assistant should wipe the ear-pieces and diaphragm with antiseptic wipes before and after use.

Comfort

Stethoscope diaphragms are usually cold. The nurse assistant should warm the diaphragm with his/her hand before applying it to the patient/resident. Cold diaphragms may startle the patient/resident.

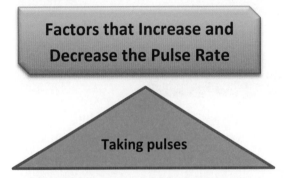

Factors that Increase and Decrease the Pulse Rate

Taking pulses

The nurse assistant should take radial and apical pulses and must count, report, and record them accurately. The radial pulse is most commonly used pulse for routine vital signs. For taking radial pulse, the nurse assistant should place his/her first 2 or 3 fingertips against the radial artery. The radial artery should be on the thumb side of the wrist. The pulse should be counted for 30 seconds and then multiplied the number by 2. This provides the number of beats per minute (pulses in 60 seconds). For example, if a nurse assistant counts 36 beats in 30 seconds. For the number of beats per minute, he/she should multiply 36 by 2 (36 × 2 = 72). The pulse would be 72 per minute. If the pulse is irregular, the nurse assistant should count it for 1 minute. In some agencies, radial pulses are measured for 1 minute. The nurse assistant should always follow agency policy. The apical pulse is slightly below the nipple, on the left side of the chest. A stethoscope should be used to count the pulse for 1 minute. The heartbeat usually sounds like a lub-dub. The nurse assistant should count each lub-dub as a single beat. It is remembered that the lub should not be counted as one beat and the dub as another.

Apical pulses are taken on patients/residents who:

- Have heart problems
- Have irregular heart rhythms
- Take medications that affect the heart

Factors that increase the pulse

a) Exercise
b) Fever
c) Shock
d) Hemorrhage
e) Pain
f) Strong emotions (fear, anger, excitement, laughter)
g) Over 100 beats/min – tachycardia

Factors that decrease the pulse

a) Sleep/rest
b) Depression
c) Athletes in good physical condition have a lower pulse, probably below 60 beats/min
d) Drugs (digitalis, morphine)
e) Below 60 beats/min – bradycardia

Respiration and Factors Affecting Respiratory Rate

Respiration means the process of breathing, in which oxygen is taken into the body (inhalation) and carbon dioxide is expelled from the body (exhalation). Each breathe involves one exhalation and one inhalation. The chest falls during exhalation and rises during inhalation. The healthy individual has 12 to 20 respirations per minute. Cardiac and respiratory problems often increase the respiratory rate. Respirations are usually regular, quiet, and effortless. Both sides of the chest should rise and fall equally. Patients/residents may alter their breathing patterns when they know their respirations are being counted. Therefore, the nurse assistant should not tell the patient/resident while counting respiratory rate. Respirations should be counted right after taking a pulse. The nurse assistant should place his/her fingers or stethoscope over the pulse site. The patient/resident assumes that the examiner is taking the pulse. To count respirations, the nurse assistant should watch the chest rise and fall and should count them for 30 seconds. He/she should multiply the number by 2 for the number of respirations in 1 minute. For example, if the examiner counts 8 breaths in 30 seconds. For the number of respirations in 1 minute, he/she should multiply 8 by 2 ($8 \times 2 = 16$). The respiratory rate would be 16/min. If an examiner notes an abnormal pattern, he/she should count respirations for 1 minute. In most of the agencies, respirations are often counted for 1 minute. The nurse assistant should always follow agency policy.

Observations when Measuring Respirations

When a nurse assistant is evaluating a patient/resident's respirations, he/she should note the following things:

Respiratory rate

The respiratory rate is the number of respirations that occur in 1 minute. It can be counted by observing the patient/resident's chest rise (inhalation) and fall (exhalation). Combination of one inhalation and one exhalation equals one respiration. The same factors that increase the pulse rate can also increase the respiratory rate (fever, exercise, pain, significant blood loss, and emotions such as fear, anger, agitation or excitement). Likewise, the factors that decrease the pulse rate may also decrease the respiratory rate (for example, certain medications, sleep, and certain conditions such as depression). In healthy adults, the normal respiratory rate is usually between 12 and 20 breaths per minute. In infants and children, the normal respiratory rate is usually faster than the adults.

Respiratory rhythm

The respiratory rhythm is the regularity with which an individual breathes. In normal breathing, the breaths should be evenly spaced.

Respiratory depth

The respiratory depth can be described as deep or shallow. Normally, an individual breathes quietly and easily. The breaths should seem as evenly spaced and effortless. Both sides of the chest should rise and fall equally. Dyspnea is the term for breathing that is difficult or seems like it is taking a lot of effort.

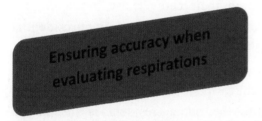

Ensuring accuracy when evaluating respirations

Respiration is one of the vital functions that can be controlled to a certain extent. Although a person breathes without having to think about it, he/she does have some control over whether his/her breaths are fast or slow, and whether they are deep or shallow. A person may have the ability to interrupt the normal pattern of breathing by holding his/her breathe. Therefore, it is best to evaluate respirations without person being aware that the examiner is doing it.

Usually, the nurse assistant evaluates a patient/resident's respirations after evaluating his/her pulse. If the examiner keeps his/her fingers on the patient/resident's wrist, the patient/resident may not be aware that the examiner is evaluating his/her respirations, which may lead to a more accurate evaluation. The examiner should count the patient/resident's respirations for 1 full minute, counting one rise and one fall of the chest for each respiration.

Altered Respiratory Function and Abnormal Breathing Pattern

Hypoxia is the most common sign of an altered respiratory function. Hypoxia means reduced oxygen supply to the cells. Without enough oxygen, cells cannot perform their functions properly. Any factor affecting respiratory function may cause hypoxia. The brain is very sensitive to sense inadequate oxygen supply. Restlessness, dizziness, and disorientation are early signs of hypoxia. Hypoxia is a serious condition that may threaten life. All body organs need oxygen to perform their proper functions. Oxygen should be administered and the cause of hypoxia should be treated.

The common signs of altered respiratory function may include:

- Hypoxia
- Anxiety and apprehension
- Fatigue
- Agitation
- Increased pulse rate
- Increased respiratory rate and depth
- Cyanosis (bluish color to the skin, lips, mucous membranes, and nail beds)
- Dyspnea
- Abnormal breathing pattern
- Shortness of breath

- Cough (note frequency and time of day)
- Hemoptysis: bloody (hemo) sputum (ptysis means to spit)
- Respirations: noisy—wheezing, wet-sounding, crowing sounds
- Chest pain (note location)

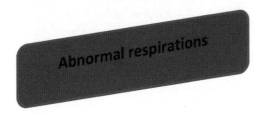

ealthy adults normally breathe 12 to 20 times per minute. Normal respirations are usually effortless, quiet, and regular. Both sides of the chest should rise and fall equally. The following breathing patterns are considered as abnormal:

Tachypnea: Rapid (Tachy) breathing (pnea). Respirations are above 20 per minute.

Bradypnea: Slow (Brady) breathing (pnea). Respirations are below 12 per minute.

Apnea: Lack or absence (A) of breathing (pnea).

Hypoventilation: Breathing (ventilation) is slow (Hypo), shallow, and sometimes irregular.

Hyperventilation: Breathing (ventilation) is rapid (Hyper) and deeper than normal.

Dyspnea: Difficult or painful (Dys) breathing (pnea).

Cheyne-Stokes respirations: Respirations gradually increase in depth and rate and then become slow and shallow. Breathing may inhibit (apnea) for 10 to 20 seconds.

Orthopnea: Breathing (pnea) deeply and comfortably only when sitting (Ortho).

Kussmaul respirations: Very deep and rapid respirations.

Taking TPR as a Combined Procedure

In health care, there are four primary measurements that may demonstrate a great deal about how a patient's body is functioning. These four measurements are called as vital signs, which may include temperature, pulse, respirations and blood pressure. Health care workers often use the medical language for talking about these vital signs. They usually talk about a patient's TPR, which stands for temperature, pulse and respiration; and BP that stands for blood pressure. Nurse assistants are usually responsible for measuring and recording the vital signs of those in their care. These measurements are always taken when a patient/resident is first admitted to a healthcare facility, at regular intervals throughout the patient/resident's stay at the facility, and before the patient/resident is discharged from the facility.

When a patient first starts receiving care, the nurse assistant may be asked to take the patient/resident's vital signs frequently because these frequent measurements may help the health care team to determine what is normal (or baseline) for that patient. After the baseline is established, the patient's primary care provider may order the patient's vital signs to be taken on a less frequent but regular basis. The frequency may vary from one patient to another. The nurse assistant may also take a patient/resident's vital signs on an "as-needed basis," such as when he/she notices a change in the patient/resident's usual condition, or when the nurse asks him/her to do so.

Accuracy is extremely important when measuring vital signs. Vital sign measurements often affect decisions that are taken about the patient/resident's clinical care. The significance of these measurements to the patient/resident's care makes it essential that the nurse assistant should measure these signs accurately, record them correctly and report any changes in them promptly to the nurse. When a nurse assistant is measuring a patient/resident's vital signs, he/she should always remember that although taking these readings may be a routine task for him/her, having these readings taken may carry special significance for the patient/resident receiving care.

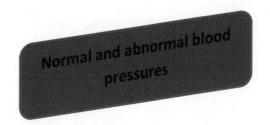

Normal and abnormal blood pressures

Blood pressure can be changed from minute to minute. Therefore, systolic and diastolic blood pressure has normal ranges i.e. Systolic pressure 90 mm Hg or higher but lower than 120 mm Hg and diastolic pressure 60 mm Hg or higher but lower than 80 mm Hg.

Blood Pressure

It is the measurement of the pressure of the circulating blood on the walls of the arteries. When the heart beats, it pumps blood into the arteries. The pressure of the blood against the unit area of the vessels' walls when the heart pumps the blood is called the systolic pressure. Systolic pressure is actually the period of heart muscle contraction. The pressure of the blood against the unit area of the vessels' walls when the heart relaxes is called the diastolic pressure. Diastolic pressure is basically the period of heart muscle relaxation. The systolic pressure is always higher than the diastolic pressure. Blood pressure is measured in mm (millimeters) of mercury (Hg). The systolic pressure is recorded and written over the diastolic pressure. For example, a systolic pressure of 115 mm Hg and a diastolic pressure of 75 mm Hg are written as 115/75 mm Hg.

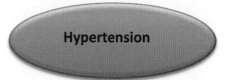

Hypertension

When the systolic pressure is 140 mm Hg or greater (hyper), or the diastolic pressure is 90 mm Hg or greater, it is called as hypertension. The nurse assistant should report any systolic measurement at or above 120 mm Hg. He/she should also report a diastolic pressure at or above 80 mm Hg.

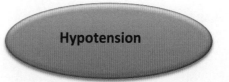

Hypotension

When the systolic pressure is less than (hypo) 90 mm Hg, or the diastolic pressure is less than 60 mm Hg, it is called as hypotension. The nurse assistant should report a systolic pressure below 90 mm Hg or a diastolic pressure less than 60 mm Hg.

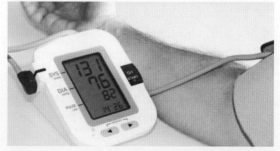

A blood pressure measurement consists of two numbers, which should be written like a fraction. The higher systolic reading goes on the top and the lesser diastolic reading goes on the bottom. For example, in the reading 115/85 mm Hg, 115 is the systolic pressure, and 85 is the diastolic pressure. In healthy adults, the normal range for blood pressure is less than 120/80 mm Hg. Hypotension is the term used to describe low blood pressure, and hypertension is the term used to demonstrate high blood pressure. A blood pressure that remains high over long period of time may damage the arteries and place stress on the heart. Therefore, it is very important for a nurse assistant to know what blood pressure is considered normal for each of the patient/resident in his/her care. Males frequently have higher blood pressures than females, and some ethnic groups may have higher blood pressures than others. In addition, blood pressure may also increase with age. When a nurse assistant is measuring a patient/resident's blood pressure, he/she should be aware that it is normal for the blood pressure to vary throughout the day, within a relatively narrow range. For example, blood pressure can be generally higher late in the day, as compared with the morning. Blood pressure may also be higher when a patient/resident is standing or sitting, as compared with when the patient/resident is lying down. Emotional stress may also increase the blood pressure. At times, the nurse assistant may be asked to measure the patient/resident's blood pressure first in one arm and then the other, or to take a series of blood pressure measurements with the patient/resident lying flat, then sitting up and then standing. The nurse assistant should always follow the nurse's instructions or the patient/resident's care plan.

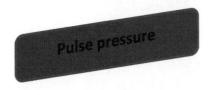

It is the difference between systolic and diastolic pressures, which can provide significant information concerning health of blood vessels. Average range of pulse pressure is usually 30-50 mmHg.

Factors that Raise and Lower Blood Pressure

Factors that raise blood pressure

a) Strong emotion
b) Sitting or standing
c) Exercise
d) Pain
e) Excitement
f) Decrease of blood vessel size
g) Digestion
h) Improperly placed cuff

Factors that lower blood pressure

a) Sleep
b) Rest
c) Depression
d) Lying down
e) Shock
f) Excessive blood loss

Equipment for Measuring Blood Pressure

The traditional way of measuring a patient/resident's blood pressure is with a sphygmomanometer and stethoscope. The sphygmomanometer consists three parts: a cuff that is placed around the patient/resident's arm, a bulb which is squeezed to fill the cuff with air, and a manometer that is a gauge for measuring the blood pressure. There are two styles of manometers available in the market.

- First is a mercury manometer, which is an upright gauge that contains a column of mercury. The mercury level shows the pressure readings.
- Second is an aneroid manometer that shows the pressure readings on a round dial with an arrow, which points to the numbers. Although the aneroid manometer contains no mercury, the unit of measure is still mm Hg (millimeters of mercury).

The fabric cuff has a rubber bladder that is connected by tubing to the bulb. A valve at the base of the bulb closes and opens to control the air flow into the bladder.

Measuring Blood Pressure

For measuring a person's blood pressure, the stethoscope is used to listen for changes in blood flow through the brachial artery of the arm. Inflating and then deflating the cuff that is wrapped around the patient/resident's arm causes changes in blood flow, which are used to identify the systolic and diastolic pressures. As the examiner pumps air into the cuff, the cuff pressure increases until it is high enough to inhibit the blood flow through the brachial artery. At this point, the examiner does not hear anything through the stethoscope. As the examiner turns the valve to deflate the cuff and releases the pressure on the brachial artery, the pressure in the cuff eventually matches the systolic blood pressure. At that point, the examiner will start to hear pulse sounds through the stethoscope. The reading on the manometer at the time that the examiner hears the first pulse sound is the systolic pressure. As the pressure in the cuff drops to equal the diastolic pressure in the artery, the sounds that the examiner hears change. The last sound that examiner hears before the pulse sounds fade away is the diastolic pressure. The electronic type displays the systolic and diastolic pressures by itself. It also displays the pulse rate. To use the device, the nurse assistant should follow the manufacturer's instructions. The nurse assistant should wrap the blood pressure cuff around the patient/resident's upper arm. An electronic sphygmomanometer measures the patient/resident's blood pressure automatically after placing the cuff on the patient/resident's arm. Some electronic instruments are completely automatic, while others need to inflate the cuff. It is not essential to use a stethoscope with an electronic sphygmomanometer.

Encouraging safety and comfort
Safety
Mercury is a dangerous and hazardous substance. Mercury manometers should be handled carefully. If one breaks, the nurse assistant should call for the nurse at once. The nurse assistant should always follow the agency's special procedures and precautions for handling all hazardous substances.

General guidelines for measuring blood pressure

- Blood pressure should not be taken on an arm:
  - With an IV infusion
  - With a dialysis access site
  - On the side of breast surgery
  - With an arm cast
  - The arm that is injured
- The nurse assistant should ask the nurse if he/she is not sure which arm to use.
- The nurse assistant should let the patient/resident rest for 10 to 20 minutes before measuring BP.
- BP should be measured with the patient/resident sitting or lying. Sometimes BP can also be measured in the standing position.
- The cuff should be applied to the bare upper arm. Clothing may affect the measurement.
- The nurse assistant should make sure that the cuff is snug. The reading would be wrong if the cuff is loose.
- A larger cuff should be used if the patient/resident is obese or has a large arm. The nurse assistant should use a small cuff if the patient/resident has a very small arm. He/she should ask the nurse what size to use as well as should check the care plan.
- The nurse assistant should make sure that the room is quiet. Talking, music, TV, and sounds from the hallway may affect an accurate measurement.

- The diaphragm of the stethoscope should be placed firmly over the brachial artery. The entire diaphragm of the stethoscope must have contact with the skin. It should not be placed under the cuff.
- The manometer should be placed where the nurse assistant can clearly see it.
- The nurse assistant should measure the systolic and diastolic pressures.
- The first sound should be expected to hear at the point where last pulse is felt. The first sound is the systolic pressure.
- The point where there is no sound or sound disappears is the diastolic pressure.
- The nurse assistant should take the BP again if he/she not sure of accuracy. He/she should wait 30 to 60 seconds to repeat the measurement. The nurse assistant should ask the nurse to take the BP if he/she is unsure of the measurement.

Observation and Reporting of the Patient/Resident's Pain

Pain or discomfort means to hurt, ache, or be sore. It is often called the fifth vital sign. Pain usually signals any tissue damage and it often causes the individual to seek clinical care. Pain is totally a personal phenomenon that differs for each individual. What aches to one individual may hurt to another. What one person calls ache, another may call it as sore. If a patient/resident complains of discomfort or pain, it means the patient/resident has pain or discomfort. Healthcare workers should believe the patient/resident.

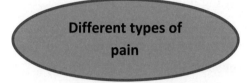

Different types of pain

There are multiple types of pain.

Acute pain

It is felt suddenly from disease, injury, trauma, or surgery. Acute pain signals any tissue damage. It lasts for a short period of time and lessens with healing.

Chronic pain

Chronic pain is a persistent pain that continues for a long period of time (months or years). It may also occur off and on and there is no longer tissue damage. Chronic pain may persist long even after healing. A common cause of chronic pain is arthritis.

Radiating pain

It is felt at the site of tissue damage and in surrounding areas. Pain from a heart attack is often felt in the left haw, left chest, left arm, and left shoulder. Gallbladder disease may cause radiating pain in the back, right upper abdomen, and the right shoulder.

Phantom pain

It is felt in a body part that is no longer there. An individual with an amputated leg may still sense leg pain.

Different signs of pain

Common signs of the pain may include:
- Increased pulse, blood pressure, and respirations.
- Moaning, sighing, groaning, or crying
- Squeezing eyes shut
- Tightening jaw
- Grinding teeth
- Holding a body part tightly
- Increased restlessness, agitation or tension
- Nausea
- Vomiting
- Increased sweating
- Difficulty moving, positioning or walking

General guidelines for observing and reporting of pain

- The nurse assistant should ask the patient/resident if he/she is still in any pain. Different types of pain can be used to assess the severity of the pain.
- The nurse assistant should ask the patient/resident to describe the characteristic features of pain, such as:
  - Location of pain
  - Frequency of pain e.g. whether pain is continuous or off and on
  - Duration of pain as how long it lasts
  - Quality of pain including its nature and type
- The nurse assistant should observe movement, facial expression, and respiration of the patient/resident to assess the severity of pain.

- The nurse assistant should also ask the patient/resident level of pain using facility policies and procedures.
- All the relevant details regarding complaints of pain should be reported to licensed nurse.

Encouraging safety and comfort

Patients/residents should be often checked and asked if the pain has been worsen or relieved. The nurse assistant should explain the patient/resident about what his/her plan to do and how it will be done. The nurse assistant should always avoid sudden or jerking movement when repositioning the patient/resident. Patients/residents should be offered backrubs (if indicated). The nurse assistant should listen to all concerns of the patient/resident carefully and should provide emotional support. A clean, comfortable, and quiet environment should be maintained by eliminating unpleasant sights, sounds, and odors from the surrounding environment.

Recording Vital Signs on Chart, Graph, Nursing Assistant Notes

Procedure for charting temperature, pulse, and respiration

The nurse assistant should record and report normal and abnormal TPR to the licensed nurse. It should be recorded on hospital flow sheets, nurse assistant notes, or graphic records. The nurse assistant should always follow his/her agency policy to record TPR. The charting of TPR and BP should be as:

1. Recording and charting temperature
2. Recording and charting pulse
3. Recording and charting respiration
4. Recording and charting blood pressure

1. Recording and charting temperature

Common sites to measure an individual's body temperature may include the mouth (an oral temperature), the rectum (a rectal temperature), armpit (an axillary temperature), ear (a tympanic temperature), and temporal artery (a forehead temperature). Body temperature is often taken in degrees. Degrees may be measured on two different temperature scales i.e. Celsius (°C) or Fahrenheit (°F). In the United States, the commonly used scale is the Fahrenheit scale.

As the variation occurs from site to site, it is significant to note the site of the measuring temperature. The nurse assistant should always follow his/her employer's policy regarding how to note the site. A routine practice is to write an "O" after the measurement if the temperature was obtained orally, an "R" if the temperature was measured rectally [example 101°F (R)], a "TY" if the temperature was obtained in the ear [example 101°F (TY)], and an "AX" if the temperature was taken in the armpit [example 101°F (AX)].

2. Recording and charting pulse

The nurse assistant should take radial and apical pulses and must count, report, and record them accurately. The radial pulse is most commonly used pulse for routine vital signs. For taking radial pulse, the nurse assistant should place his/her first 2 or 3 fingertips against the radial artery. The radial artery should be on the thumb side of the wrist. The pulse should be counted for 30 seconds and then multiplied the number by 2. This provides the number of beats per minute (pulses in 60 seconds). For example, if a nurse assistant counts 36 beats in 30 seconds. For the number of beats per minute, he/she should multiply 36 by 2 ($36 \times 2 = 72$). The pulse would be 72 per minute. If the pulse is irregular, the nurse assistant should count it for 1 minute. In some agencies, radial pulses are measured for 1 minute. The nurse assistant should always follow agency policy. The apical pulse is slightly below the nipple, on the left side of the chest. A stethoscope should be used to count the pulse for 1 minute. The heartbeat usually sounds like a lub-dub. The nurse assistant should count each lub-dub as a single beat. It is remembered that the lub should not be counted as one beat and the dub as another. Pulse readings other than radial must be noted as Apical pulse 86 (a).

3. Recording and charting respiration

Patients/residents may alter their breathing patterns when they know their respirations are being counted. Therefore, the nurse assistant should not tell the patient/resident while counting respiratory rate. Respirations should be counted right after taking a pulse. The nurse assistant should place his/her fingers or stethoscope over the pulse site. The patient/resident assumes that the examiner is taking the pulse. To count respirations, the nurse assistant should watch the chest rise and fall and should count them for 30 seconds. He/she should multiply the number by 2 for the number of respirations in 1 minute. For example, if the examiner counts 8 breaths in 30 seconds. For the number of respirations in 1 minute, he/she should multiply 8 by 2 ($8 \times 2 = 16$). The respiratory rate would be 16/min. If an examiner notes an abnormal pattern, he/she should count respirations for 1 minute. In most of the agencies, respirations are often counted for 1 minute. The nurse assistant should always follow agency policy

4. Recording and charting blood pressure

A blood pressure measurement consists of two numbers, which should be written on chart like a fraction. The higher systolic reading goes on the top and the lesser diastolic reading goes on the bottom. For example, in the reading 115/85 mm Hg, 115 is the systolic pressure, and 85 is the diastolic pressure. The nurse assistant should record and report abnormal blood pressure reading to the licensed nurse. If blood pressure reading is taken other than arm, the nurse assistant should note its location e.g. 115/85-thigh.

Helpful Resources

Baken, D. M., & Woolley, C. (2011). Validation of the distress thermometer, impact thermometer and combinations of these in screening for distress. *Psycho-Oncology*, *20*(6), 609-614. https://doi.org/10.1002/pon.1934

Bradley, R. (2007). Improving respiratory assessment skills. *The Journal for Nurse Practitioners*, *3*(4), 276-277. https://doi.org/10.1016/j.nurpra.2007.02.005

Brekke, I. J., Puntervoll, L. H., Pedersen, P. B., Kellett, J., & Brabrand, M. (2019). The value of vital sign trends in predicting and monitoring clinical deterioration: A systematic review. *PLOS ONE*, *14*(1), e0210875. https://doi.org/10.1371/journal.pone.0210875

Fillingim, R. B., Loeser, J. D., Baron, R., & Edwards, R. R. (2016). Assessment of chronic pain: Domains, methods, and mechanisms. *The Journal of Pain*, *17*(9), T10-T20. https://doi.org/10.1016/j.jpain.2015.08.010

Grodzinsky, E., & Sund Levander, M. (2019). Assessment and evaluation of body temperature. *Understanding Fever and Body Temperature*, 97-114. https://doi.org/10.1007/978-3-030-21886-7_7

Quint, M., & Thomas, S. (2009). Respiratory assessment. *Respiratory Physiotherapy*, 17-36. https://doi.org/10.1016/b978-0-7020-3003-1.50007-3

Robinson, T., & Scullion, J. (2021). Respiratory assessment. *Oxford Handbook of Respiratory Nursing*, 29-74. https://doi.org/10.1093/med/9780198831815.003.0004

Rolfe, S. (2019). The importance of respiratory rate monitoring. *British Journal of Nursing*, *28*(8), 504-508. https://doi.org/10.12968/bjon.2019.28.8.504

Schofield, P. (2015). Assessment and management of pain in older adults. *Oxford Medicine Online*. https://doi.org/10.1093/med/9780199689644.003.0012

Teixeira, C. C., Boaventura, R. P., Souza, A. C., Paranaguá, T. T., Bezerra, A. L., Bachion, M. M., & Brasil, V. V. (2015). Vital signs measurement: An indicator of safe care delivered to elderly patients. *Texto & Contexto - Enfermagem*, *24*(4), 1071-1078. https://doi.org/10.1590/0104-07072015000003970014

Wald, A., & Garber, C. E. (2017). A review of current literature on vital sign assessment of physical activity in primary care. *Journal of Nursing Scholarship*, *50*(1), 65-73. https://doi.org/10.1111/jnu.12351

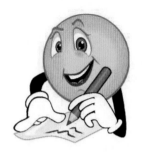

Chapter Eleven:

Nutrition

Outline

I: Basic need for food and fluids

II: Common nutrients and their food sources

III: Planning a well-balanced diet

IV: MyPlate food guidance system

V: Vegetarian diet

VI: The vegan basic four food groups

VII: Age-related changes affecting nutritional and fluid needs of the elderly

VIII: Commonly ordered therapeutic diets

IX: Procedures for feeding patients/residents

X: Influence of culture and religion on dietary practices

XI: Alternative ways to administer nutrition

Body's Need for Food and Fluids

Water and food are the basic physical needs necessary for life. The individual's diet may affect his/her physical and mental wellbeing and function. A poor diet and poor dietary habits:

- Increase the risk for infection and other diseases.
- Cause healing problems.
- Increase the risk for injuries and other accidents.

Basic Nutrition

Nutrition is the primary processes involved in the ingestion, absorption, digestion, and utilization of food and fluids by the body. Good nutrition is required for proper growth, healing, and body functions. A nutrient is a substance that is ingested, absorbed, digested, and utilized by the body. Nutrients are grouped into carbohydrates, proteins, fats, vitamins, minerals, and water. Carbohydrates, proteins, and fats provide the body fuel for energy.

A calorie is the energy value of food.

- 1 gram of fat = 9 calories
- 1 gram of protein = 4 calories
- 1 gram of carbohydrate = 4 calories

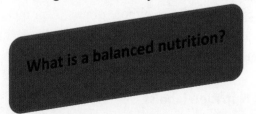

What is a balanced nutrition?

Nutrition is the biological process of taking in and utilizing nutrients, which are substances that the body requires to grow and stay healthy. Nutrients can be obtained through vitamin and mineral supplements; however, the best and main source of nutrients is through diet (the food we eat and the beverages we drink). Eating a balanced, healthy, and nutritious diet (diet that contains a wide variety of nutrients) helps to maintain proper health and may improve poor health. To get all the essential nutrients, an individual needs to eat a variety of foods. No single food or group of foods can supply all the necessary nutrients the body requires.

Common Nutrients and Their Common Food Sources

As already discussed, no food or food group can supply all essential nutrients. A well balanced and nutritious diet ensures an adequate intake of essential nutrients. Multiple types of nutrients may include the following:

Carbohydrates

Carbohydrates provide energy and fiber for bowel elimination. Carbohydrates are the major sources to supply the body with glucose, which body's most basic source of energy. The major nutritious sources of carbohydrates may include whole grains (such as whole wheat bread, oatmeal, and brown rice), vegetables and fruits. In addition to providing energy, these carbohydrates also supply fiber, a substance that aids the digestive tract function properly and decreases risk for cardiac disease and diabetes. Other less nutritious sources of carbohydrates may include white bread, table sugar, white rice and white pasta.

Proteins

Proteins are the most important nutrients required for tissue growth and repair. Proteins support the body to build muscle and other body tissues. Proteins intake and use is especially significant when an individual is healing from an injury or surgery. Proteins are also a very important source of energy for the body. The most nutritious sources of proteins may include meat, poultry, fish, eggs, beans, and dairy products.

Fats

Fats provide energy and help the body to use certain vitamins more efficiently. Fats are often a concentrated source of energy. They help to feel full and make food taste better. Fats also help to keep the body warm and protect internal organs. For good health, however, only a small amount of fats is required each day. The nutritious sources of fats may include olive oil, canola oil, peanut oil, butter, lard, margarine, meats, cheese, egg yolks, and nuts. Unneeded and extra dietary fats are stored as body fats (adipose tissues).

Vitamins and minerals

Vitamins and minerals are small molecules that are required to regulate body functions and form cells and tissues. The human body may store vitamins A, D, E, and K. Vitamin C and the B complex vitamins cannot store in the body and must be ingested daily. The lack of a certain vitamin may result in various health problems. Minerals are required for bone and tooth formation, muscle and nerve function, fluid balance, and other vital body processes. Vitamins and minerals are found in various different types of foods. The most nutritious sources of vitamins and minerals may include whole grains, vegetables and fruits, lean meats, and dairy products.

Planning a Well-Balanced Diet

A healthy and well balanced diet helps to ensure that people are consuming nutrients in the right amounts to stay healthy (or to regain health). It also helps to maintain a healthy body weight (a body weight that is not too low or too high). Being underweight or overweight puts an individual at risk for various health problems. Two major tools that are available to help people plan a healthy and well balanced diet include MyPlate and Nutrition labels.

■ MyPlate

MyPlate was established by the American government to help Americans "build a healthy plate". MyPlate mainly focuses on five major food groups (vegetables, fruits, protein foods, grains, and dairy) that supply essential nutrients. It also uses a place setting to depict how much of each food group as compared to other food groups should be eaten at each meal. MyPlate encourages individuals to choose vegetables, fruits, whole grains, lean meats and low-fat dairy, and to cut back on unhealthy fats, sodium, and added sugars.

■ Nutrition labels

It is recommended that all packaged foods should have a nutrition label to provide information about calories, serving size, the nutrients supplied by the food, and the ingredients in the food. Reading these labels may help individuals make good choices about nutrition. These labels are also an essential tool for individuals who are trying to manage their weight, because they provide significant information about the number of calories and appropriate serving sizes food contains. A calorie is the energy value of food that is used to describe the amount of energy a food supplies. Utilizing more calories than the body needs may lead to weight gain, because the extra calories are stored in the body as fat.

Although the basic principles of following a healthy and well balanced diet are the same for everyone, the number of calories and the types of nutrients an individual needs to take in each day may vary according to the person's age, gender, and specific conditions. For example:

- Males tend to need more calories than females do.
- Infants, children and teenagers have increased demands for calories and nutrients because they are growing.
- Pregnant females and females who are breastfeeding usually need more of certain types of nutrients, such as calcium and proteins.
- Individuals who are injured or ill will have different nutritional demands, depending on what type of injury or illness they have. For example, an individual who is recovering from an injury, surgery, or burn usually needs more protein and calories because the body is utilizing a great deal of energy to repair the damaged tissues.

- Older individuals who are frail usually do not require as many calories, because they are usually not very active. A dietitian (a healthcare professional who has specialized training in the field of nutrition) is generally consulted when it is essential to plan a diet for an individual with special needs.

MyPlate Food Guidance System

The MyPlate symbol encourages healthy diet planning and eating from 5 major food groups (vegetables, fruits, protein foods, grains, and dairy), which is issued by the United States Department of Agriculture (USDA). MyPlate is a nutrition guide that encourages healthy eating as well as proper physical activity. It helps individuals to make wise food choices by:

- Balancing calories
- Eating less
- Increasing certain nutrients
- Avoiding over-sized portions of foods
- Making half plate with fruits and vegetables
- Making at least half of the grains with whole grains
- Minimizing certain foods
- Selecting low-sodium foods
- Drinking fat-free or low-fat (1%) milk
- Drinking water instead of sugary drinks

The amount required from each food group depends on age, gender, and physical activity. Physical activity should be moderate or vigorous. The USDA recommends that healthy adults should do at least one of the following.

- Moderate physical activity of 2 hours and 30 minutes each week
- Vigorous physical activity of 1 hour and 15 minutes each week

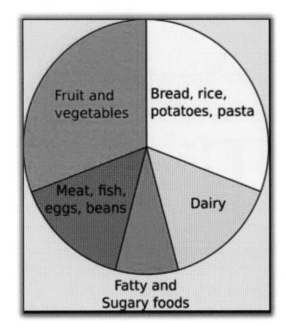

Physical activity of at least 3 days a week is the most ideal scenario. Each physical activity should be for at least 10 minutes at a time. Healthy adults should also do strengthening activities at least 2 days a week. Sit-ups, push-ups, and weight-lifting are examples.

Grains group

Foods made from rice, wheat, oats, barley, cornmeal, or other cereal grains are included in grain group. Pasta, bread, oatmeal, breakfast cereals, grits, and tortillas are examples.

- Whole grains contain the entire grain kernel. Whole wheat flour, bulgar (cracked wheat), whole cornmeal, oatmeal, and brown rice are examples of whole grains.

- Refined grains have fine texture, which are processed to remove the grain kernel. White bread, White flour, and white rice are examples of refined grains. They have lesser amount of dietary fibers as compared to whole grains.

Grains, especially whole grains, have following important health benefits:

- They reduce the risk of cardiac problems.
- They may prevent constipation.
- Grains may also help with healthy weight management.
- They may prevent certain birth defects.
- Grains contain the nutrients such as dietary fibers, several B vitamins (riboflavin, niacin, thiamin, and folate), and minerals (iron, magnesium, and selenium).

Vegetable group

Vegetables can be eaten as cooked or raw form. They may be fresh, frozen, dried, canned, or juice. The 5 major vegetable sub-groups are:

- Dark green vegetables: Dark green vegetables may include broccoli, collard greens, bok choy, dark green leafy lettuce, kale, romaine lettuce, watercress, spinach, turnips.
- Beans and peas: Black beans, chickpeas, black-eyed peas, kidney beans, lentils, pinto beans, soybeans, navy beans, split peas.
- Red and orange vegetables: They may include acorn, butternut, carrots, red peppers, sweet potatoes, pumpkin, tomatoes, and tomato juice.
- Starchy vegetables: Green bananas, green peas, corn, green bananas, green

lima beans, potatoes, plantains, taro, water chestnuts.

- Other vegetables: Artichokes, asparagus, beets, bean sprouts, Brussels sprouts, celery, cucumbers, eggplant, green beans, green peppers cabbage, cauliflower, mushrooms, parsnips, turnips, wax beans, okra, onions, zucchini.

Vegetables have following important health benefits.

- They may decrease the risk for stroke, high blood pressure, cardiovascular diseases, and diabetes.

- Vegetables may protect against certain cancers such as cancers of the mouth, stomach, and colon-rectum.
- They may reduce the risk of kidney stones and bone loss.
- Vegetables may help lower calorie intake. Most vegetables are low in calories and fats.
- They contain no cholesterol.
- Vegetables may prevent certain birth defects.
- Vegetables contain various nutrients such as potassium, folate (folic acid), dietary fiber, vitamins C and A.

Food group	Daily servings
Grains	Adult women: 5-6 oz, at least 3 oz from whole grains Adult men: 6-8 oz, at least 3-4 oz from whole grains
Fruits	Adult women: 1-2 cups Adult men: 2 cups
Dairy	Adult women: 3 cups Adult men: 3 cups
Vegetables	Adult women: 2-2.5 cups Adult men: 2.5-3 cups
Protein foods	Adult women: 5-5.5 cups Adult men: 5.5-6.5 cups

Fruit group

Fruit or pure fruit juice are included in the fruit group. Fruits may be fresh, frozen, dried, or canned. Fruits canned in syrup should be avoided because syrup contains added sugar. People should choose fruits canned in 100% fruit juice or water.

Fruits have following significant health benefits:

- They may reduce the risk for stroke, high blood pressure, cardiovascular diseases, obesity, and diabetes.

- They may also protect against certain cancers such cancers of the mouth, stomach, and colon-rectum.
- Fruits may reduce the risk of kidney stones and bone loss.
- They may help prevent constipation.
- Fruits may also help lower calorie intake because most fruits are low in calories and fats.
- Fruits usually don't have cholesterol.
- They are low in sodium and may prevent certain birth defects.

- They contain several important nutrients including potassium, dietary fibers, folate (folic acid), and vitamin C.

Dairy group

Milk and all milk products are part of the dairy group. There are many dietary products made from milk. Low-fat or fat-free products should be the best choices. The dairy group may include all fluid milk, yogurt, and cheese (Cream, butter, and cream cheese are not in this group).

Dairy group has following health benefits:
- They help to build and maintain bone mass throughout life to reduce the risk of osteoporosis.
- They may decrease the risk of cardiovascular disease, diabetes, and high blood pressure.
- Dairy group contains various essential nutrients including potassium, calcium, and vitamin D.

Protein foods group

Protein food group includes all dietary products made from poultry, meat, eggs, seafood, processed soy products, seeds, and nuts. Beans and peas are included in both protein foods group as well as the vegetable group. When choosing foods from this group, it should be remembered:
- To choose lean or low-fat poultry and meat. Higher fat choices may include chicken with skin and regular ground beef.
- Using fat for cooking may increase the calories.

- Trout, salmon, and herring are rich in substances that may decrease the risk of heart disease.
- Liver and other organ meats contain higher proportions of cholesterol.
- Egg yolks are rich with cholesterol and egg whites are cholesterol-free.
- Processed meats contain added sodium.

Oils

Oils are fats, which are liquids at room temperature. Vegetable oils used for cooking are examples. Oils may include corn oil, canola oil, and olive oil. Oils can be obtained from plants and fish. Because they have some essential nutrients, the United States Department of Agriculture (USDA) includes oils in food patterns. However, oils are basically not a food group. Adult males are allowed 6 to 7 teaspoons daily and adult females are allowed 5 to 6 teaspoons daily. Some foods are high in oil such as olives, nuts, some fishes, and avocados.

When making oil choices, it should be remembered that:
- Oils are very high in calories.
- The best oil choices come from nuts, fish, and vegetables.
- Some foods contain mainly oil like mayonnaise, soft margarine, and certain salad dressings.
- Oils obtained from plant sources do not contain cholesterol.
- Solid fats exist as solids at room temperature. Common solid fats may include milk fat, butter, beef fat (tallow, suet), pork fat (lard), stick margarine, chicken fat, and shortening.
- Solid fats and oils have about 120 calories in each tablespoon.

- Sufficient oil is usually consumed daily from fish, nuts, cooking oil, and salad dressings.

Vegetarian Diet

There are several types of vegetarian diets exist. The common characteristic of all these choices is being mainly as plant-based foods. People usually select a vegetarian diet for a variety of reasons: religious, ecological, ethnic, philosophical, economic, or ethical. Vegetarian diets have various potential health benefits, which is another important consideration for their use.

There are four major types of vegetarians exist, which may include:

Vegans
They are strict vegetarians and they exclude all animal products (fish, meat, eggs, poultry, milk, and dairy products) from their diet.

Lacto-vegetarians
They eat plant foods and dairy products (no eggs).

Ovo-vegetarians
These people eat plant foods and eggs (no dairy products).

Lacto-ovo vegetarians
They eat plant foods, dairy products, and eggs.

The Vegan Basic Four Food Groups

here are different types of vegan diets exist. Vegan diets typically exclude fish, meats, eggs, dairy, other animal products like honey. A vegan must work to balance his/her diet to make sure that he/she is receiving adequate vitamins and minerals from the food. Apart from taking evenly from each of the four vegan food groups every day, the vegan should discuss with his/her health care professional about vegan supplements for iron, vitamin B12, and other nutrients.

The most common vegan diets may include following four food groups:
1. Whole grains – 5 or more servings each day
2. Vegetables – 4 or more servings each day
3. Fruits – 3 or more servings each day
4. Legumes – 2-3 servings each day

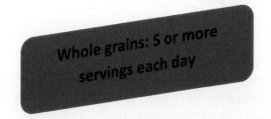

Whole grains: 5 or more servings each day

This group includes rice, bread, pasta, hot or cold cereal, millet, corn, barley, bulgur, and tortillas. Each of the meals should be around a hearty grain dish, because grains are rich in fiber and other complex carbohydrates, as well as protein, vitamin B complex and zinc. *Serving size should be: 1/2 cup hot cereal; 1 slice bread; 1 ounce dry cereal.*

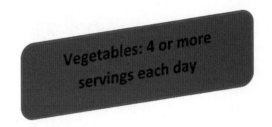

Vegetables are packed with several essential nutrients including riboflavin, iron, calcium, vitamin C, beta-carotene, fiber, and other vitamins. Dark green and leafy vegetables such as collards, kale, broccoli, turnip greens, chicory, or bok choy are especially nutritious sources of these important nutrients. Dark yellow and orange vegetables such as winter squash, sweet potatoes, carrots, and pumpkin provide extra beta-carotene. Vegans should include generous portions of a variety of vegetables in their diet. *Serving size should be: 1 cup raw vegetables; 1/2 cup cooked vegetables.*

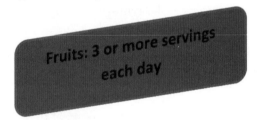

Fruits are rich in beta-carotene, fiber, and vitamin C. Vegans should include at least one serving each day of fruits that are high in citrus fruits (vitamin C). They should choose whole fruit over fruit juices, which do not contain as much fiber as whole fruit. *Serving size should be: 1 medium piece of fruit; 1/2 cup juice; 1/2 cup cooked fruit.*

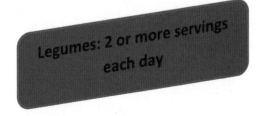

Legumes – another name for peas, beans, and lentils -- are great sources of proteins,

fibers, iron, calcium, zinc, and B vitamins. This group also includes baked and refried beans, chickpeas, tempeh, soy milk, and texturized vegetable protein. *Serving size should be: 1/2 cup cooked beans; 8 ounces soy milk; 4 ounces tofu or tempeh.*

Age-Related Changes Affecting Nutritional and Fluid Needs of Elderly

With aging, several changes occur in the gastrointestinal system, such as:

- Smell and taste becomes dull.
- Appetite and secretion of digestive juices decrease.

Fatty and fried foods are difficult to digest and may cause maldigestion. Some older persons avoid high-fiber foods that are needed for bowel elimination because high-fiber foods are difficult to chew and may irritate the intestines. Examples are celery, apricots, and fruits and vegetables with seeds and skins. Foods providing soft bulk are usually ordered for older persons with constipation or chewing problems. These foods may include whole-grain cereals and cooked vegetables and fruits. Calorie needs are also lower in older people. Energy and activity levels also become much lower with advancing age. Older people usually take several medications that may interfere with digestion, fluid balance, and nutrient use. In these people, loss of teeth, poor oral hygiene, loss of teeth, and poorly fitting dentures may result poor nutrition. Many common diseases in old age may interfere with their eating and/or the ability to use nutrients. Social isolation is also an important factor, which may interfere with appetite and the body's utilization of nutrients.

Foods that contain calcium should be preferred to prevent musculoskeletal changes. Protein should also be preferred for tissue growth and repair; however, because of cost, their diets may lack high-protein foods. A patient/resident may require nutritional supplements (such as Boost or Ensure) one to three times a day to meet their daily nutrient needs.

Elder care special notes

Older people often have multiple risk factors for malnutrition. Being on a fixed income may make it extremely hard for an older person to afford healthy food. Physical disabilities such as those caused by stroke, tooth loss, or vision loss may make it more difficult for the person to prepare, chew, or swallow the food. Emotional difficulties like depression, grief, and loneliness may cause the older person to lose interest in eating. Conditions like dementia that affect the person's memory may also cause the person to forget how and when to eat. Sensory changes such as decreased senses of smell and taste can also adversely affect a person's appetite. When caring for an older patient/resident, the nurse assistant should be alert for signs that affect the patient/resident's dietary habits (such as lack of interest in food or weight loss), and should report any concerns to the nurse right away. The nurse assistant should also pay a special attention to make meal time more enjoyable for the patient/resident.

Specific food allergies

The nurse assistant should know about the patient/resident's food allergies and should always check every tray served. Patients/residents should also be evaluated time to time for new food allergies. The nurse assistant should always check the food additive allergies such as shellfish, peanuts, and wheat along with checking for lactose intolerance.

Factors affecting patient/resident's eating and nutrition

People differ in when they eat, what they eat, and how they prepare their food. Nurse assistants can play an important role in encouraging patients/residents in their care to eat a diet that helps them to regain or maintain their health. Knowing about the factors that may affect the choices a patient/resident makes about food can help a nurse assistant to respect those choices while providing care. All this knowledge may also help a nurse assistant to identify reasons why a patient/resident may not be eating a healthy diet. Therefore, the nurse assistant can take steps to help the patient/resident eat more healthfully.

Examples of those factors that can affect what and how a patient/resident eats may include:

■ Personal likes and dislikes

Each individual has certain personal likes and dislikes when it comes to food. One individual may not like chocolate, while another may not like green beans. Usually these choices develop with age and social experiences.

■ Allergies and intolerances

Some individuals may have reactions that may range from unpleasant to life-threatening if they eat some specific foods. Therefore, patients/residents usually avoid foods that cause allergic reactions. They may also avoid foods that cause diarrhea, nausea, vomiting, gas, indigestion, or headaches.

■ Culture and religion

An individual's food choices, likes and dislikes are greatly influenced by religious practices, social customs, and the availability of ingredients. Culture influences food choices, dietary practices, and food preparation. Baking, smoking, frying, or roasting food and eating raw food are common cultural practices. Selecting, eating, and preparing food often involve religious practices. A patient/resident may follow some, all, some, or none of the dietary practices of his/her faith. The nurse assistant should respect the patient/resident's religious practices.

■ Patient/resident's budget

Individuals usually make choices about food according to what they can afford. Individuals with limited incomes often buy the cheaper carbohydrate foods. Their diets often lack certain vitamins, proteins, and minerals.

■ Willingness or ability to cook

Many people depend on restaurant meals or prepared convenience foods because they lack the time, strength, interest, or skills needed to cook.

■ Appetite

A patient/resident's desire for food or appetite may also influences greatly what and how a patient/resident eats. Physical and emotional factors may cause a patient/resident's appetite to decrease or increase. Anorexia, a loss of appetite, is a common among individuals who are receiving health care. Factors that contribute to anorexia may include nausea, pain, depression, medication side effects, or an impaired sense of smell or taste.

■ Drugs or medications

Drugs may cause loss of appetite, nausea, confusion, constipation, impaired taste, or altered GI function. They can also cause inflammation of the mouth, esophagus, throat, and stomach.

■ Chewing and swallowing problems

Teeth, mouth, and gums problems can affect chewing. Examples may include dry or sore mouth, oral pain, gums diseases, dental problems, and dentures that fit poorly. Stroke, confusion, pain, dry mouth, and diseases of the throat, mouth, and esophagus can affect swallowing.

■ Impaired cognitive function

Impaired cognitive function may adversely affect the patient/resident's ability to use eating utensils. It may affect chewing, eating, and swallowing.

■ Age

Many GI alterations may occur with aging.

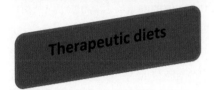

Commonly Ordered Therapeutic Diets

Therapeutic diets

It is a special diet that is ordered to support a patient/resident to maintain or regain his/her health. The patient's primary care provider orders the special therapeutic diet, and the dietitian recommends a meal plan that not only meets the demands of the diet but it also suits the patient's individual tastes and needs. When a nurse assistant is caring for a patient/resident who is receiving a therapeutic diet, he/she will need to be familiar with the type of therapeutic diet that was ordered, and also the cause why the therapeutic diet was ordered. This knowledge helps the nurse assistant to identify errors (a mix-up with meal trays) and reinforce information the nurse has provided the patient/resident about the reason for, and benefits of, the therapeutic diet. It is significant to help and encourage the patient/resident to follow any special therapeutic diet that has been ordered, because not following the therapeutic diet orders may cause health problems.

Following are some commonly ordered therapeutic diets to meet special needs of patients/residents:

Soft, mechanical, or pureed diet

Food can be prepared in special ways to make it easier for a patient/resident to swallow, chew, and digest. A soft diet includes mashed and soft foods, such as mashed potatoes and hot breakfast cereal. A mechanical diet includes foods that are ground up (such as ground meat) or chopped very small. A pureed diet includes foods that are blended to a very soft and smooth consistency, which is similar to that of pudding or a milkshake. A pureed diet may seem very unappealing, but keeping the individual foods separate from one another and having a professional attitude toward the food can help the patient/resident to accept it.

Liquid diet

A liquid diet may be ordered for a patient/resident who has digestive issues or has had recent surgery. A full liquid diet or clear liquid diet may be ordered. A clear liquid diet may include liquids that can be seen through, such as gelatin, broth, tea, clear carbonated sodas, and clear juices. A full liquid diet includes fruit juices such as grapefruit and orange juice, ice cream, strained soups, milk, and thinned cooked cereal. A liquid diet does not provide sufficient nutrition; therefore, it should be only used for 1 to 2 days.

Sodium-restricted diet

Sodium may be limited for patients/individuals with hypertension, kidney, or heart disease. Sodium-restricted diet must be prepared with no added salt, and foods that naturally have high amount of sodium (such as cured meats, pickles, lunch meat, and cheeses) should be avoided. The patient/resident is usually not permitted to add salt to foods at the table; however, the primary care provider may approve the use of a salt substitute. Sodium-restricted foods are often prepared with other spices to increase flavor and make up for the lack of salt. The average amount of sodium consumption in the daily diet should be 3000 to 5000 milligrams. The body requires no more than 2300 mg of sodium in a day. Healthy individuals normally excrete excess sodium in the urine. Liver, heart, and kidney diseases and certain drugs may cause the body to retain excessive sodium. Extra sodium in the body causes the water retention. Therefore, with excessive sodium, water is retained in excessive amount in the body. Tissues swell with excessive water. There would be excess fluid in the blood vessels and the heart needs to work harder. With heart disease, the extra workload may cause dangerous issues and even death. The physician orders the amount of sodium allowed. Sodium-restricted diets involve:

- Omitting high-sodium diets
- Not adding salt to food at the table
- Limiting the amount of salt during cooking
- Diet planning

Carbohydrate-controlled diet

This diet is ordered for patients/residents with diabetes. The dietician recommends the amount of carbohydrates, proteins, and fats the patient/resident can have each day based on the patient/resident's activity level and nutritional demands. Meals are planned so that the patient/resident's daily budget of carbohydrates, proteins, and fats is spaced throughout the day to help keep blood glucose levels steady.

Calorie-restricted diet

A diet with 1,200, 1,500, 1,800 or 2,000 calories per day can be ordered for a patient/resident who needs to control his/her weight. The dietician or primary care provider may recommend mineral supplements and multivitamins for a daily diet of 1,200 calories or fewer. For mild calorie restriction, the physician or dietician may order a regular no-concentrated-sweets (NCS) diet that only eliminates sweets, such as cookies and candy.

Heart healthy diet

A heart healthy diet is usually ordered for patients/residents with heart disease. Heart healthy diets are naturally low in unhealthy fats. Low-fat or non-fat dairy products, lean meats, vegetables, fruits, and whole grains are encouraged. Cooking techniques that involve the utilization of additional fats (such as frying) are avoided.

High-protein diet

A primary care provider or dietician may recommend this diet for patients/residents who do not eat enough protein or who require additional protein to rebuild injured tissue.

The dysphagia diet

Assisting a patient/resident who has difficulty swallowing

Dysphagia is the difficulty (dys) in swallowing (phagia).

- A slow swallow means the patient/resident has difficulty getting enough food and fluids for proper nutrition and fluid balance.
- An unsafe swallow means that food enters the airway to cause aspiration.

Aspiration is breathing food, fluid, vomitus, or an object into the lungs. Food thickness should be adjusted to meet the patient/resident's needs.

A patient/resident who has had a stroke that has resulted in speech difficulties may also have problems with swallowing food. A patient/resident who has difficulty swallowing may be on a soft diet. There may also be orders from dietician or primary care provider to use liquid thickeners.

When assisting a patient/resident who has trouble swallowing during meal time:

- The nurse assistant should remain with the patient/resident while he/she is eating.
- If the patient/resident is working with a speech therapist to relearn safe swallowing techniques, the nurse assistant should make sure that he/she is aware of these techniques so that the nurse assistant can help the patient/resident practice them.
- If liquid thickeners have been ordered, the nurse assistant should make sure that all of the liquids on the tray, including soup, are thickened before serving them.
- The patient/resident should be encouraged to chew slowly and thoroughly.
- Distractions such as watching television should be eliminated, so that the patient/resident can concentrate on eating.
- The nurse assistant should keep the patient/resident's head elevated during eating and for at least 30 minutes after eating.

Safety and comfort are significant when feeding a patient/resident with dysphagia. The nurse assistant must:

- Understand the signs and symptoms of dysphagia.
- Feed the patient/resident according to the care plan.
- Follow aspiration precautions as per care plan.
- Report changes in how the patient/resident eats.
- Observe for clinical features of aspiration such as coughing, choking, or difficulty breathing during or after meals, abnormal respiratory or breathing sounds. The nurse assistant should report these observations to the nurse at once.

Responsibilities of the Nurse Assistant

- Nurse assistants should make sure that all patients/residents receive their ordered diet properly.
- They should check arm bands against names on trays at each meal.
- They should report any issues regarding diet such as food or liquid preferences, difficulty swallowing or chewing, nausea or vomiting, food allergy, and anorexia to the nurse at once.
- The nurse assistant should open containers on tray as needed.
- They should assist physicians, nurses, and dieticians in assessing fluid balance through proper monitoring and documentation of intake and output (I & O).

- The nurse assistant should always follow the facility guidelines regarding the calculation and recording food intake.
- They should also determine the reason for any tray or food refusal, and should offer alternates to the relevant patient/resident if permitted.
- If the patient/resident refuses alternate, the nurse assistant should report refusal to licensed nurse.
- The nurse assistant should not offer any extra food or condiments to the patient/resident without checking with licensed nurse.
- Hot foods should be served as hot and cold foods as cold.
- The nurse assistant should not mix pureed foods.
- The nurse assistant should always check trays to monitor percentage of diet eaten and should always ensure an upright position of the patient/resident while eating unless otherwise ordered.

Procedures for Feeding Patients/Residents

Meal time when a patient/resident is receiving health care

Meal time can be difficult for a patient/resident who is receiving clinical care. There are various physical and emotional factors that can affect a patient/resident who is receiving clinical care to have very little or no appetite. For a patient/resident who is already ill or has a physical disability, the act of eating may need a great deal of physical effort and can be an extremely frustrating and tiring process. The patient/resident may be embarrassed about requiring help with an activity as basic as eating. There are two primary goals for meal times when a patient/resident is receiving clinical care. First, the nurse assistant should make the meal as pleasurable and positive as possible for the patient/resident. Secondly, the nurse assistant should improve or maintain the patient/resident's food intake.

Usually, achieving the first goal may help the nurse assistant to achieve the second. To make the meal more pleasurable, the nurse assistant should:

- Involve the patient/resident in decisions making regarding what to eat, when to eat, and where to eat as much as possible.
- Support traditions and rituals the patient/resident may have regarding eating and mealtimes, such as giving thanks before a meal.
- Take steps to promote the patient/resident's dignity and self-esteem throughout the meal.
- Help the patient/resident to enjoy the company of others during the meal.
- Present the meal attractively. The nurse assistant can make attractive presentation of meal by removing items from the meal tray and place them on the table. Attractive presentation like this may create a more home-like environment.
- Make a clean, pleasant, and relaxing environment for eating.

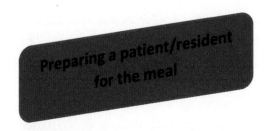

There should be more to assisting a patient/resident with meals than simply getting the meal tray and placing it down in front of him/her. Before serving the meal, there are multiple things that must be done to prepare the patient/resident for the meal. The nurse assistant should have sufficient time to accomplish the following before the meal:

- Ensuring the patient/resident's physical comfort by assisting him/her to use the bathroom and washing his/her hands before the mealtime.

- Providing oral hygiene, because a clean mouth makes food taste much better. If the patient/resident wears dentures, the nurse assistant should make sure that the dentures are clean and in place.

- The nurse assistant should assist the patient/resident with putting on glasses or inserting a hearing aid, if he/she uses these devices.

- Creating a comfortable and pleasant environment for eating. If the patient/resident will be taking the meal in his/her room, the nurse assistant should make sure the room is clean, neat, and free of odors. The nurse assistant should also make sure that there is adequate lighting.

- The patient/resident should be positioned properly for eating. In many long-term healthcare settings, residents usually go to the dining room to eat. Whether the patient/resident is eating in the dining room or in his/her room,

the nurse assistant should help the patient/resident into a comfortable, upright, sitting position, with his/her head up and hips at a 90-degree angle. This position makes it easier for the patient/resident to swallow, chew, and manage eating utensils. If the patient/resident is seated in a chair, it should be ensured that his/her feet are flat on the floor with his/her elbows or forearms on the table if he/she needs support.

- If the patient/resident would like to use a clothing protector to protect his/her clothing from spills, the nurse assistant should assist him/her with putting the clothing protector on. To protect the patient/resident's dignity, the nurse assistant should avoid referring to the clothing protector as a bib.

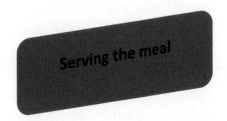

After the completion of these preparations, it is time to get the patient/resident's meal tray. The nurse assistant should make sure of delivering the right meal tray to the right patient/resident by checking the name on the card on the meal tray. If the patient/resident is on a therapeutic diet, it should be ensured that the diet noted on the card is the same one the patient/resident is supposed to be receiving. If the nurse assistant suspects that an error has been occurred, he/she should check with the nurse before serving the meal. The nurse assistant should organize his/her time so that he/she can help the patient/resident to eat shortly after delivering the tray. Foods should be served at proper temperature to make them more appealing.

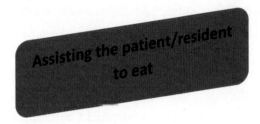

Assisting the patient/resident to eat

Many patients/residents are able to eat on their own, if a little help is provided to them with tasks such as opening cartons or identifying the location of items on the table and on the plate. The application of assistive devices for eating may further increase the patient/resident's ability to eat independently. At each meal, the nurse assistant should discuss with the patient/resident about the amount of assistance he/she requires, because he/she may have different requirements at different meals. For example, at lunchtime the patient/resident may be able to eat a sandwich by himself/herself, but at dinner time the patient/resident may require assistance for cutting his meat. The nurse assistant should always encourage patients/residents in his/her care to do as much as they can themselves. Even when a patient/resident is totally dependent on a nurse assistant to feed him/her, the nurse assistant should involve him/her in the process as much as possible (for example, by asking the patient/resident to hold his/her napkin). This helps to encourage independence and protect the patient/resident's dignity and self-esteem. It should be remembered that meals are not just about providing the food. Being in the company of other individuals and socializing is significant during the meal as well. The nurse assistant should sit down and take the time to talk with the patient/resident during the meal, even if that patient/resident cannot answer. The nurse assistant should avoid rushing the patient/resident during the meal. The patient/resident should be observed to determine whether he/she needs assistance during eating. If the patient/resident does not eat a certain food, the nurse assistance should ask him/her about the reason of not eating. Sometimes patients/residents leave part of a meal uneaten because they get too tired to finish the meal. In this case, the patient/resident may eat more if he/she is offered for help. If the patient/resident simply did not care for the food, the nurse assistance should ask if there is something else the patient/resident is needed to eat that he/she might find more appetizing. Knowing why a patient/resident did not eat part or all of a meal may help the health care team to plan future meals in such a way that will be more appealing to the patient/resident. It may also help the health care team to address other issues that may be affecting the patient/resident's appetite. When the patient/resident has finished eating, the nurse assistant should remove the dishes and tidy up the table. The patient/resident should be assisted with mouth care and changing any articles of clothing that became wet or soiled during the meal.

Paralysis, weakness, casts, and other limits can make self-feeding impossible. These patients/residents should be fed by the nurse assistant. Food and fluids should be served in the order the patient/resident prefers. Fluids should be offered during the meal. Fluids may help the patient/resident chew and swallow. Teaspoons should be used to feed the patient/resident. Teaspoons are less likely to cause injury than forks. The teaspoon should be filled by one-third (⅓) only because this portion can be chewed and swallowed easily. Some patients/residents may need smaller portions. The nurse assistant should always follow the care plan. Patients/residents who need to be fed are often embarrassed, angry, and humiliated. Some are resentful, depressed, or refuse to eat. The nurse assistant should let them do what they can. Some patients/residents can manage "finger foods" (cookies, bread, crackers). If strong enough, the nurse assistant should let them hold juice or milk cups (never hot drinks). The nurse assistant should follow activity limits ordered by the physician. The patient/resident should be encouraged to try, even if food is spilled. Visually impaired patients/residents are often very aware of food aromas. These patients/residents may know the food served. The nurse assistant should always describe what is on the tray and what

he/she is offering. Many patients/residents pray before eating. The nurse assistant should allow time and privacy for prayers, which shows respect and caring.

Meals usually provide social contact with other individuals. The patient/resident should be engaged in pleasant conversation. However, the nurse assistant should allow proper time to the patient/resident for chewing and swallowing. Also, the nurse assistant should sit facing the patient/resident. Sitting is more relaxing that shows that nursing assistants have time for the patients/residents. By facing the patients/residents, the nurse assistant can see how well the patient/resident is eating as well as he/she can also see any swallowing problems.

Encouraging safety and comfort
Safety
The nurse assistant should check food temperature. Too hot foods and fluids can burn the patient/resident. Aspiration should be prevented. The patient/resident's mouth should be checked before offering more food or fluids. The patient/resident's mouth must be empty between bites.
Comfort
The patient/resident will eat better if not rushed. The nurse assistant should sit to show the patient/resident that he/she has time. Standing communicates that the nurse assistant is in a hurry. The nurse assistant should wipe the patient/resident's hands, face, and mouth as needed during the meal. The napkin should be used and if necessary. A wet washcloth can also be used. The patient/resident then should be dried with a towel.

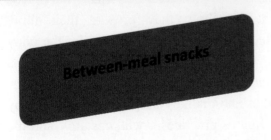
Between-meal snacks

Between-meal snacks are an important part of several special diet plans. Common snacks may include milk, juice, crackers, a milkshake, wafers, a sandwich, gelatin, cake, and custard. Snacks are usually served upon arrival on the nursing unit. The nurse assistant should provide needed utensils, a straw, and a napkin to the patient/resident. The nurse assistant should follow the same procedures and considerations for serving meals and feeding the patient/resident.

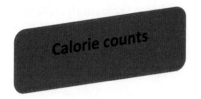

Calorie counts

Calorie records are kept for some patients/residents. On a flow sheet, the nurse assistant should note what the patient/resident ate and how much. For example, "rice, a chicken breast, a roll, beans, pudding, and 2 pats of butter were served. The patient/resident ate all the chicken, the roll, and half the rice. One pat of butter was used and the pudding and beans were not eaten." These should be noted on the flow sheet. A dietician or nurse converts these portions into calories.

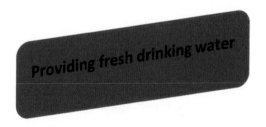

Providing fresh drinking water

Patients and residents require fresh drinking water during each shift. They also need fresh drinking water when the water mug is empty. Each patient/resident's mug should be filled as needed. The mug should be taken to an ice and water dispenser. If so, the mug should be filled with ice first and then water should be added. The nurse assistant should follow the agency's procedure for providing fresh drinking water.

Encouraging safety and comfort

Water mugs may spread infectious microorganisms. To prevent the spread of infectious microbes:

- The nurse assistant should make sure the mug is labeled with the patient/resident's name, room and bed number.
- The rim or inside of the mug should not be touched.
- The nurse assistant should not let the ice scoop touch the mug, straw, or lid.
- The ice scoop should not be placed in the ice container or dispenser. It should be placed in the scoop holder or on a towel for the scoop.
- The ice chest should be kept closed when not in use.
- The nurse assistant should make sure that the mug is clean. The mug should also be checked for cracks and chips. A new mug should be provided as needed.

Influence of Culture and Religion on Dietary Practices

Cultural background may greatly influence eating patterns. Religious beliefs and ethnic heritage often determine what individuals eat and how they prepare their food. Because eating provides food for the body as well as soul, the science of nutrition is also an art. An individual's food choices, likes and dislikes are greatly influenced by religious practices, social customs, and the availability of ingredients. Culture may influence food choices, dietary practices, and food preparation. Baking, smoking, frying, or roasting food and eating raw food are common cultural practices. Although most of the Americans think and believe that what they eat affects their health; however, nutritional considerations have a minor impact on most people's food choices than do personal food preferences influenced by ethnic heritage, region, religious beliefs, and other sociocultural factors.

Ignoring the importance of these factors in a patient/resident's food choices can undermine proper diet planning and good nutritional counselling. It should be remembered that patients/residents should be provided proper help to meet their nutritional requirements by having discussions of the wide variety and combination of foods. Selecting, eating, and preparing food often involve religious practices. A patient/resident may follow some, all, or none of the dietary practices of his/her faith. The nurse assistant should respect the patient/resident's religious practices.

Alternative Ways to Administer Nutrition

1. Enteral nutrition or tube feeding

Enteral nutrition is generally called tube feeding because the patient/resident receives nutrition (in the form of a nutrient-rich formula) and fluids through a tube that is placed directly into the stomach or intestines. If the patient/resident will only need enteral nutrition for a few days, a nasogastric or nasointestinal tube may be placed. These types of tubes are inserted through the patient/resident's nose and passed down the patient/resident's throat to the stomach or the intestines. If the patient/resident is expected to require enteral nutrition for more than a few days, a gastrostomy tube may be placed. The gastrostomy tube is inserted directly into the stomach through an incision made in the abdomen. The tube is clamped and held in place by stitches and covered with a dressing.

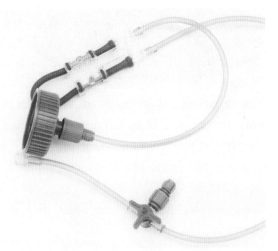

Enteral nutrition may be necessary in certain conditions that prohibit the patient/resident from taking adequate oral nourishment. Examples include inability to swallow, loss of consciousness, oral trauma, mouth surgery, esophageal or gastric cancer or trauma, or anorexia. Those suffering from conditions with increased nutritional needs, such as infection, burns, surgery, or fractures, may also need enteral nutrition.

Types of formulas

The liquid formulas for enteral nutrition contain adequate amounts of fat, protein, carbohydrate, minerals, and vitamins to maintain good nutrition. Routine formulas often provide about 1 calorie per milliliter. They are low in fiber, lactose free, and contain 14% to 16% protein. Routine formulas are also available in high-protein, and high-fiber, and high-calorie varieties. Specialized formulas marketed specifically for renal failure, liver failure, stress, diabetes, acquired immunodeficiency syndrome (AIDS), and other disorders are also available. A dietitian may help the physician to choose the right formula for a patient.

Tubes and different terminologies

The name that is given to an enteral tube may be derived from a particular device, the type of procedure used, or the insertion of the tube. There are following common types of tubes:

Nasogastric: through the nose into the stomach

Percutaneous endoscopic gastrostomy (PEG): placed through the skin

Endoscopic: placed with an instrument called an endoscope

Gastrostomy: inserted directly into the stomach

Button feeding device: a small silicone device used in place of a gastrostomy tube.

Nursing considerations

Constipation, diarrhea, delayed stomach emptying, and aspiration are major risks of tube feeding. The nurse assistant should report the following to the nurse at once.

- Nausea
- Discomfort during the feeding
- Distended (enlarged and swollen) abdomen

- Coughing
- Complaints of indigestion or heartburn
- Vomiting
- Redness, swelling, drainage, odor, or pain at the ostomy site
- Fever
- Signs and symptoms of respiratory distress
- Increased pulse rate
- Complaints of flatulence
- Diarrhea

Preventing aspiration

Aspiration is a main risk from tube feedings. It may cause pneumonia and death. Aspiration may occur:

- **During insertion**

A nasogastric tube can slip into the airway. An X-ray should be taken after insertion to check tube placement.

- **From tube movement out of place**

Sneezing, coughing, suctioning, vomiting, and poor positioning are common causes. A tube can move from the intestine or stomach into the esophagus and then into the airway. The registered nurse checks tube placement before a tube feeding. The nurse assistant should never check feeding tube placement.

- **From regurgitation**

Regurgitation is the backward flow of gastric contents into the mouth. Over-feeding and delayed stomach emptying are common causes.

To help prevent regurgitation and aspiration:

- The patient/resident should be positioned in Fowler's or semi-Fowler's position before the feeding. The nurse assistant should follow the care plan and the nurse's directions.
- Fowler's or semi-Fowler's position should be maintained after the feeding. This allows formula to move through the GI tract. The position is needed for 1 to 2 hours after the feeding or at all times.
- The left side-lying position should be avoided. It prevents the stomach contents from emptying into the small intestine.

Encouraging comfort and safety

Patients/residents with feeding tubes usually are NPO. Dry lips, dry mouth, and sore throat may cause discomfort. Sometimes gum or hard candy is allowed. These measures should be followed every 2 hours while the patient/resident is awake:

- Oral hygiene
- Lubricant for the lips
- Mouth rinsing
- Cleaning the nose and nostrils every 4 to 8 hours.
- Securing the tube to the nose.
- Securing the tube to the patient/resident's garment at the shoulder area.

2. Intravenous (IV) or parenteral therapy

Although a patient/resident's nutritional needs cannot be met using IV therapy, IV therapy is important for administering fluids. It involves injecting into a vein any number of sterile solutions that the body needs, including electrolytes and drugs. IV solutions are used on a short-term basis to maintain or restore fluid and electrolyte balance. Because it is nutritionally inadequate, simple IV therapy is generally not used for more than a few days without addition of some sort of supplementation. Parenteral or IV therapy is used when the patient/resident cannot take adequate amounts of nutrients via the enteral route.

These patients/residents include those with severe burns or a disorder of the GI tract that may inhibit absorption of nutrients. A small catheter (tube) is inserted and placed in a vein on the back of the patient/resident's hand or in the patient/resident's arm. Fluid slowly drips from the IV bag, through the IV tubing and into the catheter. Sometimes drugs may be administered through the IV tubing as well. Although nursing assistants will not be responsible for administering IV therapy, they may care for patients/residents who are receiving IV therapy.

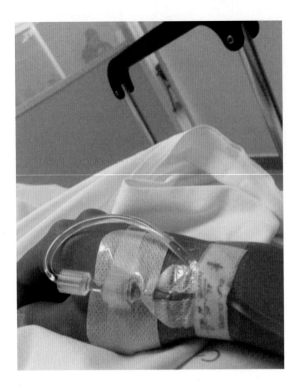

Flow rate

The physician orders the amount of fluid to administer (infuse) and the amount of time to administer it. With this information, the registered nurse figures the flow rate. The flow rate is the milliliters per hour (mL/hr) or number of drops per minute (gtt/min). The registered nurse sets the clamp for the flow rate or an electric pump can be used to control the flow rate. The flow rate is generally displayed in mL/hr. An alarm sounds if something shows wrong. The nurse assistant should tell the nurse at once if he/she hears the alarm. The nurse assistant can check the flow rate if a pump is not used. The RN tells the nurse assistant the number of drops per minute (gtt/min). To check the flow rate, the number of drops in 1 minute should be counted. The nurse assistant should tell the RN at once if:

- No fluid is dripping
- The rate is too rapid
- The rate is too slow
- The bag is close to being empty or empty

- Nurse assistants should always follow Standard Precautions and the Bloodborne Pathogen Standard.
- They should not move the needle or catheter. Needle or catheter position must be maintained. If the catheter or needle is moved, it may come out of the vein. Then fluid may flow into tissues or the flow may stop.
- They should follow the safety measures for restraints. The nurse may splint or restrain the extremity to prevent movement, or may apply a protective device. This helps prevent the catheter or needle from moving.
- The IV bag, tubing, and needle or catheter should be protected when the patient/resident walks. Portable IV stands should be rolled along next to the patient/resident.
- Proper assistance should be provided to the patient/resident with turning and re-positioning. The IV bag should be moved to the side of the bed on which the patient/resident is lying. There should always be allowed enough slack in the tubing. The needle or catheter may move from pressure on the tube.
- The nurse assistant should tell the nurse at once if bleeding occurs from the insertion site.
- The nurse assistant should report signs and symptoms of IV therapy complications. These signs and symptoms may include:
  - Local—at the IV site: Bleeding, puffiness or swelling, pale or reddened skin, hot or cold skin near

the site, blood backing up into the IV tube, and complaints of pain at or above the IV site.

- **Systemic—involving the whole body:** Fever, itching, pulse rate greater than 100 beats per minute, drop in blood pressure, cyanosis, confusion or changes in mental function, loss of consciousness, irregular pulse, decreasing or no urine output, chest pain, nausea, difficulty breathing, and shortness of breath.

multiple traumas, burns, severe infection, or multiorgan failure. TPN bypasses the digestive tract and is infused directly into the blood circulation. Several types of tubes (catheters) are used. The large catheter is surgically inserted into the central vein near the heart to permit the rich concentrated solution to be diffused rapidly into the blood circulation. Currently, TPN has grown in acceptance as both a long- and short-term therapy modality.

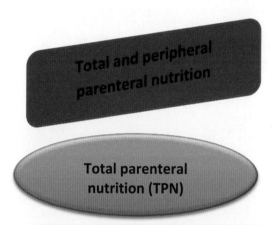

Total and peripheral parenteral nutrition

Total parenteral nutrition (TPN)

Peripheral parenteral nutrition (PPN)

It is a specifically formulated solution that is nutritionally complete to meet a specific patient/resident's nutritional demands. Total parenteral nutrition (TPN) is used when the gastrointestinal tract is not functioning properly, such as in stomach cancer, or when a patient/resident has

It contains smaller concentrations of the same ingredients applied in central vein TPN, which are administered into a peripheral vein. It is usually used to provide short term and temporary nutritional support. PPN promotes healthy weight gain and protein synthesis when oral intake is contraindicated or inadequate. Infusions given peripherally must be isotonic or hypotonic, in order to prevent dehydration and electrolyte imbalance. Thus, PPN provides much lesser calories than TPN.

Encouraging safety and comfort

The patient/resident can suffer serious harm if the flow rate is too slow or fast. The flow rate may change from:

- Position changes
- Kinked tubes
- Lying on the tube

The nurse assistant should never change the position of the clamp or adjust any controls on IV pumps. He/she should inform the nurse at once if there is a problem with the flow rate.

Helpful Resources

Andersson, A., & Bryngelsson, S. (2007). Towards a healthy diet: From nutrition

recommendations to dietary advice. *Scandinavian Journal of Food and Nutrition*, *51*(1), 31-

40. https://doi.org/10.1080/17482970701284338

Asp, N. (n.d.). Nutritional importance and classification of food carbohydrates. *Plant

Polymeric Carbohydrates*, 119-126. https://doi.org/10.1533/9781845698430.3.119

Bianchi, T. S., & Canuel, E. A. (2011). Lipids: Alkenones, polar lipids, and Ether lipids.

Chemical Biomarkers in Aquatic Ecosystems.

https://doi.org/10.23943/princeton/9780691134147.003.0011

Clinical manifestations of food allergy. (2016). *Food Allergy*, 18-37.

https://doi.org/10.1201/b15358-5

Comprehensive review of nutritional components for occupational health nurses—Part 1.

(2018). *Workplace Health & Safety*, *66*(5), 260-260.

https://doi.org/10.1177/2165079918771704

Dagnelie, P. C., & Mariotti, F. (2017). Vegetarian diets. *Vegetarian and Plant-Based Diets in

Health and Disease Prevention*, 3-10. https://doi.org/10.1016/b978-0-12-803968-7.00001-0

De Ridder, D., Kroese, F., Evers, C., Adriaanse, M., & Gillebaart, M. (2017). Healthy diet:

Health impact, prevalence, correlates, and interventions. *Psychology & Health*, *32*(8), 907-

941. https://doi.org/10.1080/08870446.2017.1316849

Havala, S., & Dwyer, J. (1993). Position of the American dietetic association: Vegetarian diets. *Journal of the American Dietetic Association*, *93*(11), 1317-1319. https://doi.org/10.1016/0002-8223(93)91966-t

Huskisson, E., Maggini, S., & Ruf, M. (2007). The role of vitamins and minerals in energy metabolism and well-being. *Journal of International Medical Research*, *35*(3), 277-289. https://doi.org/10.1177/147323000703500301

Indrani, T. (2003). Food allergy and therapeutic diet. *Nursing Manual of Nutrition and Therapeutic Diet*, 236-236. https://doi.org/10.5005/jp/books/10556_13

Indrani, T. (2017). Diet as a therapeutic agent. *Manual of Nutrition and Therapeutic Diet*, 320-320. https://doi.org/10.5005/jp/books/13041_34

KOHLMEIER, M. (2003). Fat-soluble vitamins and non-nutrients. *Nutrient Metabolism*, 457-537. https://doi.org/10.1016/b978-012417762-8/50010-7

KOHLMEIER, M. (2003). Water-soluble vitamins and non-nutrients. *Nutrient Metabolism*, 539-642. https://doi.org/10.1016/b978-012417762-8/50011-9

Lonnie, M., Hooker, E., Brunstrom, J., Corfe, B., Green, M., Watson, A., Williams, E., Stevenson, E., Penson, S., & Johnstone, A. (2018). Protein for life: Review of optimal protein intake, sustainable dietary sources and the effect on appetite in ageing adults. *Nutrients*, *10*(3), 360. https://doi.org/10.3390/nu10030360

Mangano, K. M., & Tucker, K. L. (2017). Bone health and vegan diets. *Vegetarian and Plant-Based Diets in Health and Disease Prevention*, 315-331. https://doi.org/10.1016/b978-0-12-803968-7.00017-4

Medawar, E., Huhn, S., Villringer, A., & Veronica Witte, A. (2019). The effects of plant-based diets on the body and the brain: A systematic review. *Translational Psychiatry, 9*(1). https://doi.org/10.1038/s41398-019-0552-0

Mulik, K., & Haynes-Maslow, L. (2017). The affordability of MyPlate: An analysis of SNAP benefits and the actual cost of eating according to the dietary guidelines. *Journal of Nutrition Education and Behavior, 49*(7), S99. https://doi.org/10.1016/j.jneb.2017.05.178

Proscia, A. (2014). MyPlate for healthy eating with chronic kidney disease (MyPlate education for patients with chronic kidney disease receiving hemodialysis and peritoneal dialysis treatment). *Journal of Renal Nutrition, 24*(3), e23-e25. https://doi.org/10.1053/j.jrn.2014.02.003

Skerrett, P. J., & Willett, W. C. (2010). Essentials of healthy eating: A guide. *Journal of Midwifery & Women's Health, 55*(6), 492-501. https://doi.org/10.1016/j.jmwh.2010.06.019

Tuso, P. (2013). Nutritional update for physicians: Plant-based diets. *The Permanente Journal, 17*(2). https://doi.org/10.7812/tpp/12-085

Uruakpa, F., Moeckly, B., Fulford, L., Hollister, M., & Kim, S. (2013). Awareness and use of MyPlate guidelines in making food choices. *Procedia Food Science, 2*, 180-186. https://doi.org/10.1016/j.profoo.2013.04.026

Zhang, F. F., Barr, S. I., McNulty, H., Li, D., & Blumberg, J. B. (2020). undefined. *BMJ*, m2511. https://doi.org/10.1136/bmj.m2511

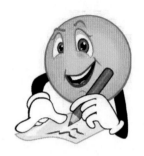

Chapter Twelve:

Emergency Procedures

Outline

I: Medical emergencies and the Nurse Assistant's role in preventing and/or responding to medical emergencies

II: Myocardial infarction

III: Heart failure

IV: Stroke

V: Fainting

VI: Seizures

VII: Insulin shock

VIII: Hemorrhage

IX: Shock

X: Respiratory distress

XI: Immediate interventions in medical emergencies

XII: Choking

XIII: Common emergency codes used in long-term care facilities

An emergency is a condition that occurs suddenly and needs immediate actions to keep an individual safe. Emergencies can be often medical in nature, involving an injury or acute illness that needs immediate intervention, in order to prevent the victim from dying or experiencing permanent long-term disabilities. Emergencies may also be environmental in nature, involving changes to an individual's environment that affect the individual's health and safety. Examples of environmental emergencies may include fires, weather emergencies (such as tornadoes, snow storms, and hurricanes) and disasters (severe events that cause widespread destruction and damage, affecting large number of people and disrupting normal functioning of the community). A nurse assistant must know how to react and respond immediately in the event of an emergency to keep the patients/residents and the visitors safe.

Medical Emergencies and the Nursing Assistant's Role

Recognizing, reacting, and responding to medical emergencies

The following steps may guide a nurse assistant's actions in an emergency and ensure his/her personal safety and the safety of others.

Recognizing the medical emergency

It is the basic and primary requirement for a nurse assistant to recognize a medical emergency. Sometimes the patient/resident who is experiencing a medical emergency will be in distress. Other times, however, a medical emergency may only be recognized by a slight change in the patient/resident's behavior or appearance. A nurse assistant should have in-depth knowledge of what is normal for each patient/resident in his/her care. A change from normal may indicate an emergency and should be reported immediately to the nurse.

Assessing the scene and patient/resident

The nurse assistant should stay calm, and should check the scene and the patient/resident. First, the nurse assistant should make sure there is nothing that could hurt himself/herself or cause further injury to the patient/resident, such as a downed wire in the area. Next, he/she should look for signals that may help him/her to understand what happened. Finally, the nurse assistant should check the patient/resident by tapping his/her shoulder or hand and shout to see if he or she is conscious.

Calling for help

The next step should be the calling for help. In a hospital setting, there is usually a code that can be dialed to call for help within the facility. In other healthcare facilities, the nurse assistant may be required to dial 9-1-1 or another emergency number. The nurse assistant should always know his/her employer's policies and procedures related to calling for help in an emergency.

Providing medical care

The nurse assistant should provide appropriate care (according to the condition and his/her level of training) until advanced clinical help arrives. The nurse assistant should help the victim rest comfortably, and should provide reassurance because the victim/patient is likely to be upset and frightened.

Reporting and recording

The observations of the nurse assistant about what happened before, during, and after the emergency are extremely important to share with other members of the health care team. These observations of the nurse assistant should be reported and shared to the nurse and should be documented on the appropriate forms, as per employer's policy. The nurse assistant should note whether the patient/victim complained any symptoms before the event, the time the symptoms initiated, and how long the symptoms remained. The nurse assistant should be specific in reporting and recording these observations. For example, "He was breathing at a rate of 28 breaths per minute" is more specific than "He was having laboured breathing." If the nurse assistant arrived on the scene to find the patient/victim in distress and unconscious or otherwise unable to describe what happened, the nurse assistant should note anything unusual that he/she observed while checking the scene and the patient/victim. The nurse assistant should also report and record exactly what he/she did to help the patient/victim.

Myocardial Infarction

Myocardial means the heart muscle and infarction refers to tissue death. A heart attack or myocardial infarction occurs when blood supply to part of the myocardium (the heart muscle) is blocked, causing the cells in that region to die. As a result, the ability of the heart to pump blood throughout the body can be greatly affected. If a large region of the heart is destructed or damaged, the heart may stop beating and the condition is called as cardiac arrest. Signs and symptoms of myocardial infarction may vary from individual to individual, and may be different in females than they are in males.

Myocardial infarction is also called as a heart attack, acute myocardial infarction (AMI), or acute coronary syndrome (ACS). A patient who is having a cardiac arrest or heart attack may show any of the following signs and symptoms:

- Chest pain, pressure, discomfort, or squeezing that usually lasts more than 3 to 5 minutes and is not relieved by changing position, resting, or taking nitroglycerin. The pain may go away and then comes back
- Pain or discomfort that spreads to one or both arms, the shoulder, the back, the jaw, the neck, or the upper part of the stomach
- Lightheadedness, dizziness, or loss of consciousness
- Trouble breathing, including shortness of breath, noisy breathing, and breathing that is rapid than normal
- A heartbeat that is slower or faster than normal, or irregular
- Nausea
- Pale, slightly bluish, or ashen skin
- A cold sweat
- A feeling of anxiety, depression, or doom
- Extreme tiredness (fatigue)

Although males most often have the classic clinical features of a heart attack (for example, chest pain), females often have more subtle signs, such as extreme fatigue, nausea, breaking out in a cold sweat, a squeezing sensation in the chest, dizziness or lightheadedness, and shortness of breath.

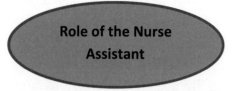

Role of the Nurse Assistant

If a nurse assistant thinks a patient/resident in his/her care is having a heart attack, he/she should stay with the patient/resident and should follow the employer's procedure for calling for help. The patient/resident should be encouraged to stay calm and remain quiet while the nurse assistant is waiting for advanced help to arrive. If the patient/resident loses consciousness, having no pulse, or stops breathing, the patient/resident may be in cardiac arrest and need immediate cardiopulmonary resuscitation (CPR) as well as defibrillation (it is delivery of an electric shock to the heart muscle to regain and restore a normal rhythm). An automated external defibrillator (AED) is commonly used for defibrillation. AED is a portable electronic device that delivers an automated defibrillation shock or deliver shock with a push of a manual button to support the heart restore an effective pumping rhythm. The proper application of an automated external defibrillator (AED) along with CPR has been shown to improve survival rates among patents/residents experiencing cardiac arrest. The nurse assistant should know the location of AEDs in his/her facility, because he/she may be required to retrieve the AED while a co-worker administers CPR in an emergency. The nurse assistant should also know where CPR breathing barrier devices (used to protect both the patient/resident being resuscitated and the nurse assistant from

the spread of microorganisms in blood, saliva, and other body fluids) are placed so he/she can access them in a hurry.

Myocardial infarction is an emergency. Efforts should be made to:

- Relieve pain
- Restore blood supply to the heart
- Stabilize vital signs
- Administer oxygen
- Calm the patient/resident
- Prevent death and other fatal complications

The patient/resident may require medical or surgical procedures to open or bypass the diseased artery. Cardiac rehabilitation is required to:

- Recover and resume normal routine activities
- Prevent another MI
- Prevent complications like cardiac failure or sudden cardiac arrest

Heart Failure

Congestive heart failure (CHF) or heart failure occurs when the weakened heart is not able to pump the blood normally. Blood backs up and tissue congestion occurs. When the left side of the heart is weakened and cannot pump blood normally, blood is backed up into the lungs. As a result, respiratory congestion occurs. The patient has cough, dyspnea, increased sputum, and gurgling sounds in the lungs. The body does not receive enough blood and oxygen. Signs and symptoms occur due to effects of poor blood flow to other organs. Poor blood flow to the brain causes

347

dizziness, confusion, and fainting. The kidneys produce less amount of urine. The skin becomes pale. Blood pressure lowers. When the right side of the heart is weakened and cannot pump blood normally, blood is backed up into the venous system. Ankles and feet become swollen. Neck veins bulge and liver congestion affects normal liver function. The abdomen becomes congested with fluid. Less amount of blood is pumped to the lungs.

Congestive heart failure is an emergency. The patient can die. There are different drugs to strengthen the heart. They also decrease the amount of fluid in the body. A sodium-controlled diet is usually ordered. Oxygen should be administered. Semi-Fowler's position is usually preferred position for breathing. Daily weight, intake and output (I&O), elastic stockings, and ROM exercises are part of the care plan for congestive heart failure patients.

Stroke

A stroke occurs when blood supply to a part of the brain is compromised or interrupted, resulting in the death of brain cells. Stroke affects the arteries that supply blood to the brain. It also is called a cerebrovascular accident (CVA) or brain attack. It occurs when one of these happens:

- An artery or vein in the brain bursts and bleeding occurs in the brain (brain hemorrhage).
- A blood clot obstructs blood flow to the brain.

Brain cells in the affected region do not receive enough nutrients and oxygen.

Brain damage occurs and functions controlled by that region of the brain are lost. Stroke or brain attack is a leading cause of disability and death among adults in the United States. The victim requires emergency care. Strokes or CVA may cause permanent brain damage; however, through the immediate interventions and restoration of blood flow to the brain, the damage can be reversed or stopped.

The signs and symptoms of a stroke may vary from individual to individual. A patient who is experiencing a stroke may show any of the following signs and symptoms:
- Slurring of speech
- Facial drooping on one side of the face (for example, the eyelid and the corner of the mouth)
- Trouble watching in one or both eyes
- Numbness or weakness in an arm or leg
- A sudden, severe headache
- Dizziness or loss of balance
- Confusion or loss of consciousness
- A generally weak appearance or abnormal behavior.

"FAST" Approach

The "FAST" check is a quick tool of checking for signs of a stroke:

F: Facial drooping

The patient should be asked to smile to see if there is weakness or drooping on one side of the face.

A: Arm

The patient should be asked to raise both arms to see if there is weakness or drooping of one of the arms.

S: Speech

The patient should be asked to say a simple sentence or phrase to check if he/she has trouble speaking or slurred speech.

T: Time

If the patient has difficulty performing any of these actions or shows other signs of stroke, the nurse assistant should call for help immediately. Prompt medical help and immediate clinical care may reduce the amount of disability the patient experiences as a result of the stroke.

If a nurse assistant thinks that a patient/resident is having a stroke, he/she should always follow his/her employer's procedure for calling help. The nurse assistant should stay with the patient/resident and should provide proper reassurance until advanced clinical help arrives. The patient/resident's breathing should be properly monitored. The nurse assistant should check any changes in the patient/resident's condition. If the patient is drooling or has trouble swallowing, the nurse assistant should place him/her on one side to keep the airway clear. It should be noted that when the patient's symptoms had started. This is significant to report because some of the medications used to manage stroke are only effective within a specific time frame after the onset of symptoms.

Warning signs of stroke may last for a few minutes. This is known as a transient ischemic attack (TIA). Blood flow to the brain is interrupted for a short period of time. A transient ischemic attack usually occurs before a stroke. The patient also may have nausea, vomiting, and memory loss. Unconsciousness, high blood pressure, noisy breathing, redness of the face, slow pulse, and seizures may occur. Hemiplegia (paralysis on one side of the body) is also an important warning sign. The patient may lose bowel and bladder control and the ability to speech. All stroke-like clinical features indicate the immediate need for emergency care.

Common warning signs of stroke may include:

- Sudden numbness or weakness of the arm, face, or leg (especially on one side of the body)
- Sudden trouble speaking, understanding, or confusion
- Sudden trouble watching in one or both eyes
- Sudden trouble walking, loss of balance, dizziness, or loss of coordination
- Sudden headache with no known cause

The effects of stroke may include:

- Loss of face, arm, hand, leg, or body control
- Hemiplegia
- Emotional changes (mood swings or crying easily, sometimes for no reason)
- Dysphagia (difficulty swallowing)
- Aphasia, slowed, or slurred speech
- Changes in touch, sight, movement, and thought
- Memory impairment
- Urinary incontinence, frequency, or urgency
- Loss of bowel control or constipation
- Frustration and depression

Rehabilitation starts at once the patient/resident may depend in part or totally on others for care. The health team assists the patient/resident regain the highest possible level of function.

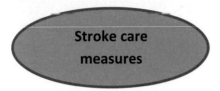

Stroke care measures

The nurse assistant should take following measures when providing care for stroke patients/residents:

- The patient/resident should be positioned in the lateral (side-lying) position to prevent aspiration.
- The bed should be kept in semi-Fowler's position.
- The patient/resident should be approached from the strong (unaffected) side. Objects should be placed on the strong (unaffected side). The patient/resident may have loss of vision on the affected side.
- The patient/resident should be turned and re-positioned at least every 2 hours.
- Assist devices should be used to turn, move, re-position, and transfer the patient/resident.
- Deep breathing and coughing should be encouraged.
- Contractures and pressure sores should be prevented.
- The nurse assistant should meet food and fluid needs. The patient/resident may need a dysphagia diet.
- Elastic stockings may be applied to prevent thrombi (blood clots) in the legs.

- The nurse assistant should assist the patient/resident with ROM exercises to prevent contractures.
- Elimination needs should be met properly. The nurse assistant should always follow the care plan for catheter care and bladder or bowel training.
- Appropriate safety precautions should be practiced.
- The call light should be placed within reach on the patient/resident's strong (unaffected) side.
- The patient/resident should be checked often if he or she cannot use the call light.
- Bed rails should be used according to the care plan.
- Appropriate steps should be taken to prevent falls and other injuries.
- The patient/resident should be encouraged to do as much self-care as possible. This may include turning, positioning, and transferring. The patient/resident should use assistive, self-help, and ambulating aids as required.
- The nurse assistant should not rush the patient/resident, because movements usually become slower after a stroke.
- The nurse assistant should follow established communication methods.
- A safety check should be completed before leaving the room.

Fainting

It is a sudden and temporary loss of consciousness due to a sudden decrease in the blood supply to the brain. Fainting may be a sign of any serious medical problem, such as a heart or nervous problem, but it can also be due to multiple factors such as hunger, fear, pain, being too warm, standing for longer periods of time, side effects of medication, fatigue, or strong emotions. An individual who is about to faint usually becomes pale, begins to sweat, loses consciousness, and finally collapse. The individual may feel weak or dizzy.

Role of the Nurse Assistant

During dizziness and before losing consciousness

- The nurse assistant should remain calm, and call for help as early as possible.
- If the patient/resident begins to faint, the nurse assistant should lower the patient/resident to the floor using good body mechanics, and should position him/her flat on his/her back.
- The patient/resident should be sitting or lying down before fainting occurs.
- If sitting, the nurse assistant should bend forward the patient/resident and place his/her head between the knees.
- If the patient/resident is lying down, his/her legs should be raised.
- The nurse assistant should loose tight clothing, such as a collar, tie, or scarf of the patient/resident.
- It should be ensured that the patient/resident is breathing.
- If the patient/resident vomits, he/she should be turned onto one side to prevent him/her from choking.
- The patient/resident will usually recover rapidly with no lasting effects; however, he/she should receive a medical assessment and general evaluation after the fainting episode.

After losing consciousness

- The patient/resident should be kept lying down if fainting has occurred.
- The nurse assistant should raise the legs of the patient/resident approximately 8-12 inches if there is no spinal, head or back injuries. If unsure, the patient/resident should be left flat on back.
- The nurse assistant should loose tight clothing, such as a collar, tie, or scarf of the patient/resident.
- The patient/resident should not be allowed to get up until symptoms have subsided for about 5 minutes.
- The nurse assistant should help the patient/resident to a sitting position after recovery from fainting and should observe the patient/resident for any changes in condition. The patient/resident's vital signs should be monitored while waiting for advanced clinical help to arrive.

Seizures

Seizures or convulsions are sudden and violent tremors of muscle groups due to an abnormal electrical activity in the brain. Seizures may lead to involuntary changes in body movement, sensation, function, awareness, or behavior. Seizures can have multiple different causes. Some patients may have epilepsy, which is a chronic seizure condition that can be controlled with medication. Other causes of seizures may include head injury during birth or from trauma, high-grade fever, brain tumors, poisoning, nervous system disorders or infection, and injuries to the brain tissue. Lack of blood supply to the brain tissue may also cause seizures. Although usually it is thought that a seizure involves convulsions and loss of consciousness; however, a person experiencing a seizure may just become very quiet with a blank stare. A patient/resident with epilepsy may have something called an aura, which is an unusual sensation or feeling before the onset of a seizure.

The major types of seizures may include:

1. Partial seizures

Only one part of the brain is involved in partial seizures. A part of the body may jerk or the patient/resident may experience a hearing or vision problem or stomach discomfort during the partial seizures. However, the patient/resident does not lose consciousness.

2. Generalized tonic-clonic seizures (grand mal seizures)

This type of seizure consists of two phases. First phase is called as the tonic phase, in which the patient/resident loses consciousness. If sitting or standing, the patient/resident may fall to the floor. The body becomes rigid because all muscles contract at once. The second phase is called as the clonic phase, in which muscle groups contract and relax. This causes twitching and jerking movements. Urinary incontinence, fecal incontinence, confusion, and headache may occur after the seizure is over on awakening.

3. Generalized absence (petit mal) seizures

This type usually remains for a few seconds. There is complete loss of consciousness along with the twitching of the eyelids and staring. No first aid is necessary for this type. However, the nurse assistant should guide the patient/resident away from dangers such as fireplaces, stairs, streets, a hot stove, fireplaces, and so on.

Emergency care for seizures: The Nurse Assistant's role

The main goal for a nurse assistant is to protect the patient/resident from injury during the seizure. Nearby furniture or other objects that the patient/resident may accidentally hit during the seizure should be removed. The nurse assistant should not try to hold or restrain the patient/resident, or put anything in the patient/resident's mouth or between the teeth to prevent the patient/resident from biting his/her tongue. After the seizure is over, the patient/resident should be placed on one side to prevent him/her from choking on secretions that may have pooled in the mouth. The patient/resident may be disoriented and drowsy or unresponsive for a short period of time. He/she may be very tired and want to rest. The nurse assistant should stay with the patient/resident until he/she is fully recovered from the seizure and completely aware of his/her surroundings.

Nobody can stop a seizure. However, the nurse assistant may protect the patient/resident from injury by following these guidelines:

- The nurse assistant should remain calm, and call for help as early as possible.
- He/she should not leave the patient/resident alone.

- The patient/resident should be lowered to the floor to protect him/her from falling.
- The time should be noted when the seizure started.
- Something soft should be placed under the patient/resident's head to prevent the patient/resident's head from striking the floor. The nurse assistant can use a cushion, pillow, or a folded blanket, jacket, or towel.
- The nurse assistant should loose tight clothing, such as a collar, tie, or scarf of the patient/resident.
- The patient/resident should be turned onto his or her side. It should be ensured that the head is turned to the side.
- It should not be tried to stop the seizure or control the patient/resident's movements.
- The time should be noted when the seizure ends.
- It should be ensured that the mouth of the patient/resident is clear of food, fluids, and saliva after the seizure.
- The nurse assistant should provide BLS if there is no breathing or no normal breathing after the seizure.

Insulin shock

Insulin shock is secondary to low blood sugar (40 mg/dL). It may be due to insulin overdose, a skipped meal, or strenuous exercise in an individual with insulin dependent diabetes mellitus (IDDM). It can also be caused by an insulin-secreting pancreatic tumor. Insulin shock is also called as hypoglycemic shock, wet shock, or diabetic shock. It may be a result of insulin overdose, a skipped meal, or strenuous exercise in a person with IDDM.

There are multiple causes of hypoglycemic shock such as skipping a meal or snack, eating too little food, exercising more than usual, vomiting, or taking too much medication. A patient/resident who is experiencing hypoglycemia may experience several signs and symptoms like shakiness, dizziness, behavioral changes (for example, argumentativeness, aggression, combativeness, or anger), cool and clammy skin, and headache.

Role of the Nurse Assistant

- The nurse assistant should remain calm, and call for help as early as possible.
- He/she should not leave the patient/resident alone

The nurse assistant should be quick to recognize the early symptoms of hypoglycemia. Carbohydrates are usually required to counteract the insulin shock in hypoglycemia. If the patient/resident is conscious, the nurse assistant should administer him/her sugar in some form of 4 oz orange juice, 4 oz regular soft drink, honey, 6 to 8 Lifesavers, or Karo syrup if instructed by the licensed nurse.

Hypoglycemia most commonly develops late at night or early in the morning when the patient/resident is asleep. During this period of time, the body still continues to absorb insulin from the injection site, although not enough amount of glucose is available for the insulin to act on it. The nurse assistant should especially pay attention to diabetic patients/resident during these times.

Hemorrhage

Life and normal body functions require a sufficient blood supply. Bleeding occurs if a blood vessel is torn or cut. If a larger blood vessel is cut or torn, there will be the greater bleeding and more blood loss. Excessive loss of blood in a short time is called as hemorrhage. Hemorrhage can be external or internal. Internal hemorrhage cannot be seen. The bleeding for the internal hemorrhage will be inside body tissues and body cavities. Shock, pain, coughing up blood, vomiting blood, and loss of consciousness are the common signs of internal hemorrhage. Severe bleeding, whether it is external or internal, is life-threatening.

Role of the Nurse Assistant

To provide care for a patient/resident who is bleeding externally, the nurse should follow the below guidelines:

- The nurse assistant should first take standard precautions by putting on gloves. If he/she thinks the blood might splatter or spray, he/she may require eye and face protection as well.
- The nurse assistant should remain calm, and call for help as early as possible.
- He/she should not leave the patient/resident alone.
- The patient/resident should be kept flat, warm, and quiet until help arrives.
- Fluids should not be administered. If not hidden by any covering or clothing, external bleeding is usually seen.

Bleeding from an artery usually occurs in spurts. There will be a slow and steady flow of blood from a vein. To control bleeding:

- The nurse assistant should remain calm and activate the EMS system.
- A sterile dressing should be directly placed over the wound or should use any clean material like towel, handkerchief, cloth, or sanitary napkin.
- A firm pressure should be applied directly over the bleeding site. Pressure should not be released until the bleeding stops. If needed, the nurse assistant should wrap an elastic bandage firmly over the dressing or material.
- The dressing or material should not be removed. If bleeding continues, the nurse assistant should apply more dressings or material on top and should apply more pressure.
- The wound should be bound when bleeding stops. The nurse assistant should be tapped or tied the dressing in place. The dressing can be tied with such things as a scarf, clothing, or a necktie.
- If the bleeding still continues and does not stop, the nurse assistant must call for help.

The nurse assistant should stay with patient/resident, and should observe him/her closely for signs that may indicate that his/her condition is worsening, such as breathing that slower or faster than normal, restlessness, and changes in skin color. The nurse assistant should provide reassurance, and should keep the patient/resident calm.

Shock

It is a condition in which the circulatory system is unable to deliver sufficient oxygen-rich blood to the body's tissues and vital organs. There are several causes of shock, including heart failure, severe allergic reactions, severe burns, massive blood loss, and severe infections that overwhelm the body. A patient/resident who is in shock may show any of the following signs or symptoms:

- Excessive thirst
- Nausea or vomiting
- Altered level of consciousness
- Irritability or restlessness
- Pale or ashen, cool, gray, moist skin
- A blue tinge to lips and nail beds (cyanosis)
- Rapid pulse and rapid breathing
- Low or falling blood pressure

The management for shock depends on the underlying cause. For example, if the shock is due to massive blood loss, the bleeding must be stopped. Shock that is resulted by a severe allergic reaction should be treated by administering epinephrine.

To provide first aid for a patient/resident who is in shock, the nurse assistant should remain calm and call for help immediately.

The nurse assistant should take any measures to address the cause of the shock. The patient/resident should be prevented from becoming chilled or overheated, and should help the patient/resident to rest comfortably. Even though the patient/resident is likely to be thirsty, the nurse assistant should not give the patient/resident anything to drink or eat. The patient/resident may need surgery, which is the safest when the stomach is empty. The nurse assistant should provide comfort and reassurance to the patient/resident until medical help arrives.

Role of the Nurse Assistant

Shock can be occurred in any patient/resident who is acutely ill or severely injured. The nurse assistant should follow below guidelines:

- The patient/resident should be kept lying down.
- If the patient/resident does not have injuries from trauma, the nurse assistant should raise the patient/resident's feet from 6 to 12 inches.
- The feet should be lowered if the position causes pain.
- An open airway should be maintained and bleeding should be controlled.
- The nurse assistant should begin CPR if cardiac arrest occurs.

Anaphylactic shock

Anaphylaxis is a life-threatening sensitivity or allergic reaction to insects, food, chemicals, and drugs. The reaction may occur within seconds. Signs and symptoms of anaphylactic reaction may include:

- An itchy rash
- Dyspnea or wheezing from a narrowed airway or a swollen tongue or throat
- Feeling of a "lump" in the throat
- A weak and fast pulse
- Pale or flushed skin
- Feeling warm
- Nausea, vomiting, or diarrhea
- A feeling of doom or dread
- Fainting or dizziness
- Signs and symptoms of shock

Anaphylactic shock is a medical emergency. The EMS system must be activated immediately and the patient needs special medications to reverse the allergic reaction. The patient should be kept lying down and the airway should be maintained. CPR should be started if cardiac arrest occurs.

Respiratory Distress

Many patients/residents have lung involvement, causing dyspnea. Position changes and stress reduction may help to provide maximum comfort for these patients/residents. Using an air conditioner to cool the room or a fan to circulate air and raising the head of the bed may help. The nurse assistant should frequently evaluate the patient/resident's vital signs and level of consciousness. Some patients/residents may need supplemental oxygen because of anxiety, fever, infection, or fluid collection. Oxygen concentrators should be recommended to use instead oxygen tanks. Medications may decrease secretions to improve respiration and thoracentesis may relieve pressure. Nebulizer and postural drainage

may help eliminate lung secretion. Surgery may help to relieve obstructions.

Signs & Symptoms of respiratory distress may include:

- Labored breathing Shortness of breath (SOB)
- Cyanosis
- Hypo/Hyperventilation
- Bradypnea/Tachypnea
- Hypoxia
- Anxiety
- confusion

Role of the Nurse Assistant

- The nurse assistant should remain calm, and call for help as early as possible.
- He/she should not leave the patient/resident alone.
- Using an air conditioner to cool the room or a fan to circulate air and raising the head of the bed may help the patient/resident.
- The nurse assistant should frequently evaluate the patient/resident's vital signs and level of consciousness.
- Some patients/residents may need supplemental oxygen because of anxiety, fever, infection, or fluid collection.
- The nurse assistant should assess vital signs while awaiting assistance from licensed nurse.
- The nurse assistance should also be prepared to gather equipment as instructed by nurse such as oxygen tank and tubing.

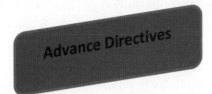

Immediate Interventions in Medical Emergencies

Advance Directives

The Omnibus Budget Reconciliation Act of 1987 (OBRA) and Patient Self-Determination Act provide patients the right to refuse or accept treatment. They also provide the right to make advance directives. Advance directive is a document stating an individual's wishes about health care when that individual cannot make his or her own decisions. Advance directives generally forbid certain health care if there is no chance of recovery. Quality of care should not be compromised because of the individual's advance directives.

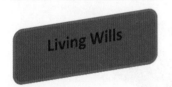

Living Wills

A living will is about measures that maintain or support life when death is likely. Ventilators, tube feedings, and resuscitation are examples. A living will may instruct physicians:

- Not to begin measures that prolong dying
- To remove certain measures that prolong dying

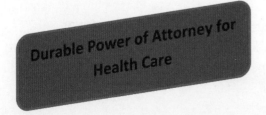

Durable Power of Attorney for Health Care

This advance directive provides the power to take health care decisions to another individual. That individual is often called a health care proxy. Generally this is a family member, lawyer, or friend. When an individual cannot take health care decisions, the health care proxy can do so. This advance directive does not cover financial or property matters.

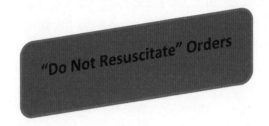

"Do Not Resuscitate" Orders

"No code" or "Do not resuscitate" (DNR) orders mean that the individual will not be resuscitated. The individual is permitted to die with dignity and peace. The provider writes the DNR order after consulting with the individual and family. The provider and family take the decision if the individual is not mentally able to do so.

Cardiopulmonary resuscitation (CPR)

Cardiopulmonary resuscitation (CPR) is an emergency lifesaving procedure which may be performed when a person stops breathing or the heart stops beating (a person in sudden cardiac arrest). CPR may help the flow of oxygen and blood to the brain and other vital organs while the medical staff try to get the heart to beat normally again.

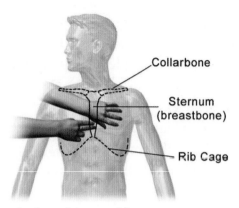

Collarbone

Sternum (breastbone)

Rib Cage

When the breathing and heart stop, oxygen and blood cannot be supplied to the body. As a result, damage of the brain and other organs occurs within minutes. CPR must be started immediately when a victim has sudden cardiac arrest (SCA). CPR supports breathing and circulation. It provides oxygen and blood to the brain, heart, and other organs until advanced emergency care arrives. CPR involves:

- Chest compressions
- Airway
- Breathing
- Defibrillation

CPR procedures need proper skill, speed, and efficiency. Chest compressions, airway, and breathing procedures should be done until a defibrillator arrives. The defibrillator should be used as soon as possible.

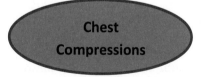

Chest Compressions

The brain, heart, and other organs must receive blood as soon as possible to prevent permanent damage. Heart stops beating in cardiac arrest and blood must be pumped through the body in any other alternate way. Chest compressions force and pump blood through the circulatory system. Before initiating chest compressions, a pulse should be checked.

The rescuer or nurse assistant should use the carotid artery on the side near him/her. To find the carotid pulse, the nurse assistant should place his/her 2 or 3 fingertips on the trachea (windpipe). The fingers should be slided down off the trachea to the groove of the neck. A pulse should be checked for at least 5 seconds but no more than 10 seconds. While checking for a pulse, the rescuer should also look for signs of circulation. It should be observed that whether the person has started breathing or is moving or coughing. The heart lies between the breastbone and the spinal column. When a firm pressure is applied to the breastbone, the breastbone is depressed. This compresses the heart between the breastbone and spinal column. For effective chest compressions, the victim must be supine on a flat, hard surface. The nurse assistant should be positioned at the victim's side and should use the heels of his/her hands, one on top of the other, for chest compressions.

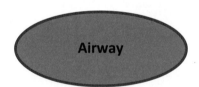

Airway

The airway (respiratory passages) must be open to restore breathing. The airway is often blocked (obstructed) during sudden cardiac arrest. The victim's tongue may fall toward the back of the throat to obstruct the airway. The two most commonly used methods for opening the airway are the head-tilt/chin-lift and modified chin lift (jaw-thrust) maneuver.

The Head-tilt/chin-lift Maneuver

The head-tilt/chin-lift maneuver is used to open the airway.

- The nurse assistant should place the palm of his/her one hand on the forehead of the victim.
- The head of the victim should be tilted back by pushing down on the forehead with his/her palm.
- The nurse assistant should place his/her other hand under the lower jaw of the victim. The nurse assistant should use his/her index and middle fingers and should not use the thumb.
- The jaw should be lifted, which will bring the chin forward.
- The nurse assistant should not close the victim's mouth. The mouth should be slightly open.

Although, the head-tilt/chin-lift is the preferred method, it can be very dangerous to use on a victim who may have a neck injury. For these victims, the modified chin-lift (jaw-thrust) maneuver should be used that allows the nurse assistant to clear the tongue of the victim from the airway with minimal neck movement, and allows rescue breaths to be administered.

For the jaw-thrust maneuver, the nurse assistant should grip firmly the angles of the lower jaw and should lift it up with his/her both hands, one on each side to move the jaw forward.

Breathing

When breathing stops, air is not inhaled. The patient must receive oxygen. If not, permanent brain, heart, and other organ damage may occur. The patient should be given two full breaths by using a barrier device. Each breath should take 1 second and the nurse assistant should see the victim's chest rise with each breath by

LLF (looking, listening and feeling) approach. Two breaths should be given after every 30 chest compressions.

Face mask is a great source for exposure protection which provides a barrier between the nurse assistant and the victim. There are different varieties of masks available in the market, some masks are equipped with a one-way valve that permit the nurse assistant's breaths to enter the victim's airway and prevent the victim's exhaled air from entering the nurse assistant's airway. These masks also protect from vomitus and blood of the victim, which may be an infection risk to the nurse assistant.

Performing Adult CPR

CPR should be done for cardiac arrest. The nurse assistant must determine if fainting or cardiac arrest has occurred. CPR should be done if the victim does not respond, or has no normal breathing. CPR can be done alone or with another co-worker. When performed alone, chest compressions and rescue breathing are done by a single rescuer. With 2 rescuers, one rescuer gives chest compressions and the other performs rescue breathing. Rescuers should switch their tasks about every 2 minutes to avoid inadequate compressions and fatigue. The second rescuer should use the AED if it is available.

Encouraging safety and comfort
CPR should never be practiced on another person as serious damage may occur while practicing CPR. Mannequins should be used to learn and practice CPR. It should

be ensured that there is a safe setting for CPR. The victim should be moved only if the setting is unsafe. The nurse assistant should not approach the victim if the scene is unsafe for him/her. The victim must be on a hard, flat surface for CPR. If the victim is in bed, a board should be placed under the victim or the victim should be moved to the floor

Recovery position

It is the position used when the victim is breathing and has a pulse but is not responding. The position helps to maintain the airway open and prevents aspiration. The victim should be logrolled into the recovery position by keeping the head, neck, and spine straight. A hand should support the head. This position should not be used if the victim might have neck injuries or other trauma.

General guidelines for an emergency situation

First aid is the basic emergency care provided to an injured or ill person before medical help arrives. The two major goals of first aid are to:
- Prevent death
- Prevent injuries from becoming worse

In an emergency situation, the Emergency Medical Services (EMS) system should be activated and below guidelines should be followed by a nurse assistant:

- Healthcare workers including nursing assistants should know their limits. They should not do more than they are able. They should not perform an unfamiliar procedure and should do what they can under the circumstances.
- They should stay calm. This helps the victim feel more secure.
- They should know where to find emergency supplies.
- They should always follow Standard Precautions and the Bloodborne Pathogen Standard to the extent possible.
- Life-threatening problems should be checked. They should also check for breathing, a pulse, and bleeding.
- The victim should not be moves as moving the victim could make an injury worse.
- The victim should be moved only if the setting is unsafe for example:
  - A building that might collapse
  - A burning car or building
  - Stormy conditions with lightning
  - In water
  - Near electrical wires
- They should wait for help to arrive if the scene is not safe enough for them to approach.
- Necessary emergency measures should be performed.
- The nurse assistant should call for help or should have someone activate the EMS system. They should not hang up until the operator has hung up. The following information should be provided:
  - Location i.e. City and street address, cross streets or roads, and landmarks
  - Phone number

- Scenario for example, heart attack, crash, fire
- How many people require help
- Situations of victims, obvious injuries, and life threatening conditions
- What aid is being provided

- The nurse assistant should not remove clothes of the victim unless it is extremely necessary. If it is necessary to remove clothing, the nurse assistant should tear or cut garments along the seams.

- The victim should be kept warm and should be covered with a blanket, coats, or sweaters.

- The nurse assistant should provide reassurance to the victim and should explain what is happening.

- Fluids should not be provided to the victim.

- The lookers should be kept away as they invade privacy and tend to stare, give advice, and comment about the victim's condition. The victim may think the situation is worse than it is.

If the patient/resident loses consciousness, having no pulse, or stops breathing, the patient/resident may be in cardiac arrest and need immediate cardiopulmonary resuscitation (CPR) as well as defibrillation (it is delivery of an electric shock to the heart muscle to regain and restore a normal rhythm). An automated external defibrillator (AED) is commonly used for defibrillation. AED is a portable electronic device that delivers an automated defibrillation shock or deliver shock with a push of a manual button to support the heart restore an effective pumping rhythm. The proper application of an automated external defibrillator

(AED) along with CPR has been shown to improve survival rates among patents/residents experiencing cardiac arrest. The nurse assistant should know the location of AEDs in his/her facility, because he/she may be required to retrieve the AED while a co-worker administers CPR in an emergency. The nurse assistant should also know where CPR breathing barrier devices (used to protect both the patient/resident being resuscitated and the nurse assistant from the spread of microorganisms in blood, saliva, and other body fluids) are placed so he/she can access them in a hurry.

Encouraging safety and comfort
Safety
During emergency conditions, contact with body fluids, blood, secretions, and excretions is more likely. The nurse assistant should always follow Standard Precautions and the Bloodborne Pathogen Standard to the extent possible. When an emergency occurs in a healthcare facility, the nurse assistant should call for the nurse at once. The nurse assistant may also need to activate the EMS system or need to take the victim's vital signs. The nurse assistant should provide assistance as instructed by the nurse.

Comfort
Mental comfort is important during emergency situations. The nurse assistant should help the victim to feel safe and secure. The nurse assistant should provide proper reassurance to the victim and should explain about the situation with a calm approach.

Foreign bodies may obstruct the airway, which is called as choking or foreign-body airway obstruction (FBAO). As a result, air cannot pass through the airways into the lungs and the body does not receive enough oxygen. It may lead to cardiac arrest. Airway obstruction can be mild, moderate, or severe. If the obstruction is not managed properly, the victim may die.

The most common cause of choking may include foreign body (such as poorly chewed pieces of meat), tongue in the unconscious patient/resident (the tongue may fall backward in the throat to block the airway), thick mucus, vomitus (aspiration of vomit), small objects, and dentures

Signs of choking may include:

- Respiratory difficulty – victim cannot breathe
- Inability to speak or cough
- High pitched sounds
- Universal choking sign in which the victim clutches throat with his/her both hands

Management of choking in children and adults

Initial step for management of choking in a child or adult is to assess whether the victim is responsive or not. Steps for effective management of choking in children and adults may include:

Following methods can be used for the management of choking in a responsive child or adult:

1. Abdominal thrusts
2. Chest thrusts
3. Back blows

The suitable method should be chosen for the victim according to circumstances. Regardless of any combination of these methods, the nurse assistant should continue interventions until:

- Foreign body dislodged
- Victim begins to breathe
- Victim becomes unresponsive

1. *Abdominal thrusts (Heimlich maneuver)*

The Heimlich maneuver is a procedure that should only be used when a victim is responsive and older than one year of age. Following are the steps to perform the Heimlich maneuver effectively:

- The nurse assistant should always stand behind the responsive victim and should wrap his/her arms around the victim's waist under the ribcage.
- The nurse assistant should put the side of his/her fist above the victim's umbilicus, in the middle of his/her belly. The nurse assistant should always avoid pressing on the lower part of the sternum.
- With the other hand, the nurse assistant should hold the first fist and press forcefully into the victim's abdomen and up toward his/her chest.
- The nurse assistant should continue to perform these thrusts until the

obstruction is relieved or until the victim becomes unresponsive.

Abdominal thrusts are good default option for most of victims; however, it is not recommended for pregnant women and obese victims. The nurse assistant should use chest thrusts in these victims.

2. *Chest thrusts*

Below steps should be followed to perform the chest thrusts effectively:

- A stable stance should be assumed behind the victim.
- The nurse assistant should make a fist and place it thumbside-in against victim's sternum.
- The fist should be grasped tightly with other hand and up to 5 quick thrusts should be delivered.
- The nurse assistant should continue to perform these thrusts until the obstruction is relieved or until the victim becomes unresponsive.

3. *Back blows*

A stable stance should be assumed behind the victim.

- The nurse assistant should clutch his/her one arm around the victim's chest and should lean the victim forward at his/her waist to maintain upper airway parallel to the ground.
- The heel of the other hand should be used to deliver 5 firm blows between the victim's shoulder blades.
- The nurse assistant should continue to perform these thrusts until the obstruction is relieved or until the victim becomes unresponsive.

Unresponsive victims: Chest compressions

In an unresponsive victim, it is recommended the following protocol for choking management:

- The nurse assistant should initiate with performing sets of 30 chest compressions same as in the CPR protocol.
- After completing each set of 30 chest compressions, the nurse assistant should look carefully inside the victim's mouth.
- If any foreign object is observed, the nurse assistant should carefully remove it by using a finger sweep.
- After observing in the mouth, or after clearing an object, the airway should be opened and should make an attempt to ventilate. If the ventilation goes in the victim's mouth, the second ventilation should be provided. If the first ventilation does not successfully go in, the victim's head should be re-positioned and the nurse assistant should attempt to give second ventilation again. If it still does not go in, the CPR sequence should be resumed, starting with 30 chest compressions and repeating this sequence until the airway is clear.

Common Emergency Codes Used in Healthcare Facilities

These are color coded indicators used in healthcare facilities to alert all staff members for potential emergency issues arising in a facility. Emergency codes include unique criteria for how nursing assistants and other staff members should respond to a specific situation, ranging from an active shooter threat to cardiac arrest.

Depending on healthcare facility's size and level of care, designation of emergency codes may vary. There are no standard conventions or definitions for the use of code designations. While code blue means a cardiopulmonary arrest at many hospitals; however, it doesn't necessarily mean the same thing everywhere. It should keep in mind that every healthcare facility or hospital has its own conventions and policies for notification of emergencies. Doctors, nursing assistants, and other staff should be trained to recognize and respond appropriately to these emergency notifications.

Code red: Fire

Code red provides an appropriate emergency response in the event of an actual or suspected fire to protect life, property and vital services. Due to the non-ambulatory nature of many patients/residents and devastating effects of fire, all employees including nursing assistants have a responsibility to respond quickly to an actual or suspected fire.

Code Red should be initiated immediately in case of any one of the following indications:

5. Watching smoke, sparks or a fire.
6. Smelling smoke or other burning material.
7. Feeling unusual heat on a door, wall, and other surfaces.
8. In response to any life/fire safety system alarm.

The Code red task force including nursing assistants performs only basic fire response operations for initial stage of fires that can be extinguished by portable fire extinguishers without the usual need for self-contained breathing apparatus or protective clothing. All employees including nursing assistants should complete an annual safety training that includes appropriate life/fire safety procedures according to their facility policies.

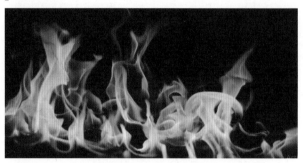

Upon discovery of suspected or actual fire:

At fire origin, R.A.C.E approach should be initiated in which first of all patients, visitors and personnel from the immediate fire area are removed from an immediate threat. Activation of the fire alarm and notification for others in the affected area to obtain assistance is the next step. Nursing assistants should follow their organizations' emergency reporting instructions. Smoke and fire should be contained by closing all doors and finally the fire should be extinguished if it is safe to do so.

S.A.F.E. Approach

S— Safety of life

A— Activation of the alarm

F — Fighting with fire (if it is safe to do so)

E — Evacuation (as necessary or instructed)

Code gray: Combative person

Code gray provides an appropriate

emergency response to situations involving a hostile, aggressive, combative, or potentially combative person. Aggressive, abusive, or combative behavior can be displayed by anyone like a patient, a patient's family member, staff, staff family members, or friends of patients and employees. Nursing assistants and other staff should effectively respond to ensure the security and safety of all persons on hospital property and minimize the number of potential injuries and assault victims.

Code yellow: Bomb threat

Code yellow provides an appropriate emergency response in the incident of a bomb threat or the finding of a suspicious device.

A code yellow denotes a bomb threat to the facility. It may include the identification of an actual bomb within the facility or just receiving a bomb threat.

If a threat is received through phone to the facility, it should be tried to get as much information as possible about the caller. Relevant questions about the threat should be asked, and share the information to other employees to activate the code yellow.

It is important to remain calm and not get angry at the person phoning in a threat. Upon the arrival of law enforcement security, the call should be turned over to them. Code yellow can be categorized into low-risk, medium risk, or high-risk threats:

A low-risk threat has the following features:

- The threat may be looking vague.

- Information is inconsistent or implausible.

- The caller may be identified easily and already has made multiple calls.

- The threat was discovered such as finding a package, not receiving an actual threat.

Medium-risk threats may have the following characteristics:

- A medium-risk threat is feasible.

- Wording may indicate the perpetrator has a possible plan for the bomb or threat.

- Time and place indications for the bomb to detonate.

- A lack of strong indicators that the perpetrator has taken preparation steps for completing the treat.

- Indications of the bomb's composition.

- There is an increased emotional state of the perpetrator, such as saying, "I'm serious," or "I'm going to do this."

High-risk threats are extremely specific and realistic. The perpetrator may give names, causes for why he/she is doing this, information about plans to indicate the bomb. The perpetrator may provide his or her identity.

Nursing assistants and other staff should follow these steps in the interim:

5. First step should be removing individuals in imminent danger from a suspected bomb or package. This may include evacuating the unit or floor if the bomb is located in a unit.

6. Contacting to authorities as soon as possible and activation the code yellow is the next step.

7. Unlike code silver, "shelter in place" is not an option in the code yellow.

   If the threat not found to be valid by law enforcement, an evacuation order may be overturned.

Code silver: Active shooter

Code silver provides an appropriate emergency response in the event involving a person with a weapon or who has taken hostages within the health facility (including an active shooter incident). The hospitals usually take all possible measures to minimize the negative impacts of a situation involving a hostage condition or person with a weapon.

Nursing assistants or anyone encountering a person brandishing a harmful weapon should:

a. Seek cover and warn others about the situation.

b. Notify the facility management of the incident with all information.

c. Provide the location in building, floor, area, and room number.

d. Describe the number of suspect(s) and any physical descriptions.

e. Provide information about any known hostages or victims.

Code blue: Medical Emergency (Adults)/Code white: Medical Emergency (Pediatrics)

Code blue or code white provides an appropriate emergency response to an eminent or suspected cardiopulmonary arrest or a medical emergency situation for an adult or pediatric patient. Code blue or code white is initiated for patients who do not have an advance healthcare directive indicating otherwise. Code blue is to be activated immediately whenever a patient eight years of age or older is found in a medical emergency or cardiac/respiratory arrest (per facility protocol). Code white is to be activated immediately whenever a patient eight years of age or younger is found in a medical emergency or cardiac/respiratory arrest (per facility protocol).

Code blue or code white is among the most easily recognized emergency codes in existence. While these codes are mostly associated with the cardiac arrest of a patient; however, these may be used to indicate any medical emergency in a health care facility, including medical emergencies of patient family members.

Depending on health facility's policies, all available staff members including nursing assistants from floors adjacent to the affected floor may be called to assist with the code blue or code white.

It is also important to make sure that nursing assistants should have the appropriate credentials for responding during a code blue. It may include ACLS (Advanced Cardiac Life Support), PALS (Pediatric Advanced Life Support), BLS (Basic Life Support) and CPR & First Aid training.

Code orange: Assistance needed or Hazardous Spill

Code Orange is the emergency code that may have facility-specific meanings. Joint Commission standards for hospitals (JCA) define code orange as an exposure to a hazardous substance or material within a health facility. However, it may also be used to indicate "attention needed" for violent patient conditions or other emergencies.

The main purpose of code orange is to provide an appropriate emergency response to an actual or suspected hazardous material spill in a manner that is safe for patients, staff, and visitors. Nursing assistants and other employees should be well familiar with the products they are using, understand how to use the products, and aware the spill precautions they should take. The clean-up of a hazardous material spill should only be done by appropriate knowledgeable and experienced nursing assistants and other personnel who have received proper training.

Helpful Resources

Arthur, W., & Kaye, G. C. (2000). The pathophysiology of common causes of syncope. *Postgraduate Medical Journal*, *76*(902), 750-753. https://doi.org/10.1136/pgmj.76.902.750

Bamford, J. (2001). Assessment and investigation of stroke and transient ischaemic attack. *Journal of Neurology, Neurosurgery & Psychiatry*, *70*(90001), 3i-6. https://doi.org/10.1136/jnnp.70.suppl_1.i3

Beyramijam, M., Khankeh, H. R., Farrokhi, M., Ebadi, A., Masoumi, G., & Aminizadeh, M. (2020). Disaster preparedness among emergency medical service providers: A systematic review protocol. *Emergency Medicine International*, *2020*, 1-5. https://doi.org/10.1155/2020/6102940

Bonanno, F. (2011). Clinical pathology of the shock syndromes. *Journal of Emergencies, Trauma, and Shock*, *4*(2), 233. https://doi.org/10.4103/0974-2700.82211

Brown, C. (2013). Increasing automated external defibrillator (AED) survival rates. *Resuscitation*, *84*, S19. https://doi.org/10.1016/j.resuscitation.2013.08.062

Da Silva, R. M. (2014). Syncope: Epidemiology, etiology, and prognosis. *Frontiers in Physiology*, *5*. https://doi.org/10.3389/fphys.2014.00471

E., D. (2013). Hypothermia for Intracerebral hemorrhage, subarachnoid hemorrhage & spinal cord injury. *Therapeutic Hypothermia in Brain Injury*. https://doi.org/10.5772/54925

Farmakis, D., Parissis, J., & Filippatos, G. (2015). Acute heart failure: Epidemiology, classification, and pathophysiology. *Oxford Medicine Online*. https://doi.org/10.1093/med/9780199687039.003.0051

Hatfield, A. (2014). Cardiopulmonary resuscitation. *Oxford Medicine Online*. https://doi.org/10.1093/med/9780199666041.003.0019

Hunter, R., Jones, M., Hurn, B. A., & Duncan, C. (1970). Impaired glucose tolerance: A late effect of insulin shock treatment. *BMJ, 1*(5694), 465-468. https://doi.org/10.1136/bmj.1.5694.465

Hurd, P. D., Lukas, S., & Hanson, A. (2018). Emergency preparedness. *Oxford Medicine Online*. https://doi.org/10.1093/med/9780190238308.003.0014

Inamdar, A., & Inamdar, A. (2016). Heart failure: Diagnosis, management and utilization. *Journal of Clinical Medicine, 5*(7), 62. https://doi.org/10.3390/jcm5070062

Khouri, G., Ozark, S., & Ovbiagele, B. (2017). Common risk factors for stroke and medical prevention therapies. *Oxford Medicine Online*. https://doi.org/10.1093/med/9780199937837.003.0103

Ko, S. (2017). Critical and medical management in acute stage of ischemic stroke. *Stroke Revisited: Diagnosis and Treatment of Ischemic Stroke*, 157-169. https://doi.org/10.1007/978-981-10-1424-6_14

ML, M. (2017). Advance directives and advance care planning. *Nursing & Healthcare International Journal, 1*(2). https://doi.org/10.23880/nhij-16000107

Ristagno, G., Pellis, T., & Li, Y. (2014). Cardiac arrest and cardiopulmonary resuscitation: Starting from basic science and bioengineering research to improve resuscitation outcome.

BioMed Research International, 2014, 1-2. https://doi.org/10.1155/2014/737542

Saleh, M., & Ambrose, J. A. (2018). Understanding myocardial infarction. *F1000Research, 7*, 1378. https://doi.org/10.12688/f1000research.15096.1

Skryabina, E., Reedy, G., Amlôt, R., Jaye, P., & Riley, P. (2017). What is the value of health emergency preparedness exercises? A scoping review study. *International Journal of Disaster Risk Reduction, 21*, 274-283. https://doi.org/10.1016/j.ijdrr.2016.12.010

Stafstrom, C. E., & Carmant, L. (2015). Seizures and epilepsy: An overview for neuroscientists. *Cold Spring Harbor Perspectives in Medicine, 5*(6), a022426-a022426. https://doi.org/10.1101/cshperspect.a022426

Surfactant therapy in the acute respiratory distress syndrome. (2016). *Acute Respiratory Distress Syndrome*, 305-330. https://doi.org/10.3109/9781420088410-19

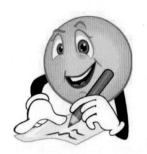

Chapter Thirteen:

Long Term Care Resident

Outline

I: Common Basic Human Needs

II: Common Community Resources for Older Adults

III: The Special Needs of Patients/Residents with Developmental and Mental Disorders

IV: The Special Needs of Patients/Residents with Alzheimer's Disease and Other Relevant

Dementias

V: Major Changes in Body Systems Associated with Aging

VI: The Basic Organization and Composition of Human Body

VII: Major Body Systems

Common Basic Human Needs

Physical needs

These are the basic and primary needs for life, such as water, oxygen, food, exercise, sleep, the ability to experience human touch, and the ability to eliminate waste products. Most of the daily responsibilities of a nurse assistant are helping patients/residents to meet their basic physical needs. For example, a nurse assistant will help patients/residents with toileting, eating, and walking or other forms of exercise. He/she will provide help to make sure that patients/residents in his/her care are able to rest by maintaining a peaceful environment and providing clean linens. The nurse assistant will also help to meet the patient/resident's need for physical contact by gently squeezing his/her hand, patting his/her arm, or giving him/her a hug.

Safety and security needs

Safety and security needs gain attention after primary needs are met. There are many different actions that can be taken to keep patients/residents safe and secure. For example, the nurse assistant may take multiple steps to prevent the spread of microorganisms that can cause infection, lock brakes of the wheels to prevent injuries, and keep a close look on patients/residents who may be confused and at higher risk for wandering away from the healthcare setting. In addition to supporting the patients/residents be safe, the nurse assistant should also help them to feel secure. Simple tasks, such as checking on each patient/resident in the care

frequently and answering requests for prompt help can develop trust of the patients/residents in the care to feel safe and secure. What makes someone feel secure and safe may vary from individual to individual, so the nurse assistant should make an effort to find out each individual's preferences. For example, one patient/resident may feel more secure with the door to his/her room closed; while another may want to leave the door to his/her room open.

Social needs

Most patients/residents need to be loved, liked, and accepted by health workers. These are called patient's social needs. Nobody wants to be ignored, to feel lonely, or to feel unloved or left out. A nurse assistant can help meet the social needs of the patients/residents in his/her care many times each day. He/she can be especially helpful when a patient/resident's family and friends cannot be with him/her. The nurse assistant should take the time to sit with the patient/resident or should talk with the patient/resident for a little while. In long-term health care facilities, there are multiple different ways to help residents to meet their social needs. For example, planned activities (such as holiday celebrations, games, and musical performances) provide residents an opportunity to meet other residents and socialize. The nurse assistant can also help residents to meet their social needs by assisting them to the dining room for meals, so that they can enjoy the company of other residents while eating.

Self-esteem needs

Individuals need to feel good about themselves, and they need to feel that they are worthy of the respect of others. Individuals who are in need of health care often feel that they cannot contribute in a meaningful way and they are no longer important for others. The loss of independence that may come with injury, illness, or advanced age can affect a patient/resident's self-esteem. Esteem is basically the feeling good about oneself. It is a sense of self-worth. Esteem is really necessary for self-actualization. Self-confidence and acceptance from others are significant components of esteem. A loss of cognitive ability (as in the case of dementia) can also affect a patient/resident's self-esteem. For a patient/resident with dementia, even simple questions may be very difficult to answer. The patient/resident's inability to answer easy questions may have a very negative impact on his/her self-esteem. The nursing assistant has a vital role to play in building resident's esteem. Through verbal and nonverbal interaction, the nursing assistant can develop resident self-esteem and confidence. A nurse assistant should help to protect and develop the self-esteem of those in his/her care by allowing them to do as much as possible independently for themselves. The nurse assistant should take an interest in the patient/resident, and should encourage him/her to talk about past accomplishments that make him/her feel proud.

Spiritual needs

Spirituality is a firm belief for something greater than oneself that supports an individual to assign purpose and meaning of life. For many individuals, organized religion is closely related to their spirituality. However, many individuals are spiritual without participating in a formal, organized religion. Spirituality is basically having an awareness of the meaning and purpose of life, and finding comfort and guidance in that awareness. Having a strong sense of spirituality can strengthen an individual's ability to cope with harsh conditions. Spiritual practices and beliefs can provide mental relief by minimizing worry and stress and increasing feelings of gratitude and hope. A nurse assistant can do many things to support and foster a patient/resident's sense of spirituality. A patient/resident may find it comforting for reading a book that is meaningful to him/her (such as a religious text or a book of poetry), engaging in a meaningful activity or ritual with him/her (such as prayer), or helping him/her with activities that strengthen his/her spirituality.

Common Community Resources for Older Adults

Area Agencies on Aging

An Area Agency on Aging (AAA) is a private or public non-profit agency, established by the state to address the concerns and needs of all older individuals at the regional and local levels.

AAAs coordinate and offer services that support older individuals remain in their homes - if that is their choice - aided by services such as homemaker assistance, meals-on-wheels, and whatever else it may require to make independent living a viable option. By providing a multiple range of options available, AAAs make it possible for older adults to choose the services and living arrangements that suit them best.

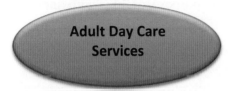

Adult Day Care Services

Adult day care centers offer a stimulating social environment for older adults while providing caregivers a vital break. Adult day care services is a planned program of activities in a professional health care setting established for older individuals who need supervised care during the day, or those older adults who are isolated and lonely. Adult day care centers enable older adults to socialize and enjoy planned routine care activities in a group setting, while still receiving needed clinical care services. At the same time, adult day care centers also provide family caregivers respite from caregiving duties while understanding that their loved one is in a safe and secure place.

Services may vary between adult care facilities, including the level of care offered. While one type of adult care center focuses mainly on recreational and social services, with a few personal care and health-related services, another type of adult care center may provide more comprehensive clinical and therapeutic services. These may include occupational, physical, or speech therapy administered by a registered nurse or other healthcare professional. Finally, a third type of adult care facility will offer specialized clinical care services for older adults with a specific health condition, such as dementia or a disability.

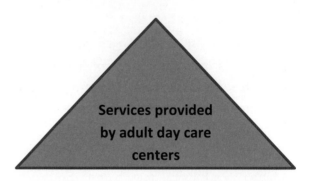

Services provided by adult day care centers

The major goals of adult day care centers may include:

Social activities

Planned social activities tend to be tailored to the individuals' abilities and health conditions, but may encompass such things like arts and crafts, musical entertainment, mental stimulation games (bingo, stretching or other gentle exercise), discussion groups, local outings, and holiday and birthday celebrations.

Nutrition

Adult day care centers provide older adults with nutritious meals, including those that accommodate special diets, along with snacks.

Personal care

Staff in day care centers can help older adults with the activities of daily living such as toilet hygiene, grooming, walking, and feeding.

Clinical services

These may vary from blood pressure monitoring, medication dispensing, hearing checks, and vision screening to symptom management and more intensive clinical or therapeutic services.

Transportation

Most of adult day care centers also provide transportation for older adults to and from the center and for any local outings.

Services for caregivers

Adult day care centers may provide counseling, help for care planning, support groups for caregivers, and caregiving education.

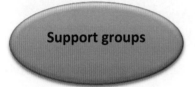

American Diabetes Association

The "Standards of Medical Care in Diabetes" of American Diabetes Association is intended to provide patients, clinicians, payers, researchers, and other interested persons with the components of diabetes care and general tools to evaluate the quality of care. The standards of medical care in diabetes recommendations must be applied in the context of excellent clinical care, with adjustments for personal preferences, comorbidities, and other care factors. Established in 1940, the American Diabetes Association (ADA) is the U.S. leading voluntary health organization whose major goal is to cure and prevent diabetes, and to improve the lives of all persons affected by diabetes.

Braille Institute or Blind Center

Braille Institute or Blind Center is a non-profit organization whose goal is to positively transform the lives of individuals with vision loss. It serves more than 37,000 individuals through a variety of multiple free programs, services, and classes at centers and community outreach locations from Santa Barbara to San Diego.

Alzheimer's Society

The Alzheimer's Society builds partnerships with all those with the shared commitment to finish Alzheimer's and other dementias, including the National Institutes of Health (NIH), National Institute on Aging, Alzheimer's organizations around the globe, universities, corporations and the biotech, pharmaceutical, and device industries. With these broad partnerships, Alzheimer's society is intended to provide healthy lifestyle for individuals with Alzheimer's and other dementias.

Parkinson's Support

American Parkinson Disease Association (APDA) and Parkinson's Foundation are the nation's leading organizations that provide information and support at every stage of Parkinson's disease. They offer resources that provide life-changing support to individuals with Parkinson's disease and their caregivers.

Multiple Sclerosis Support

The Multiple Sclerosis Association of America (MSAA) is a leading resource for the entire multiple sclerosis community. It is intended to improve lives of the individuals with multiple sclerosis and their caregivers through vital services and support.

Founded in 1970, MSAA is a national, nonprofit organization that is intended to improving lives today through ongoing direct and support services to individuals with MS, their families, and their caregivers.

Special Needs of Patients/Residents with Developmental and Mental Disorders

Seizures or convulsions are sudden and violent tremors of muscle groups due to an abnormal electrical activity in the brain. Seizures may lead to involuntary changes in body movement, sensation, function, awareness, or behavior. Seizures can have multiple different causes. Some patients may have epilepsy, which is a chronic seizure condition that can be controlled with medication. Other causes of seizures may include head injury during birth or from trauma, high-grade fever, brain tumors, poisoning, nervous system disorders or infection, and injuries to the brain tissue. Lack of blood supply to the brain tissue may also cause seizures. Although usually it is thought that a seizure involves convulsions and loss of consciousness; however, a person experiencing a seizure may just become very quiet with a blank stare. A patient/resident with epilepsy may have something called an aura, which is an unusual sensation or feeling before the onset of a seizure.

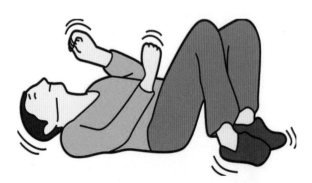

The major types of seizures may include:

Partial seizures

Only one part of the brain is involved in partial seizures. A part of the body may jerk or the patient/resident may experience a hearing or vision problem or stomach discomfort during the partial seizures. However, the patient/resident does not lose consciousness.

Generalized tonic-clonic seizures (grand mal seizures)

This type of seizure consists of two phases. First phase is called as the tonic phase, in which the patient/resident loses consciousness. If sitting or standing, the patient/resident may fall to the floor. The body becomes rigid because all muscles contract at once. The second phase is called as the clonic phase, in which muscle groups contract and relax. This causes twitching and jerking movements. Urinary incontinence, fecal incontinence, confusion, and headache may occur after the seizure is over on awakening.

Generalized absence seizures (petit mal seizures)

This type usually remains for a few seconds. There is complete loss of consciousness along with the twitching of the eyelids and staring. No first aid is necessary for this type. However, the nurse assistant should guide the patient/resident away from dangers such as fireplaces, stairs, streets, a hot stove, fireplaces, and so on.

Nobody can stop a seizure. However, the nurse assistant may protect the patient/resident from injury by following these guidelines:

- The nurse assistant should remain calm, and call for help as early as possible.
- He/she should not leave the patient/resident alone.
- The patient/resident should be lowered to the floor to protect him/her from falling.
- The time should be noted when the seizure started.
- Something soft should be placed under the patient/resident's head to prevent the patient/resident's head from striking the floor. The nurse assistant can use a cushion, pillow, or a folded blanket, jacket, or towel.
- The nurse assistant should loose tight clothing, such as a collar, tie, or scarf of the patient/resident.
- The patient/resident should be turned onto his or her side. It should be ensured that the head is turned to the side.
- It should not be tried to stop the seizure or control the patient/resident's movements.
- The time should be noted when the seizure ends.
- It should be ensured that the mouth of the patient/resident is clear of food, fluids, and saliva after the seizure.
- The nurse assistant should provide BLS if there is no breathing or no normal breathing after the seizure.

Parkinson's disease

It is one of the most common neural disorders affecting older adults. In Parkinson's disease dopamine is not produced in sufficient amounts. As a result, there is disruption of communication between the brain and the nerves that control muscle movement. A patient/resident with Parkinson's disease has shaking or repetitive motions of the muscles (muscle tremors), especially in the hands. The tremors are worse when the patient/resident is resting and reduce when the patient/resident attempts movement. As the disease gets worse over time, muscles become stiff and weak. The patient/resident may shuffle and lean forward during walking, and it can be very difficult for him/her to stop suddenly once he/she is walking. Speech may also be affected; the patient/resident may speak in a low tone without much variation. The patient/resident may lose the ability to frown, smile, or show other facial expressions.

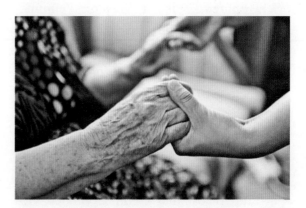

The signs and symptoms become worse with the passage of time. They may include:

- **Tremors:** The patient/resident may have trembling in the arms, hands, jaw, legs, and face.
- **Rigid, stiff muscles:** The patient/resident may have rigid and stiff muscles in the neck, arms, legs, and trunk.
- **Slow movements:** The patient/resident has a slow, shuffling gait.

- **Stooped posture and impaired balance:** It is difficult to walk for the patient/resident. Falls are a risk for these patients/residents.
- **Mask-like expression:** The patient/resident cannot blink and smile. A fixed stare is common sign.

Other common signs and symptoms may include:

- Swallowing and chewing problems
- Depression and emotional changes (fear, insecurity)
- Constipation and bladder problems
- Sleep problems
- Memory loss and slow thinking
- Slurred, monotone, and soft speech

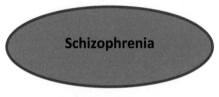

Schizophrenia

Schizophrenia is a severe, chronic, disabling neural disorder that means split (schizo) mind (phrenia). It involves:

- **Hallucinations:** Hearing, seeing, feeling, or smelling something that is not real. A patient/resident may see insects, animals, or individuals that are not real. "Tones and voices" are a common type of hallucination. "Tones and voices" may comment on behavior or order the patient/resident to do certain unrealistic things.
- **Delusions:** Delusions are false beliefs. For example, the patient/resident believes that a radio station is airing the patient/resident's thoughts. Some patients/residents have delusions of grandeur i.e. exaggerated beliefs about one's importance, power, wealth, or talents. For example, a male thinks he is Superman or a female thinks she is the Queen of England.
- **Paranoia:** Paranoia is a disorder (para) of the mind (noia). The patient/resident has suspicion and false beliefs (delusions) about another person or condition. For example, a patient/resident believes that others are harassing, cheating, spying on, poisoning, or plotting against him or her.
- **Thought disorders:** The patient/resident has trouble organizing thoughts or connecting thoughts logically. Speech may be difficult to understand or garbled. The patient/resident may suddenly stop speaking in the middle of a thought. Some patients/residents make up words that have no meaning.
- **Movement disorders:** These may include:
  - Being clumsy and uncoordinated
  - Involuntary movements
  - Grimacing
  - Unusual mannerisms
  - Sitting for hours without speaking, moving, or responding
- **Emotional and behavioral problems:** Normal body functions are impaired or absent. The patient/resident may:
  - Lose motivation or interest in daily routine activities
  - Be not able to plan or do activities
  - Seem to lack emotional responses
  - Neglect personal hygiene
  - Withdraw socially
- **Cognitive problems:** Cognitive links to remembering, understanding, and reasoning. The patient/resident may have trouble paying attention or remembering or understanding information.

Symptoms make it very hard for the patient/resident to perform daily tasks. Some patients/residents may regress. Regression means to move back to an earlier time or condition. For example, a 5-year-old child wets the bed when there is a new baby, which is a normal phenomenon. Healthy adults do not act like children or infants. Symptoms usually initiate between the ages of 16 and 30. The onset of the symptoms tends to be earlier in males than in females. Patients/residents with schizophrenia do not tend to be violent. However, if an individual becomes violent, it is often directed at family members in the home setting. Some individuals with schizophrenia attempt suicide due to extreme mental discomfort and embarrassment.

Hypochondriasis

Hypochondriasis or hypochondria is also called as illness anxiety disorder (IAD). Hypochondriasis is an overwhelming fear that anyone has a serious disease or life-threatening condition even though healthcare providers confirm that he/she has only mild symptoms or no symptoms at all. Hypochondriasis can also make individuals misinterpret their normal body sensations as signs of a serious condition or develop worries in individuals who do have a physical illness that they are sicker than they truly are. Illness anxiety disorder (IAD) is normally a chronic condition that can vary in severity. Severity usually increases in times of stress and with advancing age. Most common age for the onset of hypochondriasis is early adulthood. The excessive anxiety, not whether there is an absence or presence of illness, tends to be the most disabling.

Clinical presentation

- Excessive fear or worry over getting or having a serious illness for at least six months.
- Personal concern of mild or non-symptoms would be out of proportion.
- Misinterpreting normal body sensations.
- Persistent worry and fear of illness despite reassurance of health status by care providers.
- Frequently scheduling physician appointments for reassurance or avoiding clinical care due to fear of being diagnosed.
- Greater level of anxiety over personal health status.
- Repeatedly checking body for signs of disease.
- Avoiding individuals, areas, or activities for fear of health risks.
- Overly excessive worry about a specific illness or disease because it runs in the family.
- Frequently searching the internet for symptoms or causes of possible severe disease.
- Difficulty maintaining a job, keeping healthy relationships, and performing routine activities due to distress and anxiety.

Hypochondriasis is usually accompanied by other mental conditions such as anxiety and obsessive compulsive disorder. Alcoholism or substance abuse and dependence are also common among this population.

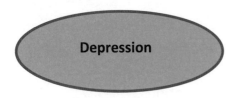

Depression

It is a persistent feeling of sadness, which involves the body, mood, and thoughts. An individual who is experiencing depression loses his/her interest in routine activities that used to give him/her pleasure. The person may demonstrate that he/she feels empty, sad, hopeless or helpless, and he/she may complain of feeling very tired all the time. The person may have crying spells. An individual who is depressed may sleep or eat too little or too much. The individual may be angry or irritable. Sometimes depression can cause physical complaints, such as stomachache, headache, or backache. An extremely depressed individual may discuss about or attempt to commit suicide. Depression can be stimulated or triggered by an event (such as the death of family member or having to leave one's home to transfer to a nursing home) but often is related to multiple events. Symptoms of depression may affect study, work, eating, sleep, and other routine activities. Some forms of depression tend to run in families. Some physical conditions may cause depression. Heart attack, stroke, cancer, and Parkinson's disease are examples. Hormonal factors may also cause depression. Pregnancy, thyroid problems, abortion, menstrual cycle, childbirth (post-partum depression), and menopause involve hormonal changes and cause depression.

Depression in older adults

Depression is common in older individuals. They have multiple losses—death of friends and family, loss of independence, and loss of body functions.

Some drugs side effects and medical conditions can cause symptoms of depression. Depression in older individuals is usually overlooked or a wrong diagnosis is made. Often older individuals are thought to have a cognitive disorder; therefore, depression is often not treated in older persons.

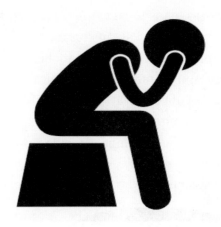

Signs and symptoms of depression in older adults

- Fatigue
- Inability to experience pleasure
- Feelings of hopelessness, uselessness, or helplessness
- Decreased sexual interest
- Increased dependency
- Anxiety
- Slow or unreliable memory
- Paranoia
- Agitation
- Focus on the past
- Thoughts of suicide or death
- Difficulty completing activities of daily living
- Changes in sleep patterns
- Poor grooming
- Withdrawal from people or interests
- Muscle aches, abdominal pain, and headaches

- Nausea and vomiting
- Dry mouth
- Loss of appetite
- Weight loss

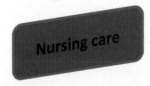

Nursing care

When a nurse assistant provides care for a patient/resident with depression, he/she should focus on maintaining the patient's safety and increasing his/her self-esteem. To accomplish this:

- The nurse assistant should encourage independence of the patient/resident to promote feelings of self-worth.
- The nurse assistant should provide appropriate positive feedback for the patient/resident and should reinforce his/her accomplishments.
- The nurse assistant should work with the patient/resident to set simple, attainable goals. The nurse assistant should be ensured to praise him/her when he/she meets the goals.
- The nurse assistant should listen when the patient/resident expresses sadness, and should allow the patient/resident to cry.
- Because the patient/resident's energy level is low, the nurse assistant should schedule his/her rest periods throughout the day.
- The nurse assistant should monitor the patient/resident's food intake to meet the nutritional needs.
- The nurse assistant should provide fluids frequently to the patient/resident, because the patient/resident may not drink sufficient fluids on his/her own.
- The nurse assistant should report all complaints of pain so that the symptoms of the patient/resident do not get overlooked.
- The patient/resident should be encouraged to use a prescribed hearing aid or eyeglasses so that he/she is more in touch with the world around him/her.
- The patient/resident should be encouraged to participate in activities, especially those that involve contact with other individuals and those that are physical as much as he/she can. However, overly stressful or tiring activities should be avoided.
- All comments about suicidal thoughts should be taken seriously and should be reported to the nurse right away.

Suicide

Suicide means the act of taking one's own life. If an individual talks or mentions about suicide, he/she should be taken seriously. The nurse assistant should call for the nurse at once and should not leave the patient/resident alone. Agencies treating patients/residents with mental health problems must identify patients/residents at risk for suicide. They must:

- Identify specific features or factors that decrease or increase the risk for suicide.
- Meet the patient/resident's immediate safety needs.
- Provide the most appropriate setting to manage the patient/resident.
- Provide crisis information to the patient/resident and his/her family. A crisis "hotline" phone number is an example.

Suicide risk factors

- Depression and other mental health problems
- Substance abuse disorder
- Prior suicide attempt
- Family history of substance abuse or a mental health disorder
- Family history of suicide
- Family violence including sexual or physical abuse
- Firearms in the home
- Incarceration
- Exposure to the suicidal behavior of others like friends, family, media figures etc.

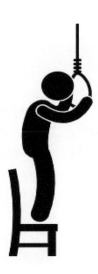

The nurse assistant should call for the nurse at once if a patient/resident mentions thoughts of suicide. A patient/resident may ask the nurse assistant not to share anyone about the suicidal thoughts. Protecting personal information is significant. But the patient/resident's safety should be the top priority. The nurse assistant should never promise that he/she will not tell anyone. The nurse assistant should report the statement to the nurse at once.

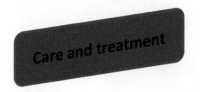

Treatment of mental health problems involves having the patient/resident explore feelings and thoughts. Psychotherapy and behavior, occupational, group, art, and family therapies are used. Often medications are ordered. The care plan reflects the patient/resident's needs that must be met. This may include physical, emotional, safety and security needs.

Communication is very important. The nurse assistant should be alert to nonverbal communication. Patients/residents with mental health diseases may respond to stress with anxiety, anger, or panic. Some patients/residents may become violent. The nurse assistant must protect himself/herself. Once he/she is safe, the health team can protect the patient/resident and others. For personal protection:

- The nurse assistant should call for help and should not try to handle the situation on his/her own.
- The nurse assistant should keep a safe distance between him/her and the patient/resident.

Intellectual impairment

There are two basic categories of impairment defined for children: intellectual disability and developmental disability. The patient/resident with intellectual disability has impairment that involves cognitive functioning, described by difficulty functioning independently and below-average intellectual abilities. Intellectual disability is also named as mental retardation, mental disability, and intellectually challenged. It can be assessed through a simple intelligence test called intelligence quotient (IQ). An average baseline normal score of IQ is about 100. Although intelligence quotient tests are widely used; however, it is known to have certain limitations. IQ tests are good indicators of academic achievement, but are greatly criticized for not being able to predict other types of intelligence. Many predictors of success in life and the working world include multiple factors such as self-confidence, motivation, interpersonal skills, creativity, intuition, persistence, and verbal and nonverbal skills. Other factors such as gender, culture, and race are also known to influence scores on standard IQ tests. Contemporary views of intellectual disability combine a person's IQ score with his/her limitations or abilities in daily life, such as social interaction, self-care, communication, and learning new skills. As a sole predictor, IQ tests cannot indicate self-esteem, successful parenting skills, or work productivity. The newer testing procedures support to determine limitations of adaptive behavior, such as the ability to use the money, language, telephone, or numbers, as well as occupational skills, social responsibility, and safety awareness. Although IQ scores should not be solely used to determine a child's abilities, the test scores should be reported so that the child can qualify for special educational support in public schools. There should be more than one type of testing procedures used to determine functional capacity.

Developmental and learning disabilities

Developmental disabilities (DDs) are assorted groups of chronic physical, psychological, sensory, cognitive, and speech impairments that are diagnosed at any time from the age of early development to 22 years of age. A developmental disability can be a physical impairment, intellectual impairment, or both. The patient/resident may have limited function in at least 3 of these areas: expressing or understanding language, self-care, mobility, learning, or self-direction. The patient/resident needs life-long assistance, help, support, guidance, and special devices. These disabilities generally persist a lifetime. Almost 2% of children under the age of 18 have some kinds of serious developmental disability.

Intellectual disability, accompanied by limitations in the ability to learn new skills, is the most common developmental disability. A learning disability is a problem in one or more of the processes involved in using or understanding language. Learning disabilities can be linked to specific aspects of learning, such as attention span, memory, or processing or sequencing of information. A learning disability not only affects school performance, but almost all aspects of a child's life. Education should be individualized to meet special needs of these children. Other DDs may include cerebral palsy, autism, attention deficit hyperactivity disorder (ADHD), hearing loss, speech and language impairment, and vision impairment. The causes for most of these disabilities are idiopathic.

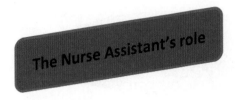
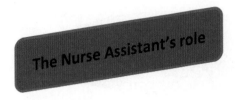
The Nurse Assistant's role

- The nurse assistant should provide an environment as normal as possible (normalization) for patients/residents with developmental and learning disabilities.
- The nurse assistant should emphasize individual strengths of the patient/resident.
- The nurse assistant should encourage independence and self-care of the patient/resident.
- Patients/residents should be treated with dignity.
- The nurse assistant should respect privacy of patients/residents,
- Patients/residents should be provided safe, secure, and structured environment.

Cerebral palsy

Cerebral palsy (CP) is a broad term used to demonstrate movement and coordination problems in children that are the result of some kind of brain damage. It may be associated with learning and intellectual deficits. Unlike other movement problems, cerebral palsy is not progressive. Symptoms of CP may appear at any time before age 2 years. Cerebral palsy is one of the most common permanent physical disabilities developed in childhood. There are many causes of brain damage of CP. During the pregnancy period, the causes may include maternal infection, fetal anoxia, pregnancy-induced hypertension, excess radiation, maternal diabetes, abnormal placental attachment, and malnutrition. The premature infant with very low birth weight is often at higher risk for developing problems that lead to CP than the full-term infant of normal birth weight. Postnatal causes may include birth trauma, brain infections (e.g., meningitis or encephalitis), head trauma, prolonged anoxia during childbirth or in very early infancy, brain tumor, and cerebral hemorrhage or clot. Severe jaundice or kernicterus in the postnatal period may cause CP because the high bilirubin levels can damage the infant's delicate brain. Mental retardation and hearing loss can also result from kernicterus.

Signs and symptoms
Clinical features of CP generally include the following to varying degrees:
- Muscle contractions
- Rapid alteration of muscle contractions and relaxations
- Muscle weakness
- Increased stretch reflexes
- Dysarthria (speech abnormalities)
- Limited range of motion
- Hearing and visual abnormalities
- Contractures
- Seizures
- Delayed motor development, such as with crawling, sitting, or walking
- Learning disabilities
- Mental abilities that range from very intelligent to severe mental retardation
- Difficulty sucking or feeding
- Scissors-like gait like crossing one foot in front of the other to walk
- Walking on toes
- Hypertension
- Underdevelopment of affected extremities

Classifications

There are four main classifications of CP:

Spastic cerebral palsy

It is the most common type of CP, representing 70%–80% of CP cases. Symptoms may include increased spasticity or muscle tone, which may affect one or more limbs. The patient/resident's muscles are stiff and movements awkward. Paralysis may be partial or full. Sensory abnormalities, such as hearing, speech, and vision deficits may also be present. The condition is usually described by a demonstration of the parts of the body that are affected. These demonstrations include spastic hemiplegia, which involves any one side of the body; spastic diplegia, which generally involves both legs; and spastic quadriplegia, which involves the whole body (trunk, face, both legs and arms).

Dyskinetic or athetoid cerebral palsy

It involves about 10%–20% of patients/residents with CP. This form of CP is characterized by slow, writhing involuntary movements, such as grimacing, twisting, and sharp jerks. These movements increase with stress and disappear during sleep. The child may have difficulty talking because of involuntary tongue and facial movements.

Ataxic cerebral palsy

It involves almost 5%–10% of patients/residents with CP. Tremors cause these patients/residents to have difficulty controlling their arms and hands when they reach for an object. Typically, they have an unsteady gait, a lack of coordination, muscle weakness, and problems with balance and depth perception. Nystagmus that is rapid, repeated movements of the eyeball may be seen in these patients/residents. During infancy period, there may be a lack of leg movements. When the child starts to walk, he/she holds the feet far apart, causing a wide gait. The child with ataxic CP is not able to make sudden or fine movements.

Mixed cerebral palsy

Almost 20% of CP cases are combinations of more than one forms of CP. The most commonly observed type of mixed CP has spasticity and athetoid movements.

Diagnosis

Cerebral palsy is primarily diagnosed by symptoms the child describes during infancy. Several critical observations can direct the healthcare providers to look closely for other symptoms. The infant who has difficulty sucking or has leg or arm tremors with voluntary movement should be evaluated for cerebral palsy. In children with cerebral palsy, infantile primitive reflexes persist past the expected period of disappearance. The infant who crosses his/her legs when lifted from behind, rather than pulling them up, is also of suspicious. Another common sign of CP is difficulty in diapering because the legs are difficult to separate. The child tends to use the hands and arms, but not the legs. Other disorders should be ruled out by CT, MRI, EEG, and nutritional studies. Visual and hearing screening is necessary to determine the extent of disability.

Treatment

There is no treatment for cerebral palsy. Preventative measures, such as wearing bike helmets and using car seats may help to minimize accidental head trauma. Disabilities linked with CP are permanent; treatment is generally multidisciplinary and aimed at preventing major complications and maximizing the child's potential. The major goal is helping the child to learn self-care activities. Appropriate educational assistance and improving communication through speech therapy is important. Physical and occupational therapy may help maintain the child's muscle strength. Splints, braces, or walkers may aid in ambulation. Orthopedic surgery is usually used to correct severe contractures.

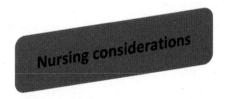

CP does not necessarily affect the length of life, but it profoundly affects the quality of life. Adaptive care devices, such as glasses, hearing aids, vision-enhancing equipment, walkers, and braces can help with mobility. Education needs to be adapted according to the capacities and needs of the child. In serious cases, institutionalization can be used instead of home care. Medications are supportive and can be used for symptomatic treatment. Muscle relaxants can minimize tremors and spasticity. Seizures can also be managed with anticonvulsants. Surgical interventions require that the nurse assistant must provide individualized pre- and postoperative care, keeping in mind the physical and mental abilities of the patient/resident, as well as the capacities of the family. The patients/resident and family teaching are very important. Nursing care is extremely important for the child as well as the adult who has CP. The child and family will need much emotional support.

Alcoholism and alcohol abuse

Alcohol minimizes brain activity and affects alertness, coordination, judgment, and reaction time. With the passage of time, heavy drinking damages the central nervous system, kidneys, heart, liver, blood vessels, and stomach. It may also cause confusion and forgetfulness. Alcoholism is when an individual has signs of physical addiction to alcohol and continues to drink. The individual continues to drink despite problems with mental and physical health and family, social, and job responsibilities. Alcohol abuse is when drinking leads to multiple problems, but not physical addiction. Alcoholism (alcohol dependence) may include:

- **Craving:** A strong desire or urge to drink.
- **Loss of control:** A person cannot control the amount of alcohol, the amount of time spent drinking, or what happens while drinking.
- **Physical dependence:** Withdrawal symptoms, which may include nausea, shakiness, sweating, and anxiety, when drinking is stopped.
- **Tolerance:** Greater quantities of alcohol are required to get "high".

Alcoholism is a chronic problem that usually lasts throughout life. Counseling and medications can be used to help the individual stop drinking. The individual must avoid all alcohol to prevent a relapse.

Alcohol effects may vary with age. Even small quantity can make older individuals feel "high." Older adults are at risk for vehicle crashes, falls, and other injuries from drinking. They have:

- Slower response times
- Vision and hearing problems
- A lower tolerance for alcohol

Older adults tend to take more prescribed medications than younger persons. Mixing alcohol with some medications can be harmful, even fatal. Alcohol can also make some health conditions worse. High blood pressure is an example.

Drug abuse and addiction

Drugs usually affect normal brain function. While they develop intense feelings of pleasure, they often have long-term effects on the brain. Changes in the brain may turn drug abuse into drug addiction.

- **Drug abuse:** It is using a drug for non-medical or non-therapeutical effects.
- **Drug addiction:** It is a chronic, relapsing brain disease. The individual has an overwhelming wish to take the drug because it affects mental awareness. The individual has to have the drug. Often higher doses are required. The individual cannot stop taking the drug without treatment. A diagnosis is generally based on three or more of the following during a 12-month time duration:
  - The drug is usually taken in larger quantities or it is taken longer than intended.

- The individual attempts to cut down or stop using the drug.
- Most of the time is spent using the drug or recovering from its effects. The individual gave up or minimized social, job, or recreational events because of drug use.
- The individual continues to use the drug and does so despite knowing that problems are caused by using the drug.
- The individual has tolerance to the drug.
- The individual requires more of the drug to get high.
- The individual has withdrawal symptoms such as anxiety, insomnia, restlessness, irritability, impaired attention, and physical illness.
- The same drug is taken to avoid or relieve withdrawal symptoms.

Drug abuse and addiction usually affect social and mental function. They are generally linked to crimes, car crashes, violence, and suicide. Work, family, school, legal, and financial issues can result. Drug abuse may involve both the legal and illegal drugs. Legal drugs are generally approved for use in the United States. Physicians prescribe them for therapeutic purposes. Illegal drugs are those drugs that are not approved for use. They are usually obtained through illegal means. A drug treatment program combines various services and therapies to meet the individual's needs. Drug abuse and addiction are chronic conditions. Relapses may occur. A short-term, single-time treatment is often not sufficient. Treatment should be a long-term process.

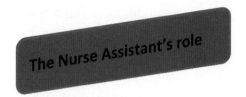

- The nurse assistant should report to the licensed nurse for any sign that the patient/resident is under the influence of alcohol or drugs.
- The nurse assistant should make sure that alcohol/drugs are not available (alcohol can be in present in products such as perfume, aftershave, cooking extracts, and cleaning products).
- The patient/resident should be observed for mental impairment, loss of coordination, or poor judgment.
- The nurse assistant should set boundaries, and should avoid being manipulated.
- The nurse assistant should be well aware of support groups such as Alcoholics Anonymous or the Mental Health Association.
- The nurse assistant should notify licensed nurse if signs of withdrawal such as:

  Alcohol: Nausea, shakiness, sweating, anxiety tremors, and agitation

  Drugs: Anxiety, insomnia, restlessness, irritability, impaired attention, runny nose, headache, pacing, poor coping mechanisms, and agitation.
- The nurse assistant should always follow the patient's/resident's care plan and should be well aware of dangerous behavior of such patients/residents.

Dealing with the agitated or aggressive patient/resident

The agitated patient/resident uses inappropriate vocal, verbal, or motor activities due to causes other than disorientation or real need. The nurse assistant should deal such patients/resident in following ways:

- The nurse assistant should report to the licensed nurse any signs of agitation including pacing, aimless wandering, screaming, cursing, biting, spitting, arguing, fighting, demanding, and talking to self.
- The nurse assistant should maintain calm and quiet atmosphere and should encourage distracting activities.
- The patient/resident should be checked for constipation or other sources of discomfort/pain.
- The nurse assistant should avoid restraints and should allow the patient/resident to walk, or rock in chair to diffuse energy.
- The nurse assistant should stand away from the agitated patient/resident. He/she should stand far enough away so that the patient/resident cannot kick or hit him.
- The nurse assistant should stand close to the door and should not become trapped in the room.
- The nurse assistant should be well aware of items in the room that can be used as weapons and should move away from such objects. Examples include phones, radios, vases, paper weights, letter openers, and belts.
- The nurse assistant should know where to find call lights, alarms, panic

- buttons, closed-circuit monitors, and other security devices.
- He/she should keep his/her hands free and should stay calm. The nurse assistant should talk to the patient/resident in a calm manner and should not raise his/her voice or argue, scold, or interrupt the patient/resident.
- The nurse assistant should be aware of his/her body language and should not point a finger or glare at the patient/resident.
- The nurse assistant should not touch the patient/resident.
- The nurse assistant should leave the room as soon as possible and should make sure the patient/resident is safe.
- The nurse assistant should tell the nurse or security officer about the matter at once. He/she should report items in the room that can be used as weapons.
- The nurse assistant should complete an incident report according to agency policy.

The Special Needs of Patients/Residents with Alzheimer's disease and other Dementias

Dementia

It is the loss of cognitive function that interferes with routine social, personal, and occupational activities. Changes in mood, personality, behavior, and communication are common in dementia. Dementia occurs when the specific areas of the brain are damaged by disease or injury. Dementia is actually a term that is used to demonstrate the group of symptoms that occur with a progressive decline in thinking and memory. A patient/resident's specific symptoms depend on what parts of the brain are damaged and how much damage there is. Dementia mostly affects older people. The disorders that cause dementia usually last for years and ultimately lead to death. As brain cells become damaged, the patient/resident gradually loses the ability to think, to remember, and to use language. Physical abilities are lost, and the patient/resident becomes totally dependent on others for routine care.

Dementia is basically not a normal component of aging. Many older individuals do not have dementia.

Early warning signs of dementia may include:

- Memory loss (forgetting names, losing things)
- Problems with routine tasks (for example, cooking, dressing, driving)
- Problems with language and communication (forgetting simple words)
- Getting lost in familiar places
- Misplacing things
- Putting things in odd places
- Mood, personality, and behavior changes
- Poor or decreased judgment

If brain changes have not occurred, some forms of dementias can be reversed. Treatable causes of dementia may include:

- Drugs and alcohol
- Delirium and depression
- Tumors
- Heart, lung, and blood vessel problems
- Head injuries
- Infection

- Hearing and vision problems

Permanent dementias

They result from irreversible changes in the brain. Permanent dementias have no cure. Function declines with the passage of time. Alzheimer's disease is the most common example of permanent dementia.

Pseudodementia

It means false (pseudo) dementia. The individual has signs and symptoms of dementia. However, there are no permanent changes in the brain. This may occur with depression and delirium. Both can be mistaken for dementia.

Causes of Permanent Dementia
- AIDS-related dementia
- Alcohol-related dementia
- Korsakoff's syndrome
- Alzheimer's disease
- Brain tumors
- Cerebrovascular disease
- Huntington's disease
- Multi-infarct dementia (MID)
- Multiple sclerosis
- Parkinson's disease
- Stroke
- Syphilis
- Trauma and head injury

Despite widespread research, there is still no treatment for dementia. Some medications may help to slow the progression of symptoms, but they do not work for every patient/resident. These medications are not beneficial in all forms of dementia and they do not prevent decline from occurring. Dementia ultimately robs the patients/residents of all memories, personality and abilities (things that make up the very essence of a patient/resident).

Delirium

It is a change in cognition that has a fast onset and is linked to chemical changes in the body. These changes may occur within a few days or even few hours. Delirium is usually reversible; however, the patient/resident may experience changes in cognition that are permanent even after the delirium is treated. Prompt identification and treatment of the underlying cause of the delirium is important to minimize the patient/resident's risk for experiencing long-term effects. Common causes of delirium may include medications and their side effects, dehydration, pain, lack of sleep, and infections.

Signs and symptoms of delirium may include:
- Feeling, seeing, or hearing something that is not there (hallucinations)
- Unable to recognize a familiar person
- Being restless, especially at night
- Failing to recognize and remember things that happened quite recently
- Wandering
- Unable to concentrate or follow instructions
- Becoming lethargic and presenting little movement or activity
- Changes in alertness (The patient/resident is usually more alert in the morning and less alert at night)
- Changes in sensation
- Changes in awareness
- Movement (very active or slow moving)
- Drowsiness
- Confusion about place or time
- Decreased short-term memory and recall. The patient/resident cannot

remember events since the delirium began

- He/she cannot remember past events
- Behaviors and thinking are without purpose
- Problems concentrating
- Speech does not make sense
- Emotional changes such as agitation, anger, anxiety, apathy, depression, euphoria
- Irritability
- Incontinence
- Restlessness

Elder care

Delirium in older adults is sometimes mistaken for dementia because some people assume that all confusion in older adults is caused by dementia. Similarly, the presence of delirium in an individual who has dementia is sometimes missed because the individual with dementia already has a change in mental processes. It is significant to recognize and report sudden changes in mental status because delirium is usually a red flag for a pending medical emergency, especially among older adults.

Depression

It is the most common mental health problem in older adults. Depression is often overlooked. Depression is generally characterized by a sad or low mood, loss of interest, and loss of energy and motivation. A patient/resident who is who is depressed may be sad or tearful, may lose interest in routine activities, may experience changes in sleeping and eating patterns, and may show increased anger or irritability.

Depression can be stimulated or triggered by an event (such as the death of family member or having to leave one's home to transfer to a nursing home) but often is related to multiple events. Symptoms of depression may affect study, work, eating, sleep, and other routine activities. Some forms of depression tend to run in families. Some physical conditions may cause depression. Heart attack, stroke, cancer, and Parkinson's disease are examples.

Hormonal factors may also cause depression. Pregnancy, thyroid problems, abortion, menstrual cycle, childbirth (post-partum depression), and menopause involve hormonal changes and cause depression.

Depression in older patients/residents

Depression is common in older individuals. They have multiple losses—death of friends and family, loss of independence, and loss of body functions. Some drugs side effects and medical conditions can cause symptoms of depression. Depression in older individuals is usually overlooked or a wrong diagnosis is made. Often older individuals are thought to have a cognitive disorder; therefore, depression is often not treated in older persons.

Alzheimer's disease

Alzheimer's disease is a brain disorder. Multiple brain cells are destroyed in Alzheimer's disease. The major functions that are affected may include:

- Memory
- Thinking
- Reasoning
- Judgment
- Language
- Behavior
- Mood
- Personality.

The patient/resident has difficulties with work and routine activities. Problems with friend, family, and social relationships occur. There is a slow and progressive decline in memory and mental function. The onset of the Alzheimer's disease is gradual. Often symptoms first appear after age of 60 years. The patient/resident can live 3 to 4 years or as long as 10 or more years. Nearly half of patients/residents age 85 and older experience Alzheimer's disease. More females than males experience AD. Females with AD usually live longer than males. Alzheimer's disease is not a normal part of aging. The cause of AD is idiopathic. A family history of Alzheimer's disease increases a patient/resident's risk of developing the disease. The most common early symptom of Alzheimer's disease is difficulty remembering newly learned things. The classic sign of Alzheimer's disease is a gradual loss of short-term memory.

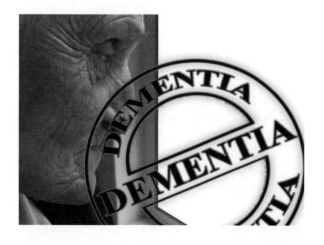

Signs of Alzheimer's disease

Warning signs of AD may include:
- The patient/resident asks the same question over and over again.
- He/she repeats the same story again and again.
- The patient/resident forgets activities that were once done regularly and with ease such as repairs, cooking, and playing cards.
- Loses the ability to balance a checkbook or to pay utility bills.
- Gets lost in common and familiar places.
- Misplaces household items.
- Wears the same clothes over and over again or neglects to bathe.
- Depends on someone else to take decisions or answer questions that he/she would have handled.

Other signs of AD may include:
- The patient/resident forgets recent conversations, events, and appointments.
- The patient/resident forgets simple directions.
- Forgets names of friends and family members and the names of common things like clock, TV, fan etc.
- Forgets simple words, cannot find the appropriate word, or loses train of thought.
- The patient/resident substitutes unusual names and words for what is forgotten.
- He/she speaks in a native language.
- Always curses or swears.
- Forgets important events and dates.

- Takes longer time to do even simple things.
- Misplaces things and puts things in odd places.
- Has difficulties keeping track of utility bills and writing checks.
- Gives away money and does not understand or recognize numbers.
- Has difficulties following conversations.
- Has problems writing and reading.
- Has difficulties driving to familiar places.
- Forgets where he/she is.
- Forgets how he/she got to a certain place.
- Does not know or understand how to get back home.
- Wanders from home.
- Cannot understand or tell time or dates.
- Cannot solve routine problems (stove burners left on, iron left on, or food burning on the stove).
- Cannot perform routine tasks such as bathing, dressing, brushing teeth, and so on).
- Distrusts other people. • Stubborn behavior. • Does not want to do routine activities and withdraws socially.
- Restless.
- Becomes fearful and suspicious.
- Sleeps more than usual.

Three stages of Alzheimer's disease: National Institute on Aging

Mild AD

- Getting lost

- Memory problems
- Problems handling money and paying utility bills
- Repeating same questions again and again
- Taking longer time to complete simple daily tasks
- Poor judgment
- Losing things or misplacing common household items in odd places
- Mood and personality changes

Moderate AD

- Increased confusion and memory loss
- Problems recognizing friends and family members
- Unable to learn new things
- Difficulties with tasks having multiple steps such as getting dressed
- Difficulties coping with new situations
- Delusions, hallucinations, and paranoia
- Impulsive behavior

Severe AD

- Relies on others for routine care
- Cannot communicate
- Sudden weight loss
- Seizures
- Skin problems and infections
- Difficulty swallowing
- Moaning, groaning, or grunting
- Increased sleeping than usual
- Lack of bladder and bowel control

Behavioral problems

Alzheimer's disease changes how an individual behaves and acts. Besides the signs and symptoms discussed above, following changes are common in AD patients:

- Wandering around and getting lost
- Sundowning
- Hallucinations
- Delusions
- Paranoia
- Catastrophic reactions
- Agitation and aggression
- Communication problems
- Screaming
- Repetitive behaviors
- Changes in intimacy and sexuality
- Rummaging and hiding things

Encouraging comfort and safety

Some problems and behaviors are not due to AD. They may be caused by injury, illness, or drugs. If the cause is not managed, it may threaten the individual's life. The nurse assistant should always report changes in behavior to the nurse.

Changes in Body Systems Associated with Aging

The Integumentary System

The skin loses its strength, elasticity, and fatty tissue layer. The skin sags and thins. Wrinkles are appeared. Secretions from oil and sweat glands usually decrease. Dry skin and itching may occur. The skin becomes fragile and easily injured. The skin's blood vessels become fragile, increasing the risk for:

- Skin breakdown
- Skin tears
- Pressure ulcers
- Bruising
- Delayed healing

Brown spots or age spots or liver spots may appear on sun-exposed areas. They are common on the hands and wrists. Loss of the fatty tissue layer of the skin affects body temperature. Socks, sweaters, lap blankets, extra blankets, and higher thermostat settings are helpful. Dry skin usually causes itching. It is easily damaged. A bath or shower twice a week is sufficient for hygiene. Partial baths should be taken at other times. Mild soaps or soap substitutes clean the genitals, underarms, and under the breasts. Often soap is not used on the arms, face, back, legs, chest, and abdomen. Creams and lotions prevent drying and itching. Deodorants may not be required because sweat gland secretion is decreased. Nails become tough and thick. Feet usually have poor circulation. A cut or nick may lead to a serious infection. The skin usually has fewer nerve endings. This affects sensing cold, heat, pain, and pressure. Burns are major risks because of fragile skin, poor circulation, and decreased sensing of cold and heat. Complaints of cold feet are common in older adults. Socks should be used to provide warmth. Hot water bottles and heating pads should not be used because of the risk for burns.

Gray or white hair is common. Hair loss may occur in men. Hair thins on older men and women—on the head, under the arms, and in the pubic area. Men and women may wear wigs. Some older adults color hair to cover graying. Facial hair (lip and chin) may occur in older women. Brushing promotes oil production and circulation.

Shampoo frequency usually decreases with age. It should be done as needed for hygiene and comfort.

The Musculoskeletal System

Muscle cells decrease in number with aging. Muscles atrophy may also occur. They also decrease in strength. Bones lose important minerals, especially calcium. Bones lose strength and become brittle and fragile. They may break easily, for example just turning in bed can cause fractures. Vertebrae shorten and joints become stiff and painful. Knee and hip joints flex (bend) slightly. These changes cause gradual loss of strength and height. Mobility also decreases. Exercise, activity, and diet help prevent bone loss and loss of muscle strength. Walking can be a good exercise. Exercise groups and range-of-motion exercises may be extremely helpful. A diet high in calcium, protein, and vitamins is required. The patients/residents should be protected from injury and falls. They should be turned and moved gently and carefully. Some patients/residents may need help and support getting out of bed as well as walking.

The Nervous System

Nerve cells are usually lost with aging. Nerve conduction and reflexes become slow. Responses are slower and blood flow to the brain is reduced. Dizziness may occur that increases the risk for falls. The nurse assistant should practice measures to prevent falls. Multiple changes occur in brain cells, which may affect personality and mental function. Blood flow to the brain is reduced and memory becomes shorter. Responses become slow and forgetfulness increases. Dizziness, confusion, and fatigue may occur. Long ago events are usually easier to recall than recent ones. Older adults who are mentally active and involved in current events show fewer mental and personality changes. Sleep patterns may change and falling asleep is harder. Older adults wake often at night and their sleep periods become shorter. Less sleep is required. Decreased blood flow and loss of energy may cause fatigue. They may nap or rest during the day. They may go to bed and get up early.

The Senses

Hearing and vision loss may occur with aging. Smell and taste become dull, along with decreasing appetite. Sensitivity and touch to pain, heat, cold, and pressure are reduced. These changes enhance the risk for injury. The patient/resident may not notice painful injuries or diseases. The nurse assistant needs to:

- Protect older patients/residents from injury.
- Assess signs of skin breakdown.
- Provide good skin care.
- Prevent skin tears and pressure sores.
- Follow safety measures for cold and heat.
-

The Circulatory System

The heart muscle may weaken with aging. With advancing age, the heart pumps blood with less force. Exercise, activity, excitement, and illness increase the body's demand for oxygen and nutrients. A weak or damaged heart cannot meet these demands. Arteries become narrow and are less elastic. Less amount of blood flows through them. Poor circulation may occur in many body parts. A weak or damaged heart works harder to pump blood through narrowed vessels. The number of red blood cells becomes reduced that can cause fatigue.

The Respiratory System

Respiratory muscles weaken with aging. Pulmonary tissue becomes less elastic. Labored, difficult, or painful breathing (dyspnea) may occur with activity. The patient/resident may lack strength to cough and clear the airway of secretions. Respiratory diseases and infections may develop, which can threaten life. Normal breathing should be promoted. Heavy bed linens should be avoided over the chest because they may prevent normal chest expansion. Re-positioning, turning, and deep breathing are important. Breathing is generally easier in semi-Fowler's position. The patient/resident should be as active as possible.

The Digestive System

Salivary glands start producing less saliva with aging, which may cause difficulty swallowing (dysphagia). Dry foods may be difficult to swallow. Secretion of digestive juices becomes reduced. Fried and fatty foods are difficult to digest. They may cause maldigestion. Ill-fitting dentures and loss of teeth may cause chewing problems. Hard-to-chew foods should be avoided. Chopped, ground, or pureed meat is easier to chew and swallow. Peristalsis may decrease with aging. The emptying of stomach and colon becomes slower, which can cause flatulence and constipation. Dry, fried, and fatty foods should be avoided to promote swallowing and digestion. Proper oral hygiene improves taste. Some patients/residents do not have teeth or dentures. High-fiber foods are difficult to chew and may irritate the intestines. They include celery, apricots, and fruits and vegetables with seeds and skins.

Patients/residents with chewing problems or constipation often require foods that provide soft bulk. They may include whole-grain cereals and cooked vegetables and fruits.

The Urinary System

The functions of kidneys decrease with aging. The kidneys may shrink (atrophy). Blood flow to the kidneys is generally reduced. Waste removal becomes less efficient. The bladder, ureters, and urethra lose elasticity tone. Bladder muscles become weaken. Bladder size decreases, storing less amount of urine. Urinary frequency or urgency may occur with advancing age. Many older patients/residents have to urinate (void) during the night. Urinary incontinence (loss of bladder control) may occur with aging. In older male adults, the prostate gland enlarges, which puts pressure on the urethra. Difficulty voiding or frequent urination may occur. Urinary tract infections are common risks. Adequate fluids are required—juices, water, milk, and gelatin. The nurse assistant should follow the care plan. Most fluids should be taken before 5:00 PM (1700). This minimizes the need to void during the night. Patients/residents with incontinence may need bladder training programs. Sometimes catheters are also required.

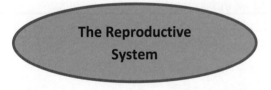

The Reproductive System

Males

The hormone testosterone may decrease slightly, which affects strength, sperm production, and reproductive tissues. These changes may affect sexual activity. An erection takes longer and the phase between erection and orgasm also becomes longer. Orgasm becomes less forceful than when younger. Erections can be lost quickly. The time between erections also becomes longer.

Females

Menopause is the time period when menstruation stops and menstrual cycles end. There should be at least one year without a menstrual period. It occurs between 45 and 55 years of age and females can no longer have children. Female hormones estrogen and progesterone also decrease. The vagina, uterus, and genitalia shrink (atrophy). Vaginal walls become thin and there is increased vaginal dryness. These changes make intercourse painful or uncomfortable. Arousal may take longer and orgasm becomes less intense.

The Basic Organization and Composition of Human Body

Anatomy and physiology

The study of the structure of the body is called anatomy. (Gross anatomy is linked with structures that can be observed with the naked eye, whereas microscopic anatomy needs the use of a microscope or other device to observe body structures.) The study of the functions of the body is called physiology. Nursing assistants requires basic knowledge of body structure as well as how these structures relate to and function with one another to maintain homeostasis. A basic understanding of normal anatomy and physiology is important before the nurse assistant can begin to understand abnormal conditions, such as injury or disease. The study of functioning disorders is known as pathophysiology.

Cells, tissues, and organs: Basic structural levels in the body

Four basic structural levels in the body are:

Cells

The basic structural and functional unit of body is the cell. Cells have the similar basic structure. Size, function, and shape may differ. Cells are extremely small and need a microscope to see them. Cells need water, food, and oxygen to live and function. The outer covering of the cell is called cell membrane. It encloses the cell and supports to hold its shape. The control center of the cell is nucleus, which directs the cell's activities. The nucleus is situated in the center of the cell, surrounded by the cytoplasm. Cytoplasm contains multiple small structures that perform several important cell functions. Protoplasm means "living substance." It refers to all structures, substances, and water within the cell. Protoplasm is a semi-liquid substance much like an egg white.

Tissues

Groups of cells with same functions combine to form tissues.

- Epithelial tissue covers external and internal body surfaces. Tissue lining the mouth, nose, respiratory tract, skin, hair, nails, glands, stomach, and intestines is epithelial tissue.
- Connective tissue anchors, supports, and connects other tissues. It is almost in every part of the body. Tendons, bones, ligaments, and cartilage are connective tissue. Blood is also a form of connective tissue.

- Muscle tissue contracts and stretches to let the body move.
- Nerve tissue carries and receives nerve impulses to the brain and spinal cord to body parts.

Organs

Groups of tissues with the similar function combine to form organs. An organ may have one or more functions. Examples of organs are the brain, heart, lungs, liver, and kidneys.

Body systems

Groups of organs that work together to perform special functions combine to form body systems.

Ten major body systems are:
1. Integumentary System
2. Respiratory System
3. Cardiovascular System
4. Musculoskeletal System
5. Endocrine System
6. Nervous System
7. Gastrointestinal System
8. Urinary System
9. Reproductive System
10. Immune System

Health is a state of physical, mental, and social well-being. Any change from the healthy state is known as disease.

The Integumentary System: Basic anatomy and physiology

The skin or integumentary system is the largest system of the body. Integument means any covering. The skin covers the whole body and has epithelial, connective, and nerve tissue. It also contains oil glands and sweat glands. There are 2 skin layers i.e. the epidermis and dermis.

- The outer layer is called epidermis. It has living and dead cells. The dead cells are situated deeper in the epidermis and pushed upward as the cells divided. Dead cells continuously flake off and are replaced by living cells. Living cells constantly die and flake off. Living cells contain pigment that provides skin its color. The epidermis contains no blood vessels and very few nerve endings.
- The inner layer is called dermis. It is primarily made up of connective tissue. Nerves, blood vessels, sweat glands, oil glands, and hair roots are found in the dermis.

The dermis and epidermis are supported by subcutaneous tissue, which is a thick layer of fat and connective tissue. Sweat glands, oil glands, hair, and nails are skin appendages.

- **Hair:** They cover the entire body, except the soles of the feet and the palms of the hands. Hair in the ears and nose and around the eyes protects these organs from insects, dust, and other foreign objects.
- **Nails:** They protect the tips of the toes and fingers. Nails support fingers to pick up and handle small objects.
- **Sweat glands:** They help the body in temperature regulation. Sweat consists of salt, water, and a small amount of wastes. Sweat is secreted through skin pores. The body is cooled through evaporation of sweat.
- **Oil glands (sebaceous glands):** Sebaceous glands are situated near the hair shafts. They secrete an oily secretion (sebum) into the space near the hair shaft. Oil moves to the skin surface. This helps to keep the hair and skin shiny and soft.

The skin has several important functions:

- It is the protective covering of the body.
- It prevents microbes and other substances from entering into the body.
- Skin prevents excessive amounts of water from leaving the body.
- It protects body organs from injury.
- Nerve endings in the skin sense both unpleasant and pleasant stimulation. Nerve endings are situated over the entire body. They sense pain, touch, cold, and pressure to protect the body from injury.
- It helps to regulate body temperature. Vasodilatation occurs when temperature outside the body is high. More blood is travelled to the body surface for cooling during evaporation. When blood vessels narrow or constrict (vasoconstriction), the body retains heat. This is because less amounts of blood reaches the skin.

- Skin stores fat and water.

Diseases and disorders

Skin lesions

Skin lesions can occur due to change in skin structure caused by any trauma, injury, aging, or disease. The signs and Symptoms of skin lesions may include:

- Rash
- Raised spots filled with fluid or pus
- Pruritus (Irregular reddened areas that itch)
- Dry crusts or scabs
- Breakdown in skin integrity

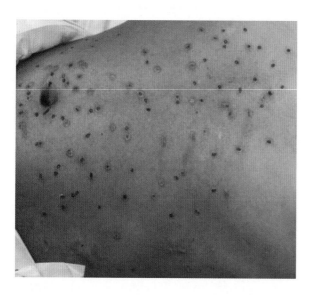

The Nurse Assistant's role

- The nurse assistant should observe and report any skin abnormalities.
- The nurse assistant should observe drainage on dressing.

- Water and soap should not be used for cleaning the drainage.
- Tepid water should be used while bathing.
- The nurse assistant should use gloves and should not remove crusts.
- The nurse assistant should always notify licensed nurse if:
  - Drainage from skin lesions
  - Sudden increase of drainage
  - Drainage with unpleasant and extremely bad odor
  - Changes in the color of drainage
  - Dressing needs changing
  - Wound has signs of red streaks, redness, pus, heat, and drainage.

The Nurse Assistant's role in the patient/resident's skin care

The nurse assistant can provide foot care, and care for dry skin and dandruff to patients/residents. Hand, foot, and nail care prevents infection, odors, and injury. Ingrown nails (nails that grow in at the side), hangnails, and nails torn away from the skin may cause skin breaks. These skin breaks can be portals of entry for microorganisms.

The nurse assistant should observe and report the following existing skin conditions and scalp to the licensed nurse:

- Alopecia
- Dandruff
- Pediculosis (lice)
- Acne

- Poison ivy or poison oak
- Insect bites or stings
- Minor burn
- Minor wounds
- Rash
- Excoriation, abrasions, skin tears
- Eczema or psoriasis

Pediculosis

It is the infestation with wingless insects (lice). Infestation means being on or in a host. Lice attach their nits (eggs) to hair shafts. Nits are oval in shape and white to yellow in color. After hatching, they bite the skin or scalp to feed on blood. Adult lice are grayish white to tan in color and about the size of a sesame seed. Lice bites may cause severe itching in the affected part.

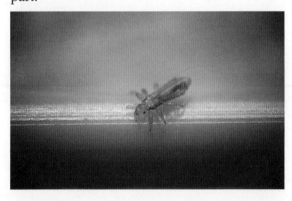

Lice can spread easily to others through head coverings, clothing, beds, bed linen, furniture, towels, sexual contact, and by sharing brushes and combs. Lice are generally treated with medicated shampoos, creams, and lotions specific for lice. Thorough bathing and washing linens and clothing in hot water are required.

- The infestation of the scalp (capitis) with lice is called Pediculosis capitis ("head lice").

- The infestation of the pubic (pubis) hair with lice is called Pediculosis pubis ("crabs").

Scabies

It is a skin problem caused by the female mite i.e. a very small spider-like organism. The female mite burrows into the skin to lay eggs. When their eggs are hatched, the female mites produce more eggs. The individual becomes infested with mites and has a rash and intense itching. Common sites for mites are between the fingers, in the underarm areas, on the thighs, around the wrists, and in the genital area. Other sites may include the breasts, buttocks, and waist. Scabies is a highly contagious condition and can be transmitted to others by close contact. Special creams and lotions can be used to kill the mites. The individual's room should be cleaned. Linens and clothing should be washed in hot water.

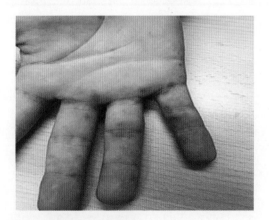

Pressure sores

Pressure sores are one of the major complications of immobility. A pressure sore is an ulcer that develops when part of a patient/resident's body presses against a hard surface (such as the seat of a chair or a mattress) for an extended period of time.

Pressure sores usually develop over bony prominences. Examples of these areas may include the back of the head, elbows, shoulder blades, hips, knees, coccyx (tailbone), ankles and heels. When a patient/resident stays in one position for too long, the weight of his/her body squeezes the tissue between the surface and the bone, which slows down blood flow to the area. Because the tissue is not receiving sufficient oxygen and nutrients, it begins to die. This loss of healthy and intact skin is called skin breakdown, which can lead to a pressure sore.

Patients/residents at risk

Patients/residents at risk for pressure sores are those who:

- Are confined to bed or wheelchair
- Need total or partial help moving
- Are agitated or having involuntary muscle movements
- Have fecal or urinary incontinence
- Are exposed to moisture—feces, urine, sweat, wound drainage, or saliva
- Have poor fluid balance or poor nutrition
- Have altered mental status
- Have problems sensing pressure or pain
- Have circulatory problems
- Are very thin or obese
- Have a healed pressure ulcer
- Taking medications that affect wound healing
- Refuse care and treatment measures
- Have health problems such as thyroid disease, kidney failure, or diabetes
- Smoke

Stages of pressure ulcer: Signs and symptoms

In patients/residents with light skin, a red or pink area is probably the first sign of a pressure sore. In patients/residents with dark skin, the skin may have no prominent color change or it may appear blue, red, or purple. Color does not fade on application of pressure. The area may feel cool or warm and firm or soft. The patient/resident may complain of burning, pain, tingling, or itching in the area. Some patients/residents do not feel anything unusual.

Stage I

An area is pale, red, or dark, and the normal color does not re-appear within a few minutes of relieving the pressure. The area may be softer, firmer, cooler, warmer, or more painful than the surrounding tissue. Detection may be more difficult in patients/residents with darker skin.

Stage II

The area may look like an open and shallow ulcer with red or pink exposed tissue at the bottom. Sometimes, instead of looking like a sore, the area may look like a blister.

Stage III

More tissue is damaged and lost. The fat that lies underneath the skin may be visible.

Stage IV

A deep crater is formed. Ulcer extends through skin and subcutaneous tissue. Bone, muscle, and underlying structures may be involved.

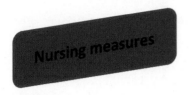

Nursing measures

Some pressure sores may be avoidable. That is, they are developed because of improper use of the nursing process. Some pressure sores unavoidable—they are developed despite efforts to prevent them. Nursing assistants should take following measures to prevent and manage them:

Sensory/mobility measures

- The pressure should be controlled by special beds or pressure-reducing devices.
- The patient/resident should be re-positioned and turned every two hours at least.
- The patient/resident should be positioned with proper support of the body and limbs.
- Active range of motion exercises should be promoted or the nurse assistant should assist patient/resident with them.
- Assistance should be provided to the patient/resident using a wheel chair to change his/her position frequently.
- The nurse assistant should prevent friction and shearing during moving, lifting, transferring, and repositioning procedures.
- The bed linens should be kept crumb free, clean, and wrinkles-free.
- It should be ensured that tubing like foley catheter does not cause pressure.
- Patients/residents should be removed from toilets and bedpans promptly.

- Circulation should be encouraged by gentle massage around red or purple area. It should not be done over red area.
- The skin should be checked every eight hours.
- Head of bed (H.O.B.) should be kept at 30 degrees as much as possible to avoid sacral and coccygeal pressure.

Elimination measures

- Skin should be kept clean and dry; powder should be applied where skin touches skin. Diaphoretic patients/residents should be frequently watched and observed.
- Incontinent patient/resident should be checked every two hours and it should be ensured that skin is dried and clean (even when applying adult incontinence garment).
- Incontinence garment should be monitored because plastic edges near skin may cause skin irritation.
- Scrubbing or rubbing should be avoided when bathing and drying the patient/resident.
- Pillows and blankets should be used to prevent skin from being in contact with skin.

Fluid status

- Limbs should be elevated limb to prevent edema.
- Compression devices, such as anti-embolic stockings and ace bandages should be properly monitored. Skin should be checked and ensured that edges do not cut into skin.

- The patient/resident should be encouraged fluids intake from 1500-2000ml/day or as per care plan.

Nutrition status

- Patients/residents should be encouraged and assisted with proper balanced diet.
- The nurse assistant should check skin folds in obese patients/residents.
- The nurse assistant should monitor bony prominences on thin patients/residents.
- Braces, casts, and clothing items should be monitored and ensured that they are not causing pressure against skin.

Use of pressure-reducing devices

The physician may order wound care products, drugs, and special equipment to promote healing. Support surfaces are used to reduce or relieve pressure. Such surfaces usually include air, foam, gel, alternating air, or water mattresses. Protective devices are generally used to prevent and manage skin breakdown and pressure sores. These devices may include:

a) Bed cradle
It is a metal frame placed on the bed and over the patient/resident. Top linens are brought over the cradle to prevent pressure on the feet, legs, and toes.

b) Heel and elbow protectors
These devices are made of pressure-relieving gel, sheepskin, foam padding, and other cushion materials. They fit the shape of elbows and heels.

c) Heel and foot elevators
These devices raise the feet and heels off of the bed. They prevent pressure as well as footdrop.

d) Gel or fluid-filled pads and cushions
These devices involve a pressure-relieving gel or fluid-filled pads. They are used for wheelchairs and chairs to prevent pressure. The outer case is vinyl and the cushion or pad is placed in a fabric cover to protect the patient/resident's skin.

e) Special beds
Some special beds have air flowing through the mattresses. The patient/resident floats on the mattress. Body weight is evenly distributed. Therefore, there is very little pressure on body parts. Some special beds also allow re-positioning without moving the patient/resident. The patient/resident is turned to the supine or prone position or the bed is tilted various degrees. Alignment does not change; however, pressure points change as the position changes. Some special beds constantly rotate from one side to another. They are useful for patients/residents with spinal cord injuries.

The Respiratory System: Basic anatomy and physiology

Oxygen is required to live. Every cell requires oxygen. Air contains almost 21% oxygen to meet the body's needs under normal conditions. The respiratory system carries oxygen into the lungs and excretes carbon dioxide. Respiration is the process of

404

supplying oxygen to the cells and removing carbon dioxide from them. Respiration involves exhalation (breathing out) and inhalation (breathing in). The terms expiration (breathing out) and inspiration (breathing in) can also be used for exhalation and inhalation.

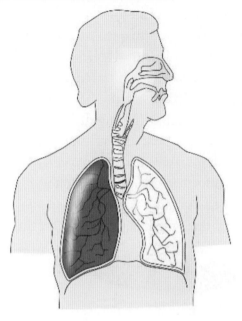

Air enters into the body through the nose. It then passes into the pharynx that is a tube-shaped passageway for both food and air. Air travels from the pharynx into the larynx (voice box). Epiglottis, a piece of cartilage, acts like a lid over the voice box. The epiglottis prevents the entry of food in the airway during swallowing. During inspiration, the epiglottis lifts up to allow air entering the larynx. Air then passes from the larynx into the windpipe (trachea). The trachea divides at its lower end into the left bronchus and the right bronchus. Each bronchus enters a lung. Upon entering the lungs, the bronchi divide multiple times into smaller branches known as bronchioles. Eventually the bronchioles further subdivide and end up in tiny one-celled air sacs called alveoli. Alveoli seem like tiny clusters of grapes. They are supplied by capillaries. Carbon

dioxide and oxygen are exchanged between the capillaries and alveoli. Blood in the capillaries carries oxygen from the alveoli. Then the oxygenated blood is returned to the left side of the heart and eventually pumped to the rest of the body. Alveoli pick up carbon dioxide from the capillaries for expiration.

The lungs are spongy tissues, which are filled with blood vessels, alveoli, and nerves. Each lung is subdivided into multiple lobes. The left lung has 2 lobes; the right lung has 3. The lungs and the abdominal cavity are separated by a muscle called the diaphragm. Each lung is covered by a double-layered sac known as pleura. One layer is attached to the chest wall and other to the lung. The pleura secrete a thin fluid that fills the space between these layers. The fluid prevents the layers from rubbing together during expiration and inspiration. A bony framework made up of the sternum, ribs, and vertebrae protects the lungs.

Diseases and disorders

Upper respiratory tract infection (URI)

It is the infection in nose, throat, and nasal sinuses. The common signs and Symptoms may include:

- Fever
- Runny nose
- Watery eyes
- Sore throat
- Cough

The Nurse Assistant's role

- The patient/resident should be encouraged to take proper rest.
- Adequate fluid intake should be encouraged.
- The nurse assistant should dispose of tissues promptly to avoid spread of the infection.
- The nurse assistant should report immediately to the licensed nurse in case of :
  - Fever
  - Dyspnea
  - Change in rhythm or rate of respiration
  - Change in mucus color from clear to yellow, green, or blood-tinged
  - Pallor, cyanosis
  - Signs that infection is moving to lungs or chest

Chronic obstructive pulmonary disease (COPD)

COPD involves 2 diseases i.e. chronic bronchitis and emphysema. These diseases interfere with oxygen and carbon dioxide exchange in the lungs. They obstruct normal air flow. Thus, less air gets into the lungs and less air leaves the lungs. Lung function is lost gradually. Cigarette smoking is the major and most important risk factor. Cigar, pipe, and other smoking tobaccos are also common risk factors. COPD has no cure and the best way to prevent COPD is stop smoking.

Chronic bronchitis

It occurs after repeated episodes of bronchitis. Bronchitis is the inflammation of the bronchi. Smoking is the major cause for chronic bronchitis. Smoker's cough in the morning is often the initial symptom. At first the cough is dry. With the passage of time, the individual coughs up mucus that may contain pus. The cough becomes more severe and frequent. The individual experiences difficulty breathing and tires easily. Mucus and inflamed air passages obstruct airflow into the lungs. The individual cannot get normal amounts of O2. The patient must stop smoking. Breathing exercises and oxygen therapy are often ordered. Respiratory tract infections should be prevented. If one occurs, the patient needs prompt treatment.

Emphysema

The alveoli become enlarge and less elastic in emphysema. They do not shrink and expand normally with breathing in and out. As a result, air is trapped in the alveoli when exhaling and the trapped air is not exhaled. With the passage of time, more alveoli are involved.

Oxygen and carbon dioxide exchange cannot occur in the affected alveoli. As more and more air is trapped in the lungs, the patient develops a barrel chest. Smoking is the major common cause for emphysema. The patient has cough and shortness of breath. Initially, shortness of breath occurs with exertion. Over time, it may occur at rest. Sputum may contain pus. Fatigue is common feature. The patient works hard to breathe in and out and the body does not get enough oxygen. Breathing is easier when the patient sits upright and slightly forward. The patient must stop smoking. Breathing exercises, respiratory therapy, medications, and oxygen therapy are ordered.

Pneumonia

It is an infection and inflammation of lung tissue. Affected lung tissues fill with fluid. CO_2 and O_2 exchange is affected. Viruses, bacteria, and other infectious microorganisms are causes. The patient becomes very ill. Signs and symptoms of pneumonia may include:

- High fever
- Chills
- Painful cough
- Chest pain on breathing
- Rapid pulse and breathing
- Shortness of breath
- Cyanosis
- Thick and white, yellow, green, or rust-colored sputum
- Nausea and vomiting
- Headache
- Tiredness
- Muscle aches

Medications are ordered for pain and infection. Fluid intake is increased for fever management and to thin secretions. Thin secretions are much easier to cough up. Oxygen and intravenous (IV) therapy may be needed. Semi-Fowler's position may ease breathing. Rest is extremely important and standard precautions should be followed. Transmission-Based Precautions should be used depending on the cause.

Tuberculosis (TB)

TB is a bacterial infection in the lungs caused by Mycobacterium tuberculosis. It is spread by airborne droplets with sneezing, coughing, singing, speaking, or laughing. Nearby individuals can inhale the bacteria. Those who have frequent and close contact with an infected individual are at risk. Tuberculosis is more likely to occur in close and crowded areas. Poor nutrition, age, and HIV (human immunodeficiency virus) infection are other risk factors. Tuberculosis can be present in the body but not cause signs and symptoms. An active TB infection may not occur for many years. Only patients with an active infection can spread the disease to others individuals. TB testing and chest x-rays can detect the disease. Signs and symptoms of tuberculosis may include loss of weight, tiredness, loss of appetite, fever, and night sweats. Sputum and cough increase over time. Chest pain occurs and sputum may contain blood. Medications for tuberculosis are given. Standard Precautions and Transmission-Based Precautions should be followed. The patient must cover the nose and mouth with tissues when coughing, sneezing, or producing sputum. Tissues should be flushed down in the toilet, or placed in a BIOHAZARD bag, or placed in a paper bag and burned. It is essential to wash hand after contact with sputum.

The Circulatory System: Basic anatomy and physiology

The circulatory system is composed of the heart, blood, and blood vessels. The blood is pumped by the heart through the blood vessels. The circulatory system has many important functions:

- Blood carries hormones, food, and other substances to the cells.

- Blood carries (transports) the gases of respiration. It carries oxygen to the cells.
- Blood removes waste products from cells and plays an important role in maintaining the body's fluid balance.
- Blood vessels and blood help to regulate body temperature. The blood brings heat from muscle activity to other body parts. Blood vessels in the skin dilate (vasodilatation) to cool the body. They constrict (vasoconstriction) to retain heat.
- The circulatory system produces and carries cells that defend the body against pathogenic microorganisms.

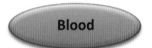

Blood

The blood consists of plasma and blood cells. Plasma is mostly watery portion that carries blood cells to other body cells. Plasma also carries multiple different substances that cells need to perform normal functions. This includes food (fats, proteins, and carbohydrates), chemicals, and hormones. Red blood cells (RBCs) are called erythrocytes.

Hemoglobin is the pigment in RBCs that carries oxygen and provides blood its red color. As red blood cells circulate through the lungs, hemoglobin picks up oxygen and carries it to the cells. When blood is bright red, hemoglobin is saturated with oxygen. As blood circulates through the body, oxygen is transported to the cells. Cells release carbon dioxide that is considered a waste product. It is picked up by the hemoglobin. RBCs filled with carbon dioxide make the blood look dark red. The body contains almost 25 trillion (25,000,000,000,000) RBCs. About 4.5 to 5 million cells are in a cubic millimeter of blood. Red blood cells live for 3 to 4 months. They are destructed by the spleen and liver as they wear out. New red blood cells are formed in the bone marrow. About 1 million red blood cells are produced every second.

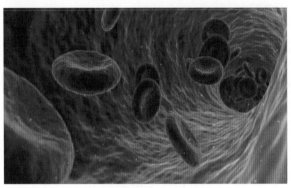

WBCs (White blood cells) are called leukocytes. They have no color. They protect the body against pathogenic microbes. There are about 5,000 to 10,000 WBCs in a cubic millimeter of blood. At the initial sign of infection, WBCs rush to the infection site and there they multiply rapidly. The number of white blood cells increases when there is an infection. WBCs are formed by the bone marrow and they live about 9 days.

Platelets are also called thrombocytes. They are needed for blood clotting. Platelets are formed by the bone marrow. There are almost 200,000 to 400,000 platelets in a cubic millimeter of blood. A platelet may live for about 4 days.

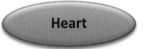

Heart

The heart is a muscle, which pumps blood through the blood vessels to the cells and tissues. The heart is situated in the middle to lower part of the chest cavity toward the left side.

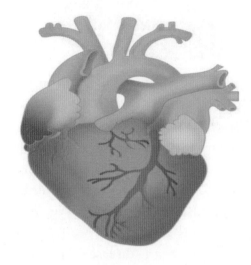

The heart is hollow with 3 layers.

- The outer layer is called pericardium. Pericardium is a thin sac covering the heart.
- The myocardium is the middle layer, which is the thick, muscular part of the heart.
- The inner layer is called endocardium. Endocardium lines the inner surface of the heart.

The heart has 4 chambers. Upper chambers are called atria and receive blood. The right atrium receives deoxygenated blood from body tissues. The left atrium receives oxygenated blood from the lungs. Lower chambers are called ventricles. They pump blood. The right ventricle pumps deoxygenated blood to the lungs for oxygen. The left ventricle pumps oxygenated blood to all parts of the body. Valves are located between the atria and ventricles. The valves permit blood flow in unilateral direction. They prevent backflow of blood into the atria from the ventricles. The tricuspid valve is located between the right atrium and the right ventricle. The mitral valve is situated between the left atrium and left ventricle. The normal heart action can be divided into two phases:

- **Diastole:** Diastole is the resting phase. Heart chambers fill with blood during this phase.
- **Systole:** Systole is the working phase. The heart contracts to pump blood through the blood vessels.

Blood vessels

Blood flows to body cells and tissues through the blood vessels. There are three groups of blood vessels i.e. arteries, veins, and capillaries. Arteries carry oxygenated blood away from the heart. Arterial blood is usually rich in oxygen. The largest artery of the body is aorta. It receives oxygenated blood directly from the left ventricle. The aorta branches into multiple other arteries that carry blood to all body parts. These arteries further branch into smaller parts within the tissues. The smallest branch of an artery is called an arteriole.

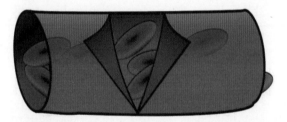

Arterioles are connected to capillaries. Capillaries are extremely tiny blood vessels. Oxygen, food, and other substances pass from capillaries into the cells. The capillaries pick up waste products (carbon dioxide) from the cells. Veins carry waste products back to the heart. Veins return blood to the heart. They are connected to the capillaries by venules. Venules are smaller veins that are branched together to form veins. The multiple veins branch together as they near the heart to form two major veins. The two major veins are the superior vena cava and the inferior vena cava, which empty into the right atrium. The inferior vena cava carries deoxygenated blood from the trunk and legs. The superior vena cava carries deoxygenated blood from the head and arms. Venous blood is dark red in color. It has very little oxygen and a great amount of carbon dioxide.

The path of blood flow is as:
- Venous blood, which is deoxygenated, empties into the right atrium.
- This blood then flows into the right ventricle through the tricuspid valve.
- The right ventricle pumps the deoxygenated blood into the lungs to pick up oxygen.
- Oxygen-rich (oxygenated) blood from the lungs enters the left atrium.
- Oxygenated blood from the left atrium passes into the left ventricle through the mitral valve.
- The left ventricle pumps the oxygenated blood into the aorta. It branches off to form multiple other arteries.
- Arterial blood is supplied to the tissues by arterioles and to the cells by capillaries.
- Cells and capillaries exchange nutrients and oxygen for carbon dioxide and waste products.
- Capillaries are connected with venules. Venules carry deoxygenated blood that has carbon dioxide and waste products.
- Venules form veins and these veins return blood to the heart.

Diseases and disorders

Coronary artery disease (CAD)

In coronary artery disease (CAD), the coronary arteries become narrow and hardened. One or all arteries are affected. The heart muscles receive less oxygen and blood. CAD is also called heart disease and coronary heart disease. The most common cause of CAD is atherosclerosis. The narrowed coronary arteries block blood flow. Blockage may be partial or total. The main complications of CAD are angina, irregular heartbeats, myocardial infarction, and sudden death. CAD is curable disease. Treatment goals are to:
- Relieve symptoms like angina pain.
- Slow or stop atherosclerosis.
- Lower the risk of formation of blood clots.
- Bypass or widen clogged arteries.
- Reduce cardiac complication and to improve overall quality of life. CAD usually requires life-style changes. Medications may be used to relieve the symptoms, decrease the heart's workload, prevent a sudden death or heart attack, or to delay the need for procedures i.e. bypass or open diseased arteries.

Myocardial infarction (MI)

Myocardial means the heart muscle and infarction refers to tissue death. In myocardial infarction (MI), blood supply to the heart muscle is suddenly stopped. Portion of the heart muscle dies and sudden cardiac death (sudden cardiac arrest) may occur. Myocardial infarction is also called:

- Heart attack
- Acute myocardial infarction (AMI)
- Acute coronary syndrome (ACS)

Signs and Symptoms

- Sudden, severe pain in chest usually demonstrated as crushing in nature
- Radiating pain to arm, neck, jaw, or back
- May present as heartburn or indigestion
- Diaphoresis, cool, and clammy skin
- Dizziness
- Pallor/cyanosis
- Dyspnea (short of breath)
- Weak, irregular pulse
- Low blood pressure
- Loss of consciousness
- Nausea, vomiting
- Anxious, restless, or feeling of impending doom
- Denial

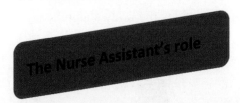

- The nurse assistant should notify licensed nurse immediately if above signs and symptoms are observes.
- he nurse assistant should remain with patient/resident, place patient/resident in comfortable position, and loose the patient/resident's clothing.
- The patient/resident should be encouraged to rest.
- The nurse assistant should reassure patient/resident that help is coming.
- Vital signs should be monitored properly.

- The patient/resident should not be provided liquids or food.
- The nurse assistant should prepare the patient/resident to transfer to acute care facility

MI is a medical emergency. Efforts should be made to:

- Relieve pain.
- Restore blood supply to the heart.
- Stabilize vital signs.
- Administer O2.
- Calm the patient/resident.
- Prevent death and life-threatening problems. The patient/resident may need medical or surgical procedures to open or bypass the diseased artery.

Cardiac rehabilitation is required. The major goals are to:

- Recover and resume routine activities.
- Prevent another MI.
- Prevent complications such as sudden cardiac arrest or heart failure.

Congestive heart failure

Congestive heart failure (CHF) occurs when the weakened heart is not able to pump the blood normally. Blood backs up and tissue congestion occurs. When the left side of the heart is weakened and cannot pump blood normally, blood is backed up into the lungs. As a result, respiratory congestion occurs. The patient has cough, dyspnea, increased sputum, and gurgling sounds in the lungs. The body does not receive enough blood and oxygen. Signs and symptoms occur due to effects of poor blood flow to other organs.

Poor blood flow to the brain causes dizziness, confusion, and fainting. The kidneys produce less amount of urine. The skin becomes pale. Blood pressure lowers. When the right side of the heart is weakened and cannot pump blood normally, blood is backed up into the venous system. Ankles and feet become swollen. Neck veins bulge and liver congestion affects normal liver function. The abdomen becomes congested with fluid. Less amount of blood is pumped to the lungs.

Congestive heart failure is an emergency. The patient can die. There are different drugs to strengthen the heart. They also decrease the amount of fluid in the body. A sodium-controlled diet is usually ordered. Oxygen should be administered. Semi-Fowler's position is usually preferred position for breathing. Daily weight, intake and output (I&O), elastic stockings, and ROM exercises are part of the care plan for congestive heart failure patients.

Anemia

It is a condition that results from a decrease in the quality or quantity of red blood cells. Signs and symptoms of anemia may include:

- Lethargy
- Pale or jaundiced
- Dyspnea
- Digestive problems
- Rapid pulse and increased respiratory rate
- Cold
- Dizzy

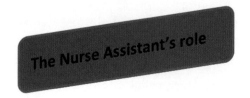

The Nurse Assistant's role

- The patient/resident should be provided nutritional meals containing increased iron like red meat and green leafy vegetables.
- The nurse assistant should notify licensed nurse if signs of bleeding or black stool are observed.
- Vital signs should be monitored properly.

The Musculoskeletal System: Basic anatomy and physiology

The musculo-skeletal system gives the basic framework for the body. It provides support for the movement. The musculo-skeletal system also protects internal organs and provides the body shape.

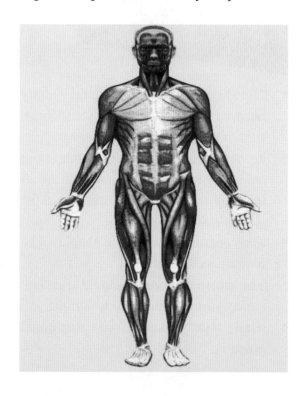

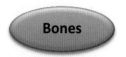

Bones

The human body contains about 206 bones. There are four major types of bones:

Long bones: They bear the body's weight. Leg bones are examples of long bones.

Short bones: They allow skill and ease in movement. Bones in the fingers, wrists, ankles, and toes are examples of short bones.

Flat bones: These bones protect the internal organs. They include the skull, ribs, pelvic bones, and shoulder blades.

Irregular bones: The vertebrae in the spinal column are examples of irregular bones. They allow multiple degrees of movement and flexibility.

Bones are rigid and hard structures. These are made up of living cells. Phosphorus and calcium are required for bone formation and strength. Bones store calcium and phosphorus for use by the body. Bones are covered by a protective covering called periosteum. Periosteum has blood vessels that supply bone cells with food and oxygen. There is a substance inside the hollow centers of the bones called bone marrow. Blood cells (including RBCs, WBCs, platelets etc.) are formed in the bone marrow.

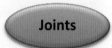

Joints

A joint is the point where two or more bones meet. They allow movement. Cartilage is connective tissue at the end of the long bones, which provides cushion for the joint so that the bone ends do not rub together. The joints are lined by synovial membrane. It secretes a fluid called synovial fluid, which acts as a lubricant for smooth movement of the joint. Bones are held together at the joint by powerful bands of connective tissue known as ligaments.

There are 3 main types of joints:

Ball-and-socket joints: They allow movement in all directions. A ball-and-socket joint is made of the rounded end of one bone and the hollow end of another bone. The rounded end of one bone fits into the hollow end of the other. The joints of the shoulders and hips are ball-and-socket joints.

Hinge joints: They allow movement in a unilateral direction. The elbow is an example a hinge joint.

Pivot joints: Pivot joints allow turning from side to side. A pivot joint joins the skull to the spine. Some joints are totally immovable. These joints connect the bones of the skull.

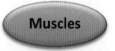

Muscles

The human body contains more than 500 muscles. Some muscles are voluntary. Others are involuntary.

Voluntary muscles: These muscles can be consciously controlled. Muscles attached to bones (skeletal muscles) are examples of voluntary muscles. Leg muscles do not work unless a person moves his/her arm; likewise for arm muscles. Skeletal muscles are striated and look striped or streaked.

Involuntary muscles: They work automatically. A person cannot control them. These muscles control the action of the blood vessels, stomach, intestines, and other body organs. They are also called smooth muscles. Smooth muscles look smooth, not striped or streaked.

Muscles have 3 major functions:
- Movement of different body parts

- Maintenance of muscle tone or posture
- Production of body heat

Diseases and disorders

Arthritis

Arthritis means inflammation of joints. In arthritis the patient/resident may experience pain, swelling, and stiffness in the affected joints. The joints are difficult to move.

Osteoarthritis: Osteoarthritis is the degenerative joint disease, which is the most common type of arthritis. Obesity, aging, and joint injury are common causes. The fingers, neck and lower back, and weight-bearing joints (knees, hips, and feet) are often affected. Joint stiffness usually occurs with rest and lack of motion. Pain occurs with motion and weight-bearing. Pain can be constant or occurs from lack of motion. Pain can affect sleep, rest, and mobility. Dampness and cold weather seem to increase symptoms. There is no cure for osteoarthritis. The osteoarthritis can be managed as:

- Medications to decrease inflammation and relieve pain.
- Use of heat relieves pain, increases blood flow, and reduces swelling. Cold applications can be used after joint use to provide comfort.
- Proper and regular exercise to decreases pain, increases flexibility, and improve blood flow. It also helps with weight control and promotes physical fitness and mental well-being. Good body mechanics, posture, and regular rest to provide comfort.

Rheumatoid Arthritis: It is a chronic inflammatory disease that causes joint pain, stiffness, swelling, and loss of function. It is more common in women and usually develops between the ages of 20 and 50. Rheumatoid arthritis may occur on both sides of the body. For example, if the left wrist is involved, so is the right wrist. The finger and wrist joints near the hand are often affected. Other joints affected are the shoulders, neck, elbows, knees, hips, ankles, and feet. Joints become warm, tender, and swollen. Fever and fatigue are common. Symptoms may be long-lasting and remain for many years. Treatment goals are to relieve pain, reduce swelling, and slow down or stop joint damage. The patient/resident's care plan may include:

- Short rest periods balanced with ROM exercises.
- Proper positioning to prevent pressure sores and contractures.
- Proper body mechanics and body alignment to reduce stress on joints.
- Healthy weight management to reduce stress on the weight-bearing joints.
- Relaxation, exercise, and regular rest to reduce stress.
- Measures to prevent falls. Medications are given for inflammation and pain relief. Cold and heat applications may be ordered. Some patients/residents may need joint replacement surgery. Emotional support may also be needed. Patients/residents with RA need to stay as active as possible.

Osteoporosis

In osteoporosis, the bone becomes porous and brittle. Bones become more fragile and break easily. Spine, wrist, hip, and rib fractures are common. Older adults are at risk. The risk for women to develop osteoarthritis increases after menopause because the ovaries are unable produce estrogen. The low levels of dietary calcium and lack of estrogen cause bone changes. Activity and exercise are needed for bone strength. Low back pain, gradual loss of height, and stooped posture are common features of osteoporosis. Fractures are a major risk. Even slight activity may cause bone fractures. They can occur from getting up from a chair, turning in bed, or coughing. Physicians often order calcium and vitamin supplements. Estrogen is usually ordered for some women.

Fractures

A fracture is a broken bone that can be of open or closed types. In open fracture (compound fracture), the broken bone comes through the skin. In case of closed fracture (simple fracture), the bone is broken but the skin remains intact. Accidents, falls, bone tumors, and osteoporosis are some common causes of fractures. Signs and symptoms of a fracture are:

- Pain
- Swelling
- Loss of movement or function
- Movement where motion should not occur
- Bone deformities
- Bruising and changes in skin color at the fracture site
- Bleeding (internal or external)

For healing of fractures, the fractured bone ends are brought into and held in normal position. It is called reduction and fixation.

Closed reduction and external fixation: In this procedure the bone is moved back into place and is not exposed.

Open reduction and internal fixation: It requires surgery. The fractured bone is exposed and moved into proper alignment. Rods, nails, screws, pins, plates, or wires keep the bone in place. After reduction, the bone ends are fixed and must not move.

The patient/resident may have a cast or traction. Walking boots, splints, and external fixators are also used.

Hip Fractures

Fractured hips are common in older patients/residents. The hip fracture requires internal fixation or total or partial hip replacement. Adduction, external rotation, internal rotation, and severe hip flexion should be avoided after surgery. Rehabilitation is usually required. Post-surgical problems may present life-threatening risks. They include urinary tract infections, respiratory complications, and thrombi (blood clots) in the leg veins. Constipation, pressure sores, and confusion are other risks.

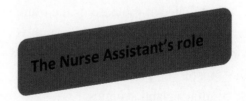

The Nurse Assistant's role

a) **Pre-surgery hip precautions**
   - The nurse assistant should avoid moving patient/resident until instructed by supervised nurse.
   - Sheet or back board should be used to move the patient/resident
b) **Post-surgery hip precautions**
   - The nurse assistant should not flex hip more than 90 degrees.
   - Affected leg should not cross over midline of body.

- The nurse assistant should not internally rotate hip on affected side.
- The nurse assistant should not do passive ROM on affected side.
- There should no weight bearing for several weeks after surgery.
- Fracture bedpan should be used.
- The nurse assistant should maintain proper hip alignment and may use trochanter roll and abduction pillow.

The Endocrine System: Basic anatomy and physiology

The endocrine system is made up of specific type of glands called the endocrine glands. The endocrine glands secrete chemical secretions called hormones into the bloodstream. These hormones regulate the activities of other glands and organs in the body. The pituitary gland is also called the master gland of the body. About the size of a cherry, it is situated at the base of the brain behind the eyes. The pituitary gland is subdivided into the anterior pituitary gland and the posterior pituitary gland. The anterior pituitary gland secretes:

Growth hormone (GH): It is needed for growth of bones, muscles, and other organs. It is required throughout life to maintain normal-sized muscles and bones. Growth is retarded if a baby is born with deficient quantities of growth hormones. Too much of the growth hormone may cause excessive growth.

Thyroid-stimulating hormone (TSH): It is required for thyroid gland function.

Adrenocorticotropic hormone (ACTH): It stimulates the adrenal glands. The anterior pituitary gland also secretes hormones that regulate development, growth, and function of the female and male reproductive systems.

The posterior pituitary gland secretes antidiuretic hormone (ADH) and oxytocin. Antidiuretic hormone prevents the kidneys from excreting excessive amounts of water. Oxytocin promotes uterine muscles contraction during childbirth.

The thyroid gland, shaped like a butterfly, is located in the neck in front of the voice box (larynx). Thyroid gland secretes the thyroid hormone to regulate metabolism. Metabolism is the burning of food for energy and heat by the cells. Too little thyroid hormone (hypothyroidism) results in slowed body processes, weight gain, and slowed movements. Too much thyroid hormone (hyperthyroidism) causes increased metabolism, weight loss, and excess energy. Some babies are born with deficient quantities of thyroid hormones. Their mental growth and physical growth are stunted. The four parathyroid glands secrete parathormone. Two are located on each side of the thyroid gland. Parathormone regulates normal calcium utilization. Calcium is required for muscle and nerve function. Insufficient calcium can cause tetany, which is a state of severe muscle contraction and spasm. If left untreated, tetany may cause death.

The thymus secretes the hormone thymosin that is important for the normal development and function of the immune system. The pancreas releases insulin to regulate the amount of sugar in the blood available for utilization by the cells.

Insulin is required for sugar to enter the cells. If there is too little insulin, sugar cannot enter the body cells. If sugar cannot enter the body cells, excess amounts of sugar may build up in the blood. This condition is known as diabetes.

There are two adrenal glands. Each adrenal gland is on the top of each kidney. The adrenal gland has two major parts: the adrenal cortex and the adrenal medulla. The adrenal medulla secretes norepinephrine and epinephrine. These hormones stimulate the body to rapidly produce energy during emergency conditions. Blood pressure, heart rate, muscle power, and energy all increase. The adrenal cortex secretes three main groups of hormones required for life.
Glucocorticoids: They regulate metabolism of carbohydrates. They also control the body's response to inflammation and stress.
Mineralocorticoids: They regulate the amount of water and salt that is absorbed and lost by the kidneys.
Sex hormones: Small amounts of female and male sex hormones are secreted. The gonads are the glands of human reproductive system. Testes (male sex glands) secrete testosterone. Ovaries (female sex glands) secrete estrogen and progesterone.

Diseases and disorders

Diabetes

In diabetes, the body cannot use or produce or use insulin properly. Insulin is required for transport of glucose from the blood into the cells. It is secreted from the pancreas. Without sufficient insulin, sugar builds up in the blood and blood sugar gets high. Cells do not have adequate glucose for energy and cannot function properly. The 3 types of diabetes are:

Type 1 diabetes
It occurs most often in children. The pancreas produces very little or no insulin. Onset of type 1 diabetes is rapid.

Type 2 diabetes
This type is more common in older adults. However, it is also becoming more common in teens, children, and young adults. Lack of exercise, being obese, and hypertension are major risk factors. The pancreas produces insulin. However, the body cannot use it properly. Onset of type 2 diabetes is slow. Infections are more frequent and wounds heal slowly.

Gestational diabetes
It develops during pregnancy. Gestational diabetes usually goes away after the baby is born. However, the mother is still at greater risk for type 2 diabetes later in life.

Signs and symptoms of Diabetes

Signs and symptoms of diabetes may include:
- Urinating often (polyuria)
- Feeling very hungry or tired (polyphagia)
- Being very thirsty (polydipsia)
- Losing weight unintentionally
- Having wounds or sores that heal slowly
- Having dry and itchy skin
- Tingling or loss of sensation in the fe

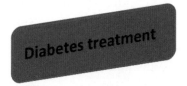

Complications of Diabetes

Diabetes must be controlled to prevent serious complications. These complications may include renal failure, blindness, nerve damage, and damage to the teeth and gums. Heart and blood vessel problems are more serious conditions. They can lead to heart attack, stroke, and slow healing. Foot and leg wounds and sores can be very serious. Infection and gangrene may occur. Amputation may be required.

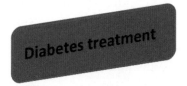

Diabetes treatment

Type I diabetes is usually treated with daily insulin therapy, exercise, and healthy eating. Type II diabetes is treated with exercise, healthy eating, and oral medications. Some patients/residents may need insulin. Obese patients/residents need to lose weight. Types 1 and 2 diabetes involves controlling cholesterol, blood pressure, and the risk factors for CAD. Good foot care is required. Blisters, corns, calluses, and other foot problems can lead to an infection, gangrene, and amputation. The patient/resident's blood sugar level can go too high or fall too low.

Blood glucose should be monitored daily or 3 or 4 time a day for:
Hypoglycemia—low blood sugar
Hyperglycemia—high blood sugar
Both conditions can lead to death if not managed.

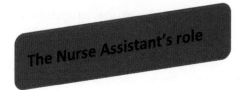

The Nurse Assistant's role

- The nurse assistant should know signs & symptoms of hyperglycemia and hypoglycemia.
- He/she should notify licensed nurse immediately if diabetic symptoms appear.
- The nurse assistant should offer snacks and meals to the patient/resident at regular intervals, and should report uneaten portions.
- The nurse assistant should be aware that stress, illness, and infection can make blood sugars high.
- Extremities (especially feet) should be observed for trauma, infection, or wounds.
- The nurse assistant should notify licensed nurse if patient/resident frequently vomits after meal.
- The patient/resident should be offered easily assimilated source of carbohydrates if signs of hypoglycemia occur.
- The nurse assistant should make sure that right and nutritious diet is given.
- Urine testing should be performed for evaluating sugar and acetone.
- There should be special foot care that may involve:
  - Feet should be washed and dried between toes daily
  - Feet should be inspected for signs of irritation
  - Toenails should be cut by licensed nurse or podiatrist only
  - Shoes and stockings should be worn at all time while out of

bed and the patient/resident should never go as barefooted
- The nurse assistant should check for anything that impairs circulation.
- It should be remembered that diet, exercise and medication are the most important parts of diabetic treatment.

The Nervous System: Basic anatomy and physiology

The nervous system directs, controls, and coordinates body functions. Its two main divisions are:

- The central nervous system (CNS), which consists of the brain and spinal cord.
- The peripheral nervous system (PNS), which involves the nerves throughout the body.

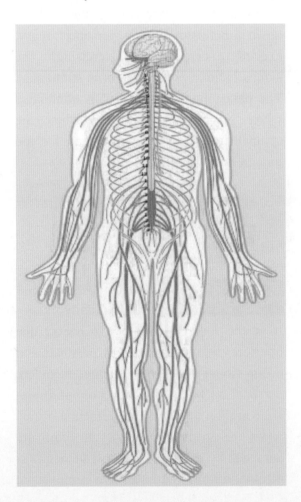

Nerves are connected to the spinal cord. Nerves carry impulses or messages to and from the brain. A stimulus stimulates a nerve impulse. A stimulus is anything that excites a body part to function, respond, or become active. A reflex is the response of the body to a stimulus. Reflexes are unconscious, involuntary, and immediate. The individual cannot control reflexes. Nerves can be easily damaged and may take a long time to heal. Some nerve fibers contain a protective covering called a myelin sheath, which also insulates the nerve fiber. Nerve fibers covered with myelin sheath conduct nerve impulses faster than those nerve fibers without it.

The central nervous system

The central nervous system (CNS) is composed of the brain and spinal cord. The brain is covered by the skull. The three major parts of the brain are the cerebrum, the cerebellum, and the brainstem. The largest part of the brain is called cerebrum. It is the center of intelligence and thoughts. The cerebrum is subdivided into two halves called left and right hemispheres. The right hemisphere controls activities on the body's left side. The left hemisphere controls the body's right side. The outside portion of the cerebrum is known as cerebral cortex. It controls the brain's highest functions. These include memory, reasoning, speech, consciousness, voluntary muscle movement, hearing, vision, sensation, and other activities.

The cerebellum coordinates and regulates body movements. It regulates balance and the smooth movements of voluntary muscles. Injury to the cerebellum may result in loss of coordination, jerky movements, and muscle weakness. The brainstem joins the cerebrum to the spinal cord. The brainstem contains the pons, midbrain, and medulla oblongata. The pons and midbrain relay messages between the medulla and the cerebrum. The medulla is located below the pons. The medulla controls breathing, heart rate, blood vessel size, coughing, swallowing, and vomiting. The brain is connected to the spinal cord at the lower end of the medulla. The spinal cord is situated within the spinal column. The spinal cord is 17 to 18 inches long. It contains pathways that conduct nerve impulses to and from the brain. Both the spinal cord and brain are covered and protected by three layers of connective tissue called meninges.

- The outer layer is located next to the skull. It is a tough protective covering and called the dura mater.
- The middle layer is the arachnoid mater.
- The inner layer is the pia mater. The space between the arachnoid mater and pia mater is the arachnoid space. The space is filled with the fluid called cerebrospinal fluid (CSF). CSF circulates around the brain and spinal cord. It protects the central nervous system. It cushions shocks that could easily injure the structures of the brain and spinal cord.

The peripheral nervous system

The peripheral nervous system consists of 12 pairs of cranial nerves and 31 pairs of spinal nerves. Cranial nerves conduct nerve impulses between the brain and the head, chest, neck, and abdomen. They conduct nerve impulses for vision, smell, touch, hearing, pain, temperature, and pressure. They also conduct impulses for involuntary and voluntary muscles. Spinal nerves carry nerve impulses from the extremities, skin, and internal structures not supplied by the cranial nerves. Some peripheral nerves form the ANS (autonomic nervous system). ANS controls involuntary muscles and certain body functions.

The functions include the blood pressure, heartbeat, intestinal contractions, and glandular secretions. These are involuntary functions that occur automatically. The autonomic nervous system is subdivided into the parasympathetic nervous system and the sympathetic nervous system. The sympathetic nervous system speeds up major body functions. The parasympathetic nervous system slows down functions. When a person is angry, excited, scared, or exercising, the sympathetic nervous system is stimulated. The parasympathetic system is stimulated when someone relaxes or when the sympathetic system is stimulated for too long period of time.

Diseases and disorders

Dementia

It is the loss of cognitive function that interferes with routine social, personal, and occupational activities. Changes in mood, personality, behavior, and communication are common in dementia. Dementia occurs when the specific areas of the brain are damaged by disease or injury. Dementia is actually a term that is used to demonstrate the group of symptoms that occur with a progressive decline in thinking and memory. A patient/resident's specific symptoms depend on what parts of the brain are damaged and how much damage there is. Dementia mostly affects older people. The disorders that cause dementia usually last for years and ultimately lead to death. As brain cells become damaged, the patient/resident gradually loses the ability to think, to remember, and to use language. Physical abilities are lost, and the patient/resident becomes totally dependent on others for routine care.

Dementia is basically not a normal component of aging. Many older individuals do not have dementia.

Early warning signs of dementia may include:

- Memory loss (forgetting names, losing things)
- Problems with language and communication (forgetting simple words)
- Getting lost in familiar places
- Problems with routine tasks (for example, cooking, dressing, and driving)
- Misplacing things
- Putting things in odd places
- Mood, personality, and behavior changes
- Poor or decreased judgment

Despite widespread research, there is still no treatment for dementia. Some medications may help to slow the progression of symptoms, but they do not work for every patient/resident. These medications are not beneficial in all forms of dementia and they do not prevent decline from occurring. Dementia ultimately robs the patients/residents of all memories, personality and abilities (things that make up the very essence of a person).

Alzheimer's disease

Alzheimer's disease is a brain disorder. Multiple brain cells are destroyed in Alzheimer's disease. The major functions that are affected may include:

- Memory
- Thinking
- Reasoning
- Judgment
- Language
- Behavior
- Mood
- Personality

The patient/resident has difficulties with work and routine activities. Problems with friend, family, and social relationships occur. There is a slow and progressive decline in memory and mental function.

Signs of Alzheimer's disease: Stages of Alzheimer's disease

Mild AD

- Getting lost
- Memory problems
- Problems handling money and paying utility bills
- Repeating same questions again and again
- Taking longer time to complete simple daily tasks
- Poor judgment
- Losing things or misplacing common household items in odd places
- Mood and personality changes

Moderate AD

- Increased confusion and memory loss

- Problems recognizing friends and family members
- Unable to learn new things
- Difficulties with tasks having multiple steps such as getting dressed
- Difficulties coping with new situations
- Delusions, hallucinations, and paranoia
- Impulsive behavior

Severe AD
- Relies on others for routine care
- Cannot communicate
- Sudden weight loss
- Seizures
- Skin problems and infections
- Difficulty swallowing
- Moaning, groaning, or grunting
- Increased sleeping than usual
- Lack of bladder and bowel control

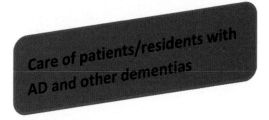

Care of patients/residents with AD and other dementias

Environment

- The nurse assistant should follow set routines.
- They should avoid changing rooms or roommates.
- Picture signs should be placed by room doors, dining rooms, bathrooms, and other areas.
- Personal items should be kept where the patient/resident can see and reach them.
- The nurse assistant should stay within the patient/resident's sight to the extent possible.
- Memory aids (large clocks and calendars) should be placed where the patient/resident can see them.
- Noise levels should be kept low.

- The nurse assistant should play music and show movies from the patient/resident's past.
- The nurse assistant should select tasks and activities that fit the patient/resident's abilities and interests.

Safety

- The nurse assistant should reassure the patient/resident that he/she is always there to help the patient/resident.
- The nurse assistant should remove sharp, harmful, and breakable objects from the area. This may include scissors, knives, dishes, glass, razors, and tools.
- The patient/resident should be provided plastic eating and drinking utensils. They help prevent cuts and breakage.
- Safety plugs should be placed in electrical outlets. Electric outlets should be covered with safety plates.
- Cords and electrical items should be kept out of patient/resident's reach.
- Electric appliances should be removed from the bathroom. Hair dryers, make-up mirrors, curling irons, and electric shavers are examples.
- The patient/resident should be provided safe storage for:
  - Personal care items (lotion, shampoo, deodorant etc.)
  - Household cleaners and drugs
  - Dangerous equipment and tools
  - Cigars, cigarettes, matches, pipes, and other smoking materials
  - Car keys
- The nurse assistant should keep childproof caps on drug containers and household cleaners.

- Knobs from stoves should be removed or safety covers should be placed on the knobs.
- The nurse assistant should remove dangerous appliances, power tools, and firearms from the home.
- The nurse assistant should supervise the patient/resident who smokes.
- Safety measures should be practiced to prevent falls, fires, burns, and poisoning
- The nurse assistant should lock doors to kitchens, utility rooms, and housekeeping closets.

Wandering

- The nurse assistant should always follow agency policy for locking doors and windows. Locks are usually at the top and bottom of doors. The patient/resident is not likely to look for a lock in such places.
- The nurse assistant should keep door alarms and electronic doors turned on and should respond to alarms at once.
- The nurse assistant should always follow agency policy for fire exits. Everybody must be able to leave the building in case of a fire.
- The nurse assistant should make sure the patient/resident wears an ID bracelet at all times.
- The nurse assistant should know the times of day the patient/resident is more likely to wander.
- The nurse assistant should follow the patient/resident's care plan for daily routine, exercise, and other routine activities. The nurse assistant should make sure food, fluid, and elimination needs are met properly.
- The patient/resident should be involved in activities such as folding napkins, dusting a table, rolling yarn, sweeping, sorting socks, sanding blocks of wood or watering plants.
- The nurse assistant should not use restraints. Restraints require a physician's order. They also tend to increase disorientation and confusion.
- The nurse assistant should not argue with the patient/resident who wants to leave. The patient/resident does not understand what the nurse assistant is saying.
- The nurse assistant should go with the patient/resident who insists on going outside. The nurse assistant should make sure he/she is properly dressed. The patient/resident should be guided inside after a few minutes.
- The nurse assistant should let the patient/resident wander in enclosed areas. The agency may have enclosed areas for walking such patients/resident.

Sundowning

- Treatments and activities should be completed early in the day.
- Patients/residents should be encouraged to exercise and activity early in the day.
- The patient/resident should be kept on a schedule. Meal times, waking up, and bedtime should involve a set routine.
- The patient/resident should be avoided to take caffeine (coffee, cola, tea, and chocolate), alcohol, and sweets late in the day. The nurse assistant should provide a calm, quiet setting late in the day.
- The nurse assistant should not restrain the patient/resident.

- Nutrition and elimination needs should be met properly. Unmet needs may increase restlessness.
- Night-lights should be used at night.
- The nurse assistant should not try to reason with the patient/resident.

Hallucinations and delusions

- The nurse assistant should make sure that the patient/resident is wearing eyeglasses and hearing aids as needed.
- The nurse assistant should not argue with the patient/resident.
- The nurse assistant should reassure the patient/resident that he/she is always there to help the patient/resident.
- The patient/resident should be distracted with some item or activity. Taking the patient/resident for a walk may be helpful.
- The nurse assistant should turn off TV or movies when disturbing and violent programs are on. The patient/resident may believe the story is real.
- The nurse assistant should provide comfort to the patient/resident if he/she seems afraid. The nurse assistant should use touch to calm and should reassure the patient/resident.
- The nurse assistant should eliminate noises that the patient/resident could misinterpret. Radio, TV, music, air conditioners, furnaces, and other things could affect the patient/resident.
- Lighting should be checked and the nurse assistant should make sure that there are no shadows, glares, or reflections.
- Mirrors should be covered or removed. The patient/resident may misinterpret his/her reflection.
- The nurse assistant should make sure the patient/resident cannot reach anything that could be used to hurt the self or others.
- The nurse assistant should report behavior changes of the patient/resident to the licensed nurse as they may signal a physical illness.

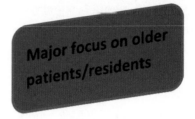

Major focus on older patients/residents

Many nursing centers have secured units for residents with Alzheimer's disease and other dementias. This means that their exits and entrances are locked. Patients/residents in these units cannot wander away. They have a very safe and secure setting to move about. Some patients/residents have aggressive behaviors that disrupt or threaten others. They need a safe and secured unit. According to the Omnibus Budget Reconciliation Act of 1987 (OBRA), safe and secured units are physical restraints. A dementia diagnosis and a physician's order are required for placement on a secured unit. At least every 90 days, the health team reviews the patient/resident's need for a safe and secured unit. The patient/resident's rights are always protected. At some point, the safe and secured unit is no longer required for safe care. For example, a patient/resident's condition progresses towards severe AD.

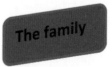

The family

The patient/resident experiencing AD may live at home or with a partner, children, or other family members. Home health care may help for these patients for a while.

Adult day care can be an option. Nursing center care is required when:

- Family members cannot meet the patient/resident's needs.
- The patient/resident no longer knows the caregiver.
- Family members experiencing health problems.
- Financial problems.
- The patient/resident's behavior presents dangers to self and others.

Diagnostic tests, physician's visits, medications, home care, assisted living, and nursing care center are costly. The patient/resident's medical care can drain family finances. Nursing center care and home care are stressful. The family has emotional, social, physical, and financial stresses. Adult children are generally in the sandwich generation. Their own children require attention while an ill parent requires care. Caring for two families is usually stressful for them. Often adult children have their jobs too. Thus, caregivers can suffer from anxiety, anger, depression, guilt, and sleeplessness. Health issues can develop. They also need to focus on their own health. They require a healthy diet, rest, and exercise. Asking friends and family members for help is important. However, asking for help is difficult for some people. Caregivers need support and encouragement. AD support groups are sponsored by nursing centers, hospitals, and the Alzheimer's Association. The Alzheimer's Association has its chapters throughout the country. Support groups offer support, encouragement, and advice. Members share their feelings, guilt, anger, frustration, and other emotions. They also share caregiving and coping ideas. Much time, energy, money, and emotion are

required to care for the patient/resident. Resentment and anger may result. Guilt feelings are very common. The family knows that the patient/resident did not choose the disorder and its signs, symptoms, and behaviors. Sometimes behaviors are much embarrassing. The family may be angry and upset that the loved one cannot show affection or love. The family is an important component of the health team. They help plan care when possible. The nurse assistant and support group may help the family in learning how to give needed care. For home care, they learn how to feed, bathe, dress, and provide oral hygiene to the patient/resident. They also learn how to provide a safe and secure setting. In nursing centers, some family members may take part in unit activities. For many patients/residents, family members may provide comfort. They also require support and understanding from the health team.

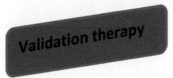

Validation therapy

The patient/resident's care plan may include validation therapy. The therapy is usually based on these principles:

- All types of behavior have some meanings.
- Development occurs in an order, sequence, and pattern. Various tasks must be completed during a stage of development. Any stage of development cannot be skipped. Each developmental stage is the basis of the next stage.
- If an individual does not successfully complete a stage of development, unmet needs and emotions may surface later in life.

- An individual may return to the past to meet such needs and emotions.
- Caregivers require listening and providing empathy.
- Attempts should not be made to correct thoughts or to bring the patient/resident back to reality.

The health team takes decision if validation therapy will be part of the patient/resident's care plan. If validation therapy is used in an agency, the nurse assistant will receive the training needed to use it correctly.

Nurse assistants' statistics show that at least half of the residents who live in nursing homes have dementias. Sometimes these residents may live on a special unit for dementia care, and other times they usually live among the general facility population. In either case, the nurse assistant who works in those facilities faces caring for multiple residents with dementias at the same time.

Patients/residents with dementia require constant supervision and frequent redirection. Meeting their basic physical care needs is often difficult because of their challenging behaviors. In addition, the nurse assistant often feels burden due to workload and feeling as if there is never sufficient support to get the job done.

Many nurse assistants are not just caregivers at work but they are also caregivers for children or other family members when off duty. Like family caregivers, nurse assistants may fall victim to the physical and emotional toll of care.

Nurse assistants should know his/her limits. They should stay alert and should recognize when to ask for help so that they do not find themselves in a situation where they are overwhelmed. Also, they should be alert for possible signs of stress in their co-workers. They can help relieve some of that stress by stepping in to assist. It is also significant for them to find ways for coping their own stress. Activities such as listening to music, exercising, getting together with friends, or engaging themselves in hobbies can help them to relieve their stress. Activities should not be expensive or time consuming. It is always possible to find something enjoyable that fits their lifestyle. The main thing is to find what works and to commit to it so they can function at their best whether they are caring for residents at work or caring for their family at home.

Parkinson's disease

It is a slow, progressive disorder with no treatment. People over the age of 50 are at more risk. It is one of the most common neural disorders affecting older adults. In Parkinson's disease, a chemical in the brain called dopamine is not produced in sufficient amounts. Dopamine is required for normal functioning of the nerves that control movement. As a result, there is disruption of communication between the brain and the nerves that control muscle movement.

A patient/resident with Parkinson's disease has shaking or repetitive motions of the muscles (muscle tremors), especially in the hands. The tremors are worse when the patient/resident is resting and reduce when the patient/resident attempts movement. As the disease gets worse over time, muscles become stiff and weak. The patient/resident may shuffle and lean forward during walking, and it can be very difficult for the patient/resident to stop suddenly once he/she is walking. These factors put the patient/resident at risk for falling. As the muscles of the face are affected, the patient/resident may have trouble swallowing and chewing, and he/she may drool. Speech may also be affected; the patient/resident may speak in a low tone without much variation. The patient/resident may lose the ability to frown, smile, or show other facial expressions.

The signs and symptoms become worse with the passage of time. They may include:

- **Tremors:** The patient/resident may have trembling in the arms, hands, jaw, legs, and face.
- **Rigid, stiff muscles:** The patient/resident may have rigid and stiff muscles in the neck, arms, legs, and trunk.
- **Slow movements:** The patient/resident has a slow, shuffling gait.
- **Stooped posture and impaired balance:** It is difficult to walk for the patient/resident. Falls are a risk for these patients/residents.
- **Mask-like expression:** The patient/resident cannot blink and smile. A fixed stare is common sign.

Other common signs and symptoms may include:

- Swallowing and chewing problems
- Constipation and bladder problems
- Sleep problems
- Depression and emotional changes (fear, insecurity)
- Memory loss and slow thinking
- Slurred, monotone, and soft speech

When a nurse assistant provides care for a patient/resident who has Parkinson's disease, he/she should focus on promoting independence, safety, good nutrition, and mobility of the patient/resident. Care strategies for a patient/resident with Parkinson's disease may include the following:

- The nurse assistant should avoid rushing the patient/resident as muscle tremors usually increase when the patient/resident becomes anxious.
- The patient/resident should be encouraged to use assistive devices as needed.
- The patient/resident should be encouraged to exercise within his/her capabilities and according to his/her care plan. Exercise and activity can help prevent worsening of balance and stiffness problems.
- When the patient/resident is walking, the nurse assistant should remind him/her to take big steps. A patient/resident with Parkinson's disease has to make a conscious effort to do what comes naturally to individuals who can control their movements.
- The nurse assistant should use a high toilet or elevated toilet seat set on top of a regular toilet seat to make it easier for him/her to sit down on, and get up from, the toilet.
- Many patients/residents with Parkinson's disease work with a speech therapist to learn safe techniques for swallowing, speaking, and eating. The nurse assistant should remind the patient/resident to use these techniques and should check to ensure that he/she uses them properly.
- The nurse assistant should offer small and frequent meals and snacks to

patients/residents. Patients/residents with Parkinson's disease usually lose weight because they tire before finishing a meal. They may also feel embarrassment by spilling food or by how slowly they eat.

- The nurse assistant should be aware that Parkinson's disease can affect the muscles used for speech, which makes it hard for the patient/resident to express himself/herself. The patient/resident should be provided proper time to respond to a question or request. When appropriate, the nurse assistant should prefer asking questions that can be answered with a simple "no" or "yes" that may make it easier for the patient/resident to express himself/herself.
- Patients/residents should be provided proper emotional support.

Seizures

Seizures or convulsions are sudden and violent tremors of muscle groups due to an abnormal electrical activity in the brain. Seizures may lead to involuntary changes in body movement, sensation, function, awareness, or behavior. Seizures can have multiple different causes. Some patients may have epilepsy, which is a chronic seizure condition that can be controlled with medication. Other causes of seizures may include head injury during birth or from trauma, high-grade fever, brain tumors, poisoning, nervous system disorders or infection, and injuries to the brain tissue. Lack of blood supply to the brain tissue may also cause seizures.

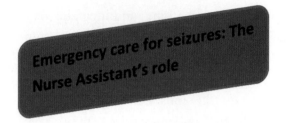

Emergency care for seizures: The Nurse Assistant's role

The main goal for a nurse assistant is to protect the patient/resident from injury during the seizure. Nearby furniture or other objects that the patient/resident may accidentally hit during the seizure should be removed. The nurse assistant should not try to hold or restrain the patient/resident, or put anything in the patient/resident's mouth or between the teeth to prevent the patient/resident from biting his/her tongue. After the seizure is over, the patient/resident should be placed on one side to prevent him/her from choking on secretions that may have pooled in the mouth. The patient/resident may be disoriented and drowsy or unresponsive for a short period of time. He/she may be very tired and want to rest. The nurse assistant should stay with the patient/resident until he/she is fully recovered from the seizure and completely aware of his/her surroundings.

Nobody can stop a seizure. However, the nurse assistant may protect the patient/resident from injury by following these guidelines:

- The nurse assistant should remain calm, and call for help as early as possible.
- He/she should not leave the patient/resident alone.
- The patient/resident should be lowered to the floor to protect him/her from falling.
- The time should be noted when the seizure started.

428

- Something soft should be placed under the patient/resident's head to prevent the patient/resident's head from striking the floor. The nurse assistant can use a cushion, pillow, or a folded blanket, jacket, or towel.
- The nurse assistant should loose tight clothing, such as a collar, tie, or scarf of the patient/resident.
- The patient/resident should be turned onto his or her side. It should be ensured that the head is turned to the side.
- It should not be tried to stop the seizure or control the patient/resident's movements.
- The time should be noted when the seizure ends.
- It should be ensured that the mouth of the patient/resident is clear of food, fluids, and saliva after the seizure.
- The nurse assistant should provide BLS if there is no breathing or no normal breathing after the seizure.

The sense organs

The five major senses are hearing, sight, smell, taste, and touch.

1. Receptors for taste

They are situated in the tongue and are called taste buds.

2. Receptors for smell

Receptors for smell are located in the nose.

3. Touch receptors

Touch receptors are situated in the dermis, especially in the fingertips and toes.

4. The eye

Receptors for vision are located in the eyes. The eye can easily be injured. Bones of the skull, eyelashes and eyelids, and tears protect the eyes from injury.

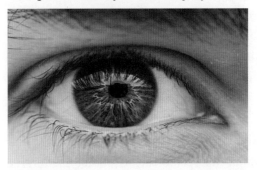

The eye has three major layers:

a) The sclera, the white portion of the eye, is the outer layer. It consists of tough connective tissue.

b) The choroid is the second layer of the eye. The ciliary muscle, blood vessels, and the iris make up the choroid. The iris provides the eye its color. The opening in the center of the iris is the pupil. Pupil size changes with the amount of light entering the eye. The pupil narrows (constricts) in bright light. It widens (dilates) in dim or dark places.

c) The retina is the inner layer of the eye. The retina has receptors for vision and the nerve fibers of the optic nerve.

Light passes into the eye through the cornea, which is the transparent portion of the outer layer that lies over the eye. Light rays pass to the lens, which is located behind the pupil. The light is then reflected to the retina and carried to the brain by the optic nerve. The aqueous chamber separates the lens from the cornea. The aqueous chamber is filled with a fluid called aqueous humor. The aqueous humor helps the cornea keep its position and shape. The vitreous humor is located behind the lens. It is a gelatin-like substance that maintains the eye's shape and supports the retina.

Eye disorders

Vision loss may occur at all ages. Vision loss may range from mild loss to complete blindness. Blindness is the absence of vision that can be sudden or gradual. One or both eyes are affected. The following can be common eye problems.

Cataract: It is a clouding of the lens. The normal lens is clear. Cataract is derived from the Greek word means waterfall. Attempting to see is just like looking through a waterfall. A cataract may occur in one or both eyes. Surgery is the only option to cure the cataract. Signs and symptoms may include:

- Blurry, cloudy, or dimmed vision
- Colors seem faded. Purples and blues are hard to see.
- Glares and sensitivity to light.
- Poor vision at night and halos around lights.
- Double vision in the affected eye.
- Age-related macular degeneration (AMD) that blurs central vision.
- Diabetic retinopathy, which is a complication of diabetes.

Glaucoma: It results when fluid builds up in the affected eye and causes extra pressure on the optic nerve. Accumulated fluid damages the optic nerve is, which leads to vision loss and eventually blindness. Glaucoma can be developed in one or both eyes. Peripheral vision is lost. The patient/resident sees through a tunnel and sees halos around lights. Medications and surgery can control glaucoma and may prevent further damage; however, prior damage cannot be reversed.

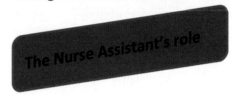

The Nurse Assistant's role

- The nurse assistant should announce himself/herself by name while entering the room.
- The patient/resident should be encouraged for television or radio listening.
- The nurse assistant should be extra careful in explaining what he/she is doing.
- The nurse assistant should describe the food he/she is going to feed them; is it cold or hot? The nurse assistant should also describe food placement like the hands of a clock.
- The nurse assistant should not disrupt environment. He/she should keep ADL supplies in same place and should not move furniture unless necessary.

5. The ear

The ear is a sense organ for hearing and balance. It has three main parts: the external ear, middle ear, and inner ear. The outer part (external ear) is called the auricle or pinna. Sound waves are guided through the auricle into the auditory canal. Glands in the auditory canal release a thick and waxy substance called cerumen. The auditory canal extends almost one inch into the tympanic membrane (eardrum).

The tympanic membrane separates the external and middle ear. The middle ear is a tiny space. It contains the eustachian tube and three tiny bones called ossicles. The eustachian tube joins the middle ear and the throat. Air enters the eustachian tube to equalize pressure on both sides of the eardrum. The ossicles amplify sound waves received from the eardrum and transmit these sound waves to the inner ear. The three ossicles are:

The malleus
Malleus looks like a hammer.

The incus
Incus seems like an anvil.

The stapes
It looks like a stirrup.

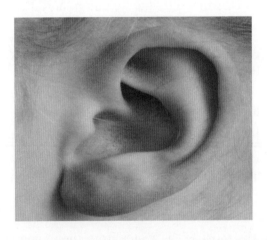

The inner ear contains semicircular canals and the cochlea. The cochlea seems like a snail shell. It contains fluid that carries sound waves from the middle ear to the acoustic nerve. The acoustic nerve then carries these sound waves to the brain. The three semicircular canals are involved with balance. The semicircular canals sense the head's position and changes in position. They transmit messages to the brain, in order to maintain the balance.

Otosclerosis

Otosclerosis is a term derived from Oto meaning "of the ear" and sclerosis meaning "abnormal hardening of body tissue." The problem is caused by abnormal bone remodeling in the middle ear. Otosclerosis is the abnormal growth of stapes in the MIDDLE ear. This bone prevents structures within the ear from functioning properly and causes hearing loss. For some patients/residents with otosclerosis, the hearing loss may become more severe.

Otosclerosis usually develops gradually. Otosclerosis is one of the most common causes of conductive deafness.

Signs and symptoms
One of the initial symptoms of otosclerosis is tinnitus (ringing in the ears) that is accentuated in quiet surroundings. It may occur for some time before the patient/resident notices a hearing loss. The patient/resident may not notice that he/she is gradually losing the ability to hear, until ordinary conversation and communication becomes difficult to hear—especially when people speak in low voices or there is background noise. Use of hearing aid or surgery may help the patient/resident with this condition.

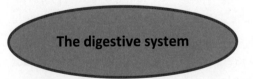

The digestive system

The process of breakdown of complex food particles physically and chemically into simple ones that can be absorbed by the cells. The digestive system is also called the GI (gastro-intestinal) system. The GI system

431

also removes solid wastes from the body. It involves the GI tract (alimentary canal) and the accessory organs of digestion.

The alimentary canal (GI tract) is a long tube, which extends from the mouth to the anus. The major parts of the alimentary canal are the mouth, pharynx, esophagus, stomach, small intestine, and large intestine. Accessory organs are the tongue, teeth, salivary glands, gallbladder, liver, and pancreas. Digestion starts in the oral cavity (mouth), which receives food and prepares it for digestion. Using chewing motions, the teeth cut, grind, and chop food into small particles for swallowing and digestion. The tongue helps in chewing and swallowing. Taste buds on the tongue's surface have nerve endings to allow sweet, bitter, sour, and salty tastes to be sensed. Salivary glands in the mouth release saliva, which moistens food particles to ease swallowing and begin digestion. During swallowing, the tongue forces and pushes food into the pharynx.

The pharynx is a muscular tube. The process of swallowing continues as the pharynx contracts. Contraction of the pharynx forces and pushes food into the esophagus. The esophagus is a long muscular tube that is about 10 inches long. The esophagus extends from the pharynx to the stomach. Involuntary muscle contractions push food down the esophagus through the GI tract (peristalsis). The stomach is a pouch-like, muscular bag. It is situated in the upper left area of the abdominal cavity. Strong gastric muscles churn and stir food to break it up into even smaller particles. The stomach is lined by a mucous membrane. It contains gastric glands that secrete gastric juices.

Food is mixed and churned with these gastric juices to produce a semi-liquid substance called chyme. Through peristalsis, the chyme is forced and pushed from the stomach into the small intestine. The small intestine is almost 20 feet long and has 3 parts. The first part is called the duodenum. In duodenum, more digestive juices are added to the chyme to form bile. Bile is a greenish liquid produced in the liver and stored in the gallbladder. Juices from the small intestine and pancreas are added to the chyme. Digestive juices break down food chemically so it can be properly absorbed. Peristalsis moves the chyme through the other two parts of the small intestine i.e. the jejunum and the ileum.

There are multiple tiny projections called villi line the small intestine, which absorb the digested food into the capillaries. Most food absorption occurs in the jejunum and the ileum. Some chyme remains undigested. Undigested chyme moves from the small intestine into the large intestine or colon. The large intestine absorbs most of the water from the chyme and remaining semi-solid material is known as feces. Feces contain a very small quantity of water, solid waste products, and some mucus and germs. These remaining semi-solid materials are the waste products of digestion. Through the peristalsis, feces pass through the colon into the rectum and pass out of the body through the anus.

The digestive system rids the body of solid waste products. The lungs remove carbon dioxide from the body. Water and other waste substances leave the body through sweat.

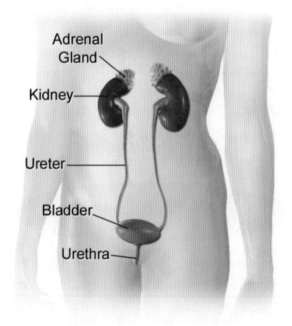

Adrenal Gland
Kidney
Ureter
Bladder
Urethra

The urinary system:

- Removes waste substances from the blood.
- Maintains water balance and homeostasis within the body.
- Maintains electrolyte balance.
- Sodium is required for fluid balance. The body retains water if sodium levels are too high. Loss of sodium (through diarrhea, vomiting, and some medications) can result in dehydration.
- Calcium and potassium are required for the proper function of cardiac and skeletal muscles.
- Maintains acid-base balance.

The kidneys are a pair of bean-shaped organs in the upper abdominal cavity. They are situated against the back muscles on each side of the spine. The kidneys are protected by the lower edge of the rib cage. Each kidney contains over a million tiny nephrons. A nephron is the basic functional unit of the kidney. Each nephron consists of a convoluted tubule, which is a tiny coiled tubule. Each convoluted tubule contains a Bowman's capsule at one end. The capsule is partly surrounded by a cluster of capillaries called a glomerulus. Blood moves through the glomerulus and is filtered by the capillaries. The watery portion of the blood is squeezed into the Bowman's capsule and then passes into the tubule.

Most of the water and other required substances are re-absorbed by the blood. The rest of the remaining fluid and the waste materials form urine in the tubule. Urine passes through the tubule to a collecting tubule. All collecting tubules are drained into the renal pelvis in the kidney. A long tube called the ureter is attached to the renal pelvis. Each ureter is almost 10 to 12 inches long and carry urine from the kidneys to the urinary bladder. The urinary bladder is a muscular, hollow bag, which is located toward the front in the lower portion of the abdominal cavity.

Urine is stored in the urinary bladder until the need to urinate is sensed. This usually occurs when there is about a 250 mL (half pint) of urine in the bladder. Urine passes from the urinary bladder through the urethra. The opening at the ending part of the urethra is called the meatus. Urine is a clear, yellowish fluid that passes from the body through the meatus.

Diseases and disorders

Urinary tract infection (UTI)

UTIs are the most common infections. Microorganisms can enter the urinary system through the urethra. Catheterization, sexual intercourse, urological exams, immobility, poor perineal hygiene, and poor fluid intake are common causes. UTI is a common healthcare-associated infection.

Cystitis

It is a bladder infection caused by bacteria. Urinary frequency, difficult or painful urination, urgency, blood or pus in the urine, foul-smelling urine, and fever may occur. Antibiotics are ordered to treat infection. Fluid intake is encouraged. If untreated, cystitis may lead to pyelonephritis and other serious complications.

Pyelonephritis

It is inflammation of the kidney pelvis. Cloudy urine may contain mucus, pus, and blood. Fever, chills, back pain, and nausea or vomiting may occur. Signs and symptoms are same as of cystitis. Treatment involves administration of antibiotics and fluid intake.

Urinary incontinence

It is the loss of control of urine. Signs and symptoms may include:

- Unable to control urination
- Stress incontinence: urination when exerting little pressure (Coughing, sneezing, standing up)

The Nurse Assistant's role

It may include:

- Proper bowel and bladder training
- The call light should be answered promptly
- The nurse assistant should be positive when changing soiled linen or garments
- Proper perineal care should be provided
- Liquids should be avoided after dinner

The Reproductive System

Human reproduction results from the union of a female sex cell and a male sex cell. The female and male reproductive systems are different to allow the process of reproduction.

The male reproductive system

The testicles (testes) are the male sex glands. Sex glands are also called gonads. The two testes are oval or almond-shaped sex glands. Male sex cells are called sperm cells that are produced in the testes. The male sex hormone, Testosterone, is produced in the testes. Testosterone is required for reproductive organ function. It is also required for the development of the male secondary sex characteristics such as facial hair, axillary and pubic hair, and hair on the chest, arms, and legs. Shoulder and neck sizes increase. The testes are embedded in a sac called the scrotum. The scrotum is made of muscle and skin. Sperms move from the testis to the epididymis (epididymis is a coiled tube on the sides and top of the testis). From the epididymis, sperms move through another tube called the vas deferens. Each vas deferens joins a seminal vesicle. There are two seminal vesicles that store sperm and produce semen. Semen is a fluid that brings sperm from the male reproductive tract. The ducts of the seminal vesicles combine to form the ejaculatory duct. The ejaculatory duct passes through the prostate gland. The prostate gland is situated just below the urinary bladder and shaped like a donut. The prostate gland secretes fluid into the semen. As the ejaculatory ducts leave the prostate, they meet the urethra. The urethra travels through the prostate gland. The urethra is the outlet for semen and urine. The urethra is contained within the penis, which is outside of the body. The glans is located at the end of the penis. The urethra opens at the end of the glans penis. A fold of skin called prepuce or foreskin is situated at the end of the penis. The penis contains erectile tissue. When a male is sexually stimulated, blood fills the erectile tissue. The penis enlarges and becomes erect and hard. The hard and erect penis can enter a female's vagina. There are two pea-sized Cowper's glands under the prostate. They produce a colorless and clear fluid before ejaculation (release of semen). This clear fluid cleanses the urethra, protects sperm from destruction and damage, and provides lubrication for sexual intercourse. With ejaculation, semen containing sperms is released into the vagina.

Prostate enlargement

The prostate is a male gland. It is located in front of the rectum and just below the bladder. The prostate surrounds the urethra and it is about the size of a walnut. The prostate enlarges as the male grows older. This is called benign prostatic hyperplasia (BPH). Benign is a term means non-malignant, hyper means excessive, and plasia means formation or development. BPH is also called benign prostatic hypertrophy. After age of 60 years, older adults mostly experience some symptoms of BPH. The enlarged prostate presses against the urethra to cause obstruction of urine flow. Bladder function is lost gradually. These problems are common:

- A weak urinary stream
- Frequent voidings of small amounts of urine
- Urgency and dribbling or leaking of urine
- Frequent voiding at night
- Urinary retention.

The doctor may order medications to shrink the prostate or inhibit its growth. Some laser and microwave treatments destroy the enlarged prostate tissue. Surgery may also be an option to remove enlarged tissue.

The female reproductive system

The female sex glands are two almond-shaped glands called ovaries. An ovary is located on each side of the uterus in the abdominal cavity. The ovaries contain eggs or ova. Eggs or ova are the female sex cells. One egg (ovum) is released monthly during the female's reproductive years. Release of an ovum from the ovary is called ovulation. The ovaries release the female hormones estrogen and progesterone. Estrogen and progesterone are required for reproductive system function. They are also required for the development of secondary sex characteristics in the female such as increased breast size, axillary and pubic hair, slight deepening of the voice, and rounding and widening of the hips.

When an ovum is released from an ovary, it moves through a fallopian tube. There are two fallopian tubes, one on each side. The fallopian tubes are attached at one end to the uterus. The ovum moves through the fallopian tube to the uterus. The uterus is a muscular, hollow organ shaped like a pear. It is located in the center of the pelvic cavity just behind the urinary bladder and in front of the rectum. The major part of the uterus is the fundus. The narrow section or neck of the uterus is the cervix.

Endometrium is the tissue that lines the uterus. The endometrium has multiple small blood vessels. If sex cells from the female and male unite into one cell, that cell implants into the endometrium. There the cell grows into an unborn baby (fetus) and receives proper nourishment. The cervix of the uterus is projected into a muscular canal called the vagina, which opens to the outside of the body. It is located just behind the urethra. The vagina receives the male penis during sexual intercourse. It is also a part of the birth canal. Glands within the vaginal wall keep it wet and moistened with secretions. The Bartholin's glands are examples of such glands. In younger females, the external opening of the vagina is partially closed by

a membrane called the hymen. The hymen is ruptured when the female has intercourse for the first time.

The external genitalia of females are called the vulva. The mons pubis is a rounded-shaped fatty pad over a bone called the symphysis pubis. It is covered with hair in the adult female. The labia minora and labia majora are two folds of tissue on each side of the vaginal opening. The clitoris is a tiny organ composed of erectile tissue. It becomes hard when stimulated during sexual intercourse. The breasts (mammary glands) secrete milk after childbirth. The mammary glands are on the outside of the chest. They are made up of fat and glandular tissue. The milk is drained into ducts that open onto the nipple.

Menstruation

The endometrium is rich in blood for nourishment of the cell that grows into a fetus. If pregnancy does not occur, the menstruation process begins. Menstruation is the process in which the uterine lining (endometrium) breaks up and is discharged from the body through the vagina. Menstruation occurs about every 28 days. Therefore it is known as menstrual cycle. The first day of the menstrual cycle starts with menstruation. Blood flows from the uterus through the vagina. Menstruation generally lasts 3 to 7 days. The next phase is the ovulation phase that occurs on or about day 14 of the cycle. An egg or ovum matures in an ovary and is released during ovulation phase. Meanwhile, the female hormones (estrogen and progesterone) are secreted by the ovaries. These hormones thicken the endometrium for pregnancy. If pregnancy does not occur, the female hormones decrease in amount. This causes the reduction of the blood supply to the endometrium. The endometrium breaks up and it is discharged through the vaginal opening. Another menstrual cycle begins in the same way.

Fertilization

For reproduction, a female sex cell (ovum) must unite with a male sex cell (sperm). The uniting of the ovum and sperm into one cell is called fertilization. Both the sperm and ovum have 23 chromosomes each. When the two cells unite, the fertilized cell (zygote) has 46 chromosomes. During sexual intercourse, millions of sperm are deposited through the vaginal opening into the vagina. Sperm move up the cervix, through the uterus, and into the fallopian tubes. If an ovum and a sperm unite in a fallopian tube, fertilization occurs. The fertilized cell moves down the fallopian tube to the uterus. After a short period of time, the fertilized cell is implanted into the thick endometrium and grows during pregnancy.

Cystocele

It is the weakening of muscles between vagina and bladder. Signs and symptoms of cystocele may include: Urinary incontinence, urinary urgency, dribbling of urine, and frequent urinary tract infections 2) Rectocele: Weakening of muscles between wall of rectum and vagina is called as rectocele. Signs and symptoms of rectocele may include hemorrhoids, constipation, and prolapsed uterus.

Sexually transmitted diseases (STDs)

A sexually transmitted disease (STD) is spread by vaginal, oral, or anal sex. Some patients do not have signs and symptoms or are unaware of an infection. Others know about the condition but do not seek treatment because of embarrassment. STDs often occur in the rectal and genital areas. They may also occur in the mouth, ears, throat, nipples, eyes, tongue, and nose. Use of condom helps to prevent the spread of STDs, especially the HIV (human immunodeficiency virus) and AIDS (acquired immunodeficiency syndrome). Some STDs can also be spread through skin breaks, by direct contact with infected body fluids (semen, saliva, blood), or by contaminated needles or blood. Standard Precautions and the Bloodborne Pathogen Standard should always be followed while handling these patients/residents.

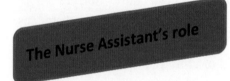

The Nurse Assistant's role

- The nurse assistant should be aware that virus can be killed by 10:1 water to bleach solution.
- Secondary infections should be prevented through proper measures.
- The nurse assistant should report new symptoms and complaints of discomfort immediately to licensed nurse and should provide comfort measures to the patient/resident.

The Immune System

The immune system provides protection to the body from disease and infection. Abnormal body cells may grow into tumorous cells. Sometimes the body produces such substances that can cause the body to attack itself. Microbes

437

(viruses, bacteria, and other germs) can cause an infection. The immune system provides defense against threats inside and outside the body. The immune system provides the body immunity. Immunity means that an individual has protection against a disorder or condition. The individual will not get or be affected by the disorder.

- Specific immunity is the reaction of the body to a certain threat.
- Non-specific immunity is the reaction of the body to anything it does not recognize as a normal body material.

There are some special substances and cells to develop immunity, which may include:

Antibodies: These are normal body substances that recognize other substances. Antibodies are involved in destroying unwanted or abnormal substances.

Antigens: Antigens are the substances that cause an immune response. Antibodies recognize and bind with antigens to destroy unwanted substances and to produce more antibodies.

Phagocytes: Phagocytes are the WBCs (white blood cells) that digest and destroy microbes and other unwanted substances.

Lymphocytes: They are the WBCs that produce antibodies. Lymphocyte production increases as the body responds against an infection.

B lymphocytes (B cells): B lymphocytes cause the production of antibodies that circulate in the plasma. These antibodies may react to specific antigens to provide immunity.

T lymphocytes (T cells): T lymphocytes destroy invading cells. Killer T cells secrete poisons near the invading cells. Some T lymphocytes may attract other cells. The other cells destroy the invaders.

When the body feels an antigen from an unwanted substance, the immune system starts acting against the unwanted antigens. Lymphocyte and phagocyte production increases. Phagocytes destroy the invaders through phagocytosis. The lymphocytes produce specific antibodies that recognize and destroy the unwanted substances.

Acquired Immunodeficiency Syndrome (AIDS)

AIDS is caused by the human immunodeficiency virus (HIV) in which the virus attacks the immune system and destroys the body's ability to fight against infections and certain cancers. HIV is spread through body fluids such as semen, blood, vaginal secretions, and breast milk. HIV is not spread by tears, sweat, saliva, coughing, sneezing, insects, or casual contact. AIDS can be spread mainly by:

- Unprotected vaginal, anal, or oral sex with an infected person. "Unprotected" mean without a new latex or polyurethane condom.
- Syringe and needle sharing among IV drug users.
- HIV-infected mothers. New born babies can become infected during pregnancy, through breast-feeding, and shortly after birth.

Signs and symptoms of AIDS
- Loss of appetite
- Cough

- Depression
- Diarrhea
- Lack of energy
- Fatigue
- Fever
- Headache
- Memory loss, confusion, and forgetfulness
- Brown, pink, red, or purple spots or blotches on the tongue
- Night sweats
- Pneumonia
- Shortness of breath
- Rashes or flaky skin
- Red, brown, pink, or purple spots or blotches on the skin, nose, or eyelids
- Painful or difficult swallowing
- Swollen glands of neck, underarms, and groin
- Vision loss
- Weight loss

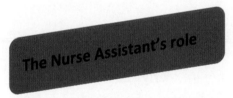

Some HIV-infected individuals have symptoms within a few months. Others may be symptom-free for more than 10 years. However, they carry the HIV and spread it to others. Individuals with AIDS are at risk for TB, pneumonia, Kaposi's sarcoma, and nervous system damage. Loss of coordination, paralysis, memory loss, mental health problems, and dementia signal nervous system damage. Many new medications help to slow the spread of HIV in the body. They also minimize severe complications and prolong life. AIDS has no cure and no vaccine at present. It is a life-threatening condition. The nurse assistant may care for patients/residents with AIDS or for patients/residents who are HIV carriers. The nurse assistant may have contact with the patient/resident's blood or body fluids. He/she should protect himself/herself and others and should follow Standard Precautions and the Bloodborne Pathogen Standard. A patient/resident may have the HIV virus but no symptoms. In some patients/residents, HIV or AIDS is not yet diagnosed.

Other nursing considerations may include:
- The patient/resident should be provided daily hygiene.
- Proper oral hygiene should be provided before meals and at bedtime. It should be ensured that the patient/resident uses a toothbrush with soft bristles.
- Oral fluids should be provided as ordered by licensed nurse.
- The nurse assistant should measure and record intake and output.
- The patient/resident should perform deep breathing exercises as ordered.
- The nurse assistant should practice proper measures to prevent pressure sores.
- The patient/resident should be assisted with range-of-motion exercises and ambulation as ordered.
- The patient/resident should be encouraged to perform self-care as much as possible.
- The patient/resident should be encouraged to be as active as possible.
- The nurse assistant should change linens, gowns, or pajamas as often as needed.
- The nurse assistant should be a good listener and should provide emotional support to the patient/resident.

Helpful Resources

Agasti, T. (2011). Anatomy and physiology of respiratory system. *Textbook of Anaesthesia for Postgraduates*, 17-17. https://doi.org/10.5005/jp/books/11339_2

Barnes, P. (2006). Chronic obstructive pulmonary disease | Overview. *Encyclopedia of Respiratory Medicine*, 429-439. https://doi.org/10.1016/b0-12-370879-6/00072-7

Birinder, P. (2014). Etiology and pathogenesis of Parkinson's disease. *Textbook of Movement Disorders*, 42-42. https://doi.org/10.5005/jp/books/12347_6

Dhingra, N., & Bhagwat, D. (2011). Benign prostatic hyperplasia: An overview of existing treatment. *Indian Journal of Pharmacology*, *43*(1), 6. https://doi.org/10.4103/0253-7613.75657

Fong, T. G., Tulebaev, S. R., & Inouye, S. K. (2009). Delirium in elderly adults: Diagnosis, prevention and treatment. *Nature Reviews Neurology*, *5*(4), 210-220. https://doi.org/10.1038/nrneurol.2009.24

Guo, Q., Wang, Y., Xu, D., Nossent, J., Pavlos, N. J., & Xu, J. (2018). Rheumatoid arthritis: Pathological mechanisms and modern pharmacologic therapies. *Bone Research*, *6*(1). https://doi.org/10.1038/s41413-018-0016-9

Hooton, T. (2010). Urinary tract infections in adults. *Comprehensive Clinical Nephrology*, 629-640. https://doi.org/10.1016/b978-0-323-05876-6.00051-4

Imms, C., & Gibson, N. (2017). An overview of evidence-based occupational and physiotherapy for children with cerebral palsy. *Cerebral Palsy*, 165-192. https://doi.org/10.1007/978-3-319-67858-0_17

Kanter, J. W., Busch, A. M., Weeks, C. E., & Landes, S. J. (2008). The nature of clinical depression: Symptoms, syndromes, and behavior analysis. *The Behavior Analyst, 31*(1), 1-21. https://doi.org/10.1007/bf03392158

Kruse, M., & Schulz, S. C. (2016). Overview of schizophrenia and treatment approaches. *Schizophrenia and Psychotic Spectrum Disorders*, 3-22. https://doi.org/10.1093/med/9780199378067.003.0001

Lock, M. (2013). Making and remaking Alzheimer disease. *The Alzheimer Conundrum*. https://doi.org/10.23943/princeton/9780691149783.003.0002

Mafi, M. (2018). Review of "Diabetes mellitus: The epidemic of the century". https://doi.org/10.14322/publons.r2314592

Meeta, M. (2013). Osteoporosis—An overview. *Postmenopausal Osteoporosis: Basic and Clinical Concepts*, 1-1. https://doi.org/10.5005/jp/books/11789_1

Sabat, S. R. (2018). Dementia. *Alzheimer's Disease and Dementia*. https://doi.org/10.1093/wentk/9780190603106.003.0001

Saleh, M., & Ambrose, J. A. (2018). Understanding myocardial infarction. *F1000Research*, *7*, 1378. https://doi.org/10.12688/f1000research.15096.1

Siegler, E. L., Lama, S. D., Knight, M. G., Laureano, E., & Reid, M. C. (2015). Community-based supports and services for older adults: A primer for clinicians. *Journal of Geriatrics*, *2015*, 1-6. https://doi.org/10.1155/2015/678625

Stafstrom, C. E., & Carmant, L. (2015). Seizures and epilepsy: An overview for neuroscientists. *Cold Spring Harbor Perspectives in Medicine*, *5*(6), a022426-a022426. https://doi.org/10.1101/cshperspect.a022426

Taormina, & Gao. (2013). Maslow and the motivation hierarchy: Measuring satisfaction of the needs. *The American Journal of Psychology*, *126*(2), 155. https://doi.org/10.5406/amerjpsyc.126.2.0155

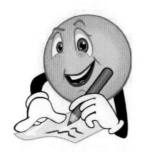

Chapter Fourteen:

Rehabilitative Nursing

Outline

I: Rehabilitation: Basic Introduction

II: Goals of Restorative Care

III: The Rehabilitation Team

IV: Assisting with Rehabilitation and Restorative Care

V: Activities of Daily Living (ADLs)

VI: Common Comfort and Adaptive Devices

VII: Steps to Prevent Complications from Immobility

VIII: Range of Motion Exercises

IX: Devices Used to Promote Ambulation for Patients/Residents with Physical and/or Visual Impairment

X: Relationship Between the Patient/Resident's Self-Esteem and Family Involvement in Care

XI: Documentation and the Nurse Assistant's Role in Care Planning

Rehabilitation: Basic Introduction

Injury, disease, birth defects, and surgery may affect body function. Often multiple functions of the body are lost. A disability is any lost, absent, or impaired mental or physical function. Some disabilities are short-term, whereas others may be permanent. Routine activities are difficult or seem impossible. The individual may depend partially or totally on others for basic needs. The degree of disability depends on how much function is possible.

Rehabilitation is the process of restoring the individual to his/her highest possible level of physical, social, psychological, and economic function. The major goal of rehabilitation is to improve abilities and function at the highest level of independence. Some individuals have the goal of returning to work. For others, self-care is the main goal. Sometimes improved function is not fully possible. Then the goal becomes to prevent further loss of function for the highest possible quality of life. Some individuals have suffered strokes, amputations, fractures, or other diseases and injuries. Some have had joint replacement surgeries. All need to regain proper function. Some individuals must adjust to a long-term disability. Some may need home care or nursing center care.

Restorative nursing

Some individuals are very weak. Many of them even cannot perform daily functions. Restorative nursing care is the type of care that helps patients/residents regain strength, health, and independence. With progressive illnesses and diseases, disabilities increase. Restorative nursing:

- Helps maintain the highest possible level of function.
- Prevents unnecessary decline in function.

Restorative nursing care promotes:
- Self-care
- Elimination
- Positioning
- Mobility
- Communication
- Cognitive function

Many patients/residents may need both restorative nursing and rehabilitation. In many healthcare agencies, they mean the same thing. Both focus on the individual as a whole.

Some healthcare agencies may have restorative aides. A restorative aide is a nursing assistant with special training in rehabilitation skills and restorative nursing. These nursing assistants assist the nursing and health teams as needed. Required training may vary among states. If there are no state requirements, the agency usually provides required training.

The Nurse Assistant's role in providing restorative care

Restorative care is carried out primarily by the nursing staff; however, a nurse assistant can play an important role in providing restorative care. This is a very important and essential part of a nurse assistant's job, because he/she is the member of the health care team who will spend the most time with the patient/resident each day. The nurse assistant can provide restorative care by encouraging and helping the patient/resident to do as much for himself/herself as he/ she is able, and by providing care according to the patient/resident's care plan.

The physical care such as repositioning patients/residents and helping them to get out of bed and walk is important for helping these patients/residents to maintain or regain their physical health, strength and abilities. In addition, when a patient/resident is encouraged to do something for himself/herself, it may help to maintain the patient/resident's physical abilities as well as his/her sense of independence, which is essential for the patient/resident's dignity and emotional health.

Some of the patients/residents may need to learn new ways to do old things so that they can do as much for themselves as possible. Another important aspect of providing restorative care is helping and encouraging patients/residents to practice these new skills. Often, the patient/resident will work with other members of the health care team (such as an occupational therapist, physical therapist, or speech therapist) to learn these new skills, but the nurse assistant will be responsible for helping the patient/resident to practice the skills on an ongoing basis. For example, a physical therapist may teach a patient/resident how to walk with a walker, but the nurse assistant will be responsible for encouraging the patient/resident to use the walker, and making sure that he/she is correctly using the walker.

Getting positive results from restorative care may take a long time. An important part of a nurse assistant's job is observing and reporting even the smallest changes in a patient/resident's abilities. What a nurse assistant observes depends on the goals that are written in the patient/resident's care plan. The nurse assistant may have to watch to observe how far the patient/resident walks, how much he/she eats, or how far he/she can bend a joint.

It is critical to note changes in the patient/resident's abilities in measurable terms, such as amount, distance, or length of time. The nurse assistant should also take note of how much effort it took for the patient/resident to complete the task. The nurse assistant should listen to the patient/resident's comments, and should observe physical signs, such as sweating, difficulty in breathing, or the number of times the patient/resident must stop and rest before continuing. The nurse assistant should always remember to report and record the restorative care that he/she provides, and his/her observations about the patient/resident's progress or setbacks. This information may help the other health care team members adjust the patient/resident's care plan as necessary.

In many healthcare facilities that receive Medicare funding, accurate documentation is also necessary to make sure that the patient/resident continues to be eligible for therapy and other services as required, and that the healthcare facility receives proper reimbursement for the services provided.

The rehabilitation principles are mainly based on early recognition and individualized planning for each patient/resident. When Maslow's hierarchy of needs is applied to rehabilitation, the patient/resident in the acute stage of injury or illness initially needs assistance with basic survival requirements, such as maintaining a patent airway and a sufficient oxygenation level, obtaining water and food, and eliminating waste substances.

Next, activities of daily living (ADLs) should be addressed, such as being able to dress, feed, bathe oneself, the ability of independent movement, and being able to communicate effectively. Later, the patient/resident learns to work toward self-actualization and to be a contributing and creative member of society.

Rehabilitation presents multiple opportunities and challenges for members of the healthcare team. The major goals of all rehabilitation nursing are to assist patients/residents to approach normal functioning as much as possible, to minimize the patient/resident's limitations, and to maximize his/her capabilities. Special emphasis should be placed on quality of life of the patient/resident.

Goals of Restorative Care

The patients/residents in a healthcare facility require nursing care because they are injured, ill, or very frail. Because of mental disability, physical disability or both, their ability to care for themselves is reduced. One of the major goals of the nursing care is to help patients/residents maintain the abilities they still have, and to help them regain the abilities they have lost as much as possible.

Restorative care supports a patient/resident become as fully functional and independent as possible, which increases the patient/resident's ability to enjoy life. Practicing the restorative care principles is significant with all of the patients/residents in a nurse assistant's care, no matter where he/she works. However, if a nursing assistant is working in a facility that receives Medicare funding, providing restorative care is a particularly important part of his/her job. To fulfil Omnibus Budget Reconciliation Act (OBRA) requirements, the health care staff including the nurse assistants must identify each patient/resident's risk factors for functional decline, and should take appropriate steps to maintain the patient/resident's existing abilities and prevent any future loss of abilities from occurring. The nurse assistant should provide restorative care that is essential to achieving these goals.

Self-care

Self-care is a major goal of the restorative care. Activities of daily living (ADL) are the routine activities generally done during a normal day in an individual's life. ADL include oral hygiene, bathing, eating, dressing, elimination, and moving about. The health team including the nurse assistant assesses the patient/resident's ability to perform ADL. The need for self-help devices should also be considered. Sometimes the wrists, hands, and arms are affected. Self-help devices are often required in these cases. Equipment should be changed, made, or bought to meet the patient/resident's needs.

- Eating devices include plate guards, glass holders, and silverware with curved handles or cuffs. Some devices are attached to splints.
- Electric toothbrushes which have back-and-forth brushing motions can be used for oral hygiene.
- Adaptive devices for hygiene encourage independence.
- Self-help devices are useful for dressing, cooking, phone calls, writing, and other routine tasks.

Mobility

The patient/resident may require crutches or walkers, braces, or canes. Physical and occupational therapies are common for nervous and musculo-skeletal problems. Some patients/residents need wheelchairs. If possible, they may learn wheelchair transfers to and from the bed, bathtub, toilet, chair, and sofa, and in and out of vehicles. Prosthesis is an artificial replacement for a missing body part. The patient/resident learns how to use the artificial leg or arm. The main goal is for the device to be like the missing body part in appearance and function.

Nutrition

Dysphagia (difficulty swallowing) may occur after a stroke. The patient/resident may need a dysphagia diet. When possible, the patient/resident learns exercises to improve swallowing. Some patients/residents cannot swallow and need enteral nutrition.

Communication

Aphasia may occur after a stroke. Aphasia is the partial or total loss of the ability to understand or use language. Communication devices and speech therapy are helpful in these cases.

Psychological and social aspects

An illness or disability can affect appearance and function. Relationships and self-esteem may suffer. Some patients/residents may feel unwhole, unattractive, unclean, useless, or undesirable. They may deny the disability and expect therapy to correct the disability. Some patients/residents are angry, depressed, and hostile. A good behavior is important. The patient/resident must accept his/her limits and be motivated. The focus should be on abilities and strengths. Frustrations and despair are common. Progress may be slow and learning a new skill is a reminder of the disability. Emotions and old fears may recur. The nurse assistant should remind patients/residents of their progress. They need help accepting limits and disabilities. The nurse assistant should provide support, reassurance, and encouragement to patients/residents. Social and psychological needs are part of the care plan. Spiritual support may help some patients/residents.

The Rehabilitation Team

Rehabilitation is a team effort. The patient/resident and the family are the key team member. The rehabilitation team may include the physician, physiatrist, advanced practice nurse or certified rehabilitation nurse, and therapists (physical, occupational, speech, recreation, music, sexual), as well as the vocational counselor, social worker, and psychologist.

The patient/resident's case manager (care manager) is becoming an increasingly critical member of the rehabilitation team. Team meetings and conferences are held regularly during the rehabilitation process so that all team members can establish common goals. The family is usually involved in team conferences or family meetings. The main focus should be on regaining function and independence.

The rehabilitation team meets often to discuss the patient/resident's progress. The rehabilitation plan can be changed as needed. The patient/resident and family attend the meetings when possible. Families provide encouragement and support. Often they help with home care of the patient/resident. The nurse assistant mainly focuses on promoting the patient/resident's independence. Preventing decline in function is also a major goal.

Assisting with Rehabilitation and Restorative Care

- The nurse assistant should follow the care plan and the nurse's instructions.

- The nurse assistant should follow the patient/resident's daily routine and should provide him/her safety.
- Privacy and personal choice are very essential. The nurse assistant should protect the patient/resident's rights.
- He/she should report early signs and symptoms of complications such as contractures, pressure ulcers, and bowel and bladder problems.
- The patient/resident should be kept in good alignment at all times.
- The nurse assistant should turn and re-position the patient/resident as directed.
- Safe transfer methods should be used.
- Proper measures should be practiced to prevent pressure ulcers.
- ROM exercises should be performed as instructed.
- Assistive devices should be applied as ordered.
- The required self-help devices should be provided.
- The nurse assistant should not pity the patient/resident.
- The patient/resident should be encouraged to perform ADL to the extent possible.
- The nurse assistant should give the patient/resident proper time to complete tasks. He/she should not rush the patient/resident.
- The nurse assistant should provide praise when even a little progress is made from the patient/resident.
- The nurse assistant should provide emotional support and reassurance to the patient/resident.
- The nurse assistant should always try to understand and appreciate the patient/resident's situation, concerns, and feelings.

- The nurse assistant should practice the methods developed by the rehabilitation team. This helps him/her better assist the patient/resident.
- The nurse assistant should practice the task that the patient/resident must do. This helps him/her guide and direct the patient/resident.
- The nurse should know how to apply the patient/resident's self-help devices.
- He/she should also know how to use the patient/resident's equipment.
- The nurse assistant should stress what the patient/resident can do. He/she should focus on abilities and strengths and should not focus on disabilities and weaknesses of the patient/resident.
- It should be remembered that muscles will atrophy if not used. And contractures may develop.

Activities of Daily Living (ADLs)

It is very important to encourage patients/residents to become as independent as possible. The nurse assistant should assist patients/residents by providing them physical care and encouragement and by helping them with self-care. It is important for all patients/residents to perform as much self-care as possible. When the rehabilitation team has thoroughly assessed the patient/resident and determined what functional capacity is realistic, a comprehensive plan of retraining in ADLs is initiated.

Functional ADLs

The basic functional ADLs (FADLs) may include routine activities of self-care, such as bathing, dressing, toileting, mobility, transfer, and eating. Because of disability, adaptations may be required so the patient/resident can perform self-care activities. Not all patients/residents will be able to care for themselves or to live independently.

Instrumental ADLs

Instrumental ADLs (IADLs) are more complex living skills, such as laundry, food preparation, taking medicines, and financial management. These IADLs may or may not be achievable by individual patients/residents. One important IADL is being able to purchase prepare meals and groceries. Healthcare staff including the nurse assistant maintains an ADL record that informs all team members of the rehabilitation team of the activities the patient/resident is able to do and those that he/she is attempting. Nursing care plans are usually updated on continuous basis with improvements or regressions in progress.

Common Comfort and Adaptive Devices

Comfort devices

Supportive or comfort devices are generally used to support and maintain the patient/resident in a certain position.

Foot-boards

They prevent plantar flexion that can lead to footdrop. In plantar flexion, the foot is usually bent. Footdrop occurs when the foot falls down at the ankle. The foot-board should be placed so the soles of the feet are flush against it. Foot-boards also keep top linens off the toes and feet.

Trochanter rolls

They prevent the legs and hips from turning outward (external rotation). A bath blanket should be folded to the desired length and rolled up. The loose end should be placed under the patient/resident from the hip to the knee. Then the roll should be tucked alongside the body.

Splints

Splints keep the wrists, elbows, fingers, thumbs, ankles, and knees in normal position. They are usually secured in place with Velcro.

Bed cradles

They keep the weight of top linens off the toes and feet. The weight of top linens can cause pressure sores and footdrop.

Trapeze

A trapeze can be used to raise the upper body off the bed.

Heel and elbow protectors

They are made of foam padding, sheepskin, pressure-relieving gel, and other cushion materials. They fit the shape of elbows and heels.

Heel and foot elevators

These raise the feet and heels off of the bed. They prevent pressure sores and footdrop.

Gel or fluid-filled pads and cushions

Gel or fluid-filled pads and cushions involve a pressure-relieving gel or fluid. They can be used for wheelchairs and chairs to prevent pressure. The outer case is vinyl. The cushion or pad is placed in a fabric cover to protect the patient/resident's skin.

Special beds

Some special beds have air flowing through the mattresses. The patient/resident floats on the mattress. Body weight is evenly distributed. There is very little pressure on body parts. Some special beds allow re-positioning without moving the patient/resident. The patient/resident is turned to the supine or prone position or the bed is tilted various degrees. Alignment is not changed. Pressure points change with the change in the position. There is very little friction. Some special beds constantly rotate from side to side. They are beneficial for patients/residents with spinal cord injuries.

Other equipment

Trochanter rolls, foot-boards, pillows, and other positioning devices are used to keep the patient/resident in good alignment.

Dressings

Sometimes dressings are also used. The wound should be moist enough to promote quick healing. If too moist, the dressing may interfere with healing. If a pressure sore has drainage, a dressing that absorbs drainage should be used. The dressing usually absorbs slough. The slough is removed with the removal of the dressing.

Canes and Walkers

Many patients/residents can achieve mobility just by using a walker or cane for support. Multiple different types of canes are available. Many patients/residents paint or decorate their canes or use fancy canes to express their individuality. Various different varieties of walkers are also available. Each patient/resident should be evaluated to determine which type of walker will be the most safe and comfortable to use. It is very important to encourage the patient/resident to move independently as much as possible.

Splints and Braces

Patients/residents may require special splints or braces to support affected limbs or to maintain correct positioning. The medical specialty that deals in the fabrication of splints and braces is called orthotics. Splints are available in two major forms:

Resting splints: They hold the body part stationary and protect the hand or limb from becoming contracted.

Dynamic hand splints: Dynamic (moving) hand splints enable patients/residents to function more easily than would be possible without them.

Some splints can be attached to sling-type devices, one on each finger. These permit the patient/resident with hand and arm weakness or paralysis to use the hands. Some splints are combined with a hook device for grasping objects. Braces are often used to the legs for support, especially for patients/residents with hemiplegia or paraplegia (lower limb paralysis). In some cases, a special brace can be used to support a joint after an injury or reconstructive surgery. The brace should be adjusted to permit limited movement, which helps to protect the joint while it heals. This special type of brace can also be used on a permanent basis to support a weak joint.

Many patients/residents who would otherwise be immobilized are able to walk with the aid of braces. Physical therapists teach patients/residents to apply and remove braces, and nursing assistants should reinforce this teaching. If a patient/resident has quadriplegia (all four extremities and possibly the trunk paralyzed), he/she may require a neck or back brace. This patient/resident may also use a special type of inflatable trousers (exoskeleton) to maintain an upright posture and to prevent vascular collapse. Many patients/residents also need special shoes or shoe inserts. Some patients/residents will require breathing assistance on a permanent basis.

Artificial Limbs

Patients/residents who have had a part or all of a leg or arm amputated are often fitted with artificial limbs. The specialty that deals with the fabrication and adjustment of prostheses is called prosthetics. The nurse assistant may be familiar with the arm prosthesis that resembles a "hook." This prosthesis gives movement and control similar to normal thumb–finger opposition. Leg prosthesis is usually fitted over the amputation stump that permits the patient/resident to walk and participate in sports. Current technology has so much advanced the science of prosthetics. Artificial hands are also available that seem much like a natural hand, but still have the flexibility of the hook prosthesis. Some prostheses are electronic or/and computer-driven.

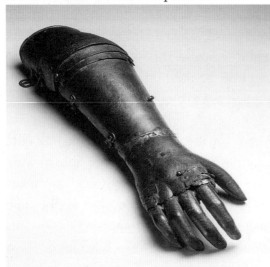

Steps to Prevent Complications from Immobility

Complications of immobility

Neurological

- Stress
- Depression
- Changes in behavior
- Sleep disturbances

Respiratory

- Stasis pneumonia
- Atelectasis

Circulatory

- Thrombophlebitis
- Pulmonary embolism

Musculoskeletal

- Contractures

- Osteoporosis (demineralization due to lack of weight bearing)
- Muscle atrophy

Integumentary

- Pressure sores

Gastrointestinal

- Constipation
- Anorexia

Genito-urinary

- Kidney stones
- Urinary tract infection

Psychological

- Loneliness
- Depression

Causes of immobility

- Are confined to bed or wheelchair
- Need total or partial help moving
- Are agitated or having involuntary muscle movements
- Prolonged illness c. Immobility due to injury d. Surgery
- Have fecal or urinary incontinence
- Are exposed to moisture—feces, urine, sweat, wound drainage, or saliva
- Have poor fluid balance or poor nutrition
- Have altered mental status
- Have problems sensing pressure or pain
- Have circulatory problems
- Are very thin or obese
- Have a healed pressure ulcer

- Taking medications that affect wound healing
- Refuse care and treatment measures
- Have health problems such as thyroid disease, kidney failure, or diabetes
- Smoking

Preventive methods

Turning/repositioning

Turning patients/residents onto their sides can prevent complications such as contractures and pressure sores. Several procedures and care measures also need the side-lying position. Many older patients/residents have arthritis in their hips, spines, and knees. Thus, less painful and logrolling is preferred for turning these patients/residents.

TCDB

It is turning, coughing, and deep-breathing exercises.

Body alignment

When walking, lifting, or performing any activity, correct body alignment is necessary to maintain the balance. When an individual's body is in proper alignment, all the muscles work together for the most efficient and safest movement (without muscle strain). Body stretching as high as possible produces correct alignment. This can be established through proper posture. When a person is in standing position, the weight is a bit forward and is held up on the outside part of the feet. Again, the back is straight, the head is erected, and the abdomen is tucked in (It should be remembered that the patient/resident in bed should be in almost the same position as if he/she were standing).

Range of motion

The movement of a joint to the maximum possible extent without causing pain or discomfort is called the range of motion (ROM) of the joint. Range-of motion exercises may involve moving the joints through their complete range of motion. They should be usually done at least two times a day.

Other preventive measures may include:
- Supportive devices
- Proper skin care
- Encouraging independence
- Toileting
- Bowel and bladder training
- Elastic stockings
- Ambulation

Range of Motion Exercises

The movement of a joint to the maximum possible extent without causing pain or discomfort is called the range of motion (ROM) of the joint. Range-of motion exercises may involve moving the joints through their complete range of motion. They should be usually done at least two times a day.

Active range of motion exercises: These are done by the patient/resident.

Passive range of motion exercises: The nurse assistant moves the joints of the patient/resident through their range of motion.

Active-assistive range of motion exercises: The patient/resident performs the exercises with some assistance.

Joint Movements may include:

Abduction: It is moving a body part away from the mid-line of the body.

Adduction: Adduction is moving a body part toward the mid-line of the body.

Opposition: It is touching an opposite finger with the thumb.

Flexion: Flexion is bending a body part.

Extension: Extension is straightening a body part.

Hyperextension: It is excessive straightening of a body part.

Dorsiflexion: It is bending the toes and foot up at the ankle.

Plantar flexion: Plantar flexion is bending the foot down at the ankle.

Rotation: Rotation is turning the joint.

Internal rotation: It is turning the joint inward.

External rotation: It is turning the joint outward.

Pronation: Pronation is turning the joint downward.

Supination: Supination is turning the joint upward

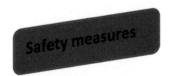

- The patient/resident should be covered with a bath blanket for warmth and privacy.
- The nurse assistant should exercise only the joints the nurse tells him/her to exercise.
- The nurse assistant should expose only the body parts being exercised.
- Proper body mechanics should be used.

- The part being exercised should be supported.
- The joint should be moved slowly, smoothly, and gently.
- The nurse assistant should not force a joint beyond its present range of motion.
- The nurse assistant should not force a joint to the point of pain.
- The patient/resident should be asked if he/she has pain or discomfort.

Encouraging comfort and safety

ROM exercises may cause injury if not performed properly. Joint injury, muscle strain, and pain are possible. The patient/resident should be reminded to tell the nurse assistant if he/she has pain during the procedure. ROM exercises to the neck may cause severe injury if not performed properly. Some agencies may provide special training to nursing assistants before performing such exercises. Many other agencies may not allow nursing assistants do them. The nurse assistant should always know his/her agency's policy. The nurse assistant should perform ROM exercises to the neck only if allowed by his/her agency and if the nurse instructs him/her to do so. In many agencies, only physical therapists are allowed to do neck exercises.

Helping a patient/resident with passive Range-of-Motion exercises

The nurse assistant should provide assistance for passive ROM exercises in following ways:

1. Hands should be washed properly.
2. The nurse assist should gather all supplies.
3. The nurse assistant should knock, greet the patient/resident and should ensure his/her privacy.
4. The procedure should be explained thoroughly to the patient/resident.
5. Equipment should be adjusted for proper body mechanics and safety: the bed should be raised to a comfortable working height. It should be ensured that the wheels on the bed are locked.
6. The head of the bed should be lowered as low as the patient/resident can tolerate. The nurse assistant should make sure the patient/resident is in the supine position (lying on the back) and in good body alignment.

Exercise of the Shoulder

7. With one hand, the nurse assistant should hold the patient/resident's wrist and should put his/her other hand under the elbow. The nurse assistant should provide this support throughout the following motions.
8. **Flexion and extension:** With the patient/resident's arm by his/her side and the palm down, the nurse assistant should raise the patient/resident's arm straight up and then should move it alongside the ear and then should lower the arm to the patient/resident's side. It should be repeated at least 5 times.
9. **Abduction and adduction**: With the patient/resident's arm by his/her side and the palm up, the nurse assistant should move the patient/resident's arm out away from the body. Then the arm should be turned to the patient/resident's side. It should be repeated at least 5 times.
10. **Horizontal abduction and adduction:** The nurse assistant should hold the patient/resident's arm out away from the body with the palm up. The elbow should be bent, touching the patient/resident's hand to the opposite shoulder. Then the patient/resident's elbow should be straightened, returning the hand to its original position. It should be repeated at least 5 times.
11. **Rotation**: The patient/resident's arm should be bent and should be positioned the elbow so that it is at the same height as the shoulder. The hand should be moved up toward the patient/resident's head and then down. It should be repeated at least 5 times.

Exercise of the Elbow

12. With one hand, the nurse assistant should hold the patient/resident's wrist and should put his/her other hand under the elbow. The nurse assistant should provide this support throughout the following motions.
13. **Flexion and extension:** With the patient/resident's arm by his/her side with the palm up, the nurse assistant should bend the patient/resident's arm at the elbow so that the hand

moves toward the shoulder on the same side. The arm should be straightened back down to the hip. It should be repeated 5 times.

Exercise of the Wrist

14. The nurse assistant should hold the patient/resident's wrist with the palm down with one hand and the patient/resident's fingers with his/her other hand. The nurse assistant should provide this support throughout the following motions.

15. **Flexion and extension**: The nurse assistant should bend the patient/resident's elbow so that the forearm is at a right angle to the bed. The wrist should be bent to move the patient/resident's hand forward, and then the wrist should be straightened to move the hand backward. It should be repeated at least 5 times.

16. **Radial and ulnar deviation**: With the patient/resident's hand still raised off the mattress, the nurse assistant should gently tilt the patient/resident's hand toward the thumb. Then his/her hand should be tilted the other way, toward the patient/resident's little finger. It should be repeated at least 5 times.

Exercise the Fingers and Thumb

17. The patient/resident's hand should be raised off the mattress. The nurse assistant should hold the patient/resident's wrist with one hand and the fingers with his/her other hand. The nurse assistant should provide this support throughout the following motions.

18. **Flexion and extension:** Each of the fingers (one at a time) and the thumb should be bent to touch the palm. Then each of the fingers (one at a time) and the thumb should be extended. It should be repeated at least 5 times.

19. **Abduction and adduction**: The nurse assistant should hold the patient/resident's thumb and index finger together in one of his/her hands. With the other hand, the middle finger should be spread away from the index finger. The middle finger should be moved to the index finger and should hold the middle finger, index finger and thumb together. The ring finger should be moved away from the other three fingers (thumb, index and middle), then back to them. The nurse assistant should hold all four fingers and then should move the little finger away from the other four fingers (thumb, index, middle and ring), then back to them. Now the nurse should do this in the other direction. The nurse assistant should hold the little finger and ring finger together and should move the middle finger away and back. This should be completed with the index finger and thumb. It should be repeated at least 5 times.

20. **Thumb flexion and extension**: The nurse assistant should bend the patient/resident's thumb toward the palm, and then should return it to its natural position. It should be repeated at least 5 times.

21. **Thumb opposition**: The tip of the thumb should be touched to each finger. It should be repeated at least 5 times.

Exercise of the Hip and Knee

22. The nurse assistant should put his/her one hand under the patient/resident's knee and his/her other hand under the ankle. The nurse assistant should provide this support throughout the following motions.

23. **Flexion and extension:** The patient/resident's knee should be bent and should be moved it up toward the head to flex the knee and hip, then the patient/resident's knee should be straightened, extending the knee and hip. The patient/resident's leg should be lowered to the bed. It should be repeated at least 5 times.

24. **Abduction and adduction**: The patient/resident's leg should be moved out away from his/her body. Then the leg should be returned to the patient/resident's side. It should be repeated at least 5 times.

25. **Hip rotation**: Keeping the patient/resident's leg straight, the nurse assistant should turn the leg inward and then outward to rotate the hip. It should be repeated at least 5 times.

Exercise the Ankle

26. The nurse assistant should put one hand under the patient/resident's ankle and should grasp the foot of the patient/resident with his/her other hand. The nurse assistant should provide this support throughout the following motions.

27. **Dorsiflexion and plantar flexion:** The nurse assistant should gently push the patient/resident's foot backward toward his/her head and then forward toward the mattress. It should be repeated at least 5 times.

28. **Inversion and eversion**: The nurse assistant should turn the patient/resident's foot inward and then outward. It should be repeated at least 5 times.

Exercise the Toes

29. The nurse assistant should put one hand under the patient/resident's foot and should provide this support throughout the following motions.

30. **Flexion and extension**: The nurse assistant should place his/her other hand on the top of the foot, over the toes. The toes should be curled downward and then should be straightened them.

31. **Abduction and adduction**: Starting with the big toe and the one next to it, the nurse assistant should hold the two toes together and should move the middle toe away from them. The nurse assistant should continue spreading the toes in the same way he/she spreads the fingers of hands. It should be repeated at least 5 times.

32. It should be ensured the patient/resident's comfort and proper body alignment.

33. Hand should be properly washed, and observations should be reported and recorded at the end of the procedure.

Ambulation

The act of walking is termed as ambulation. Some patients/residents are unsteady and weak due to any illness, injury, bed rest, or surgery. They need support for walking. After bed rest, activity increases gradually and in steps. Initially, the patient/resident sits on the side of the bed (dangles), followed by sitting in a bedside chair. Next the patient/resident walks in the room and then in the hallway. The nurse assistant should follow the care plan when helping a patient/resident walk. They should use a gait (transfer) belt if the patient/resident is weak or unsteady. The patient/resident may also use hand rails along the wall.

Walking increases flexibility of the most of the body's muscles and joints. It improves gastrointestinal and respiratory function. Ambulating also minimizes the risk for complications of immobility. However, even a very short period of immobility may reduce a patient/resident's tolerance for ambulating. If necessary, the nurse assistant should make use of appropriate equipment and assistive devices to assist in patient handling and movement.

Before helping with ambulation, the nurse assistant needs following information from the nurse supervisor and the care plan:
- How much help the patient/resident needs?
- Is the patient/resident using a walker, cane, crutches, or a brace?
- Areas of weakness—right leg or arm, left leg or arm?
- How far to walk?
- What observations to record and report?
- How well the patient/resident can tolerate the activity?
- Shuffling, limping, sliding, or walking on tip-toes?
- Complaints of discomfort or pain?
- Complaints of orthostatic hypotension—dizziness, weakness, spots before the eyes, faintness?
- The distance walked?
- When to report the recorded observations?
- What patient/resident concerns to report at once?

Helping the patient/resident to walk

The nurse assistant should follow the below procedure to assist a patient/resident walk:

24. The nurse assistant should knock before entering the patient/resident's room.

25. After proper introduction, explaining the procedure, and proper hand hygiene, following items should be arranged for further procedure:
- Robe and non-skid footwear
- Towel or paper to protect bottom linens
- Gait (transfer) belt

26. The bed should be adjusted to a safe and comfortable level for the patient/resident. The nurse assistant should always follow the care plan. Bed wheels should be locked with lowering the bed rail if up.

27. Top linens should be fan-folded to the foot of the bed.

28. Paper or towel should be placed under the patient/resident's feet.

29. The nurse assistant should help the patient/resident to sit on the side of the bed (dangling).

30. It should be ensured that the patient/resident has put and fastened the shoes. The patient/resident's feet should be flat on the floor.

31. The nurse assistant should help the patient/resident to put on the robe.

32. The gait belt should be applied at the waist over clothing.

33. Proper support should be provided to the patient/resident in standing. The gait belt should be grasped at each side. If no gait belt, the nurse assistant should place his/her arms under the patient/resident's arms around to the shoulder blades.

34. The nurse assistant should stand at the patient/resident's weak side while he/she gains balance. The belt should be held at the side and back. If not using a gait belt, the nurse assistant should place one arm around the back and the other at the elbow to support the patient/resident.

35. The patient/resident should be encouraged to stand erect with the head up and the back straight.

36. The patient/resident should be provided proper help and support to walk. The nurse assistant should walk to the side and slightly behind the patient/resident on his/her weak side. Support should be provided with the gait belt. If not using a gait belt, the nurse assistant should place his/her one arm around the back and the other at the elbow to support the patient/resident.

37. Patient/resident should be encouraged to use the hand rail on his/her strong side. He/she should also be encouraged to walk normally. The heel should strike the floor first. The patient/resident should be discouraged from shuffling, walking, or sliding on tip-toes.

38. The nurse assistant should walk at the required distance if the patient/resident tolerates the activity. The patient/resident should not be rushed during walking.

39. The patient/resident should be provided proper help in returning to bed. The gait belt should be removed and the head of the bed should be lowered down. The patient/resident should be assisted to move at the center of the bed.

40. Shoes and the paper towel over the bottom sheet should be removed.

41. Comfort should be provided to the patient/resident.

42. The call light should be placed within reach.

43. Bed rails should be adjusted at a safe and comfortable level.

44. The robe and shoes should be returned to their proper place.

45. The patient/resident should be unscreened and safety check of the room should be completed before leaving the room.

46. The nurse assistant at the end should report and record his/her observations.

Devices Used to Promote Ambulation for Patients/Residents with Physical and/or Visual Impairment

Following things should be assessed to determine if patient/resident can be more independent

- Physical strength
- Special training programs
- Use of assistive devices
- Financial resources of patients/residents
- Cognitive abilities and level of motivation
- Mental status
- Mental health

Patient/resident's transfer

Patients/residents are moved to and from chairs, beds, wheelchairs, commodes, toilets, shower chairs, and stretchers. The amount of help required and the method used may differ, based on the patient/resident's dependency level. The room should be properly arranged to allow enough space for a safe transfer. The chair, wheelchair, or other device should be placed correctly.

Gait belts

Transfer belts also known as gait belts are most commonly used to:

- Support patients/residents during their transfers.
- Re-position patients/residents in wheelchairs and chairs.

Assistive devices

Crutches

Crutches are the walking aids used when the patient/resident cannot use one leg or when one or both legs need to gain stability and strength. Some patients/residents with permanent leg weakness can use crutches. Falls are a major risk. The nurse assistant should follow these safety measures:

- The crutch tips should be thoroughly checked. They must not be torn, worn down, or wet. Worn or torn crutch tips should be replaced. Wet tips should be properly dried with paper towels.
- Crutches should be checked for any flaws. Wooden crutches should be evaluated for cracks and metal crutches for bends.
- All bolts should be tightened.
- It should be ensured that the patient/resident wear street shoes. The shoes must be flat with non-skid soles.
- It should be ensured that clothes of the patient/resident fit well. Loose clothes may get caught between the underarms and crutches. Loose skirts and long clothes can hang forward and may block the patient/resident's view of the feet and crutch tips.
- The nurse assistant should practice safety rules to prevent falls.
- Crutches should be kept within the patient/resident's reach. They should be placed at the patient/resident's chair or against a wall.

Walkers

Walkers provide more support than canes. Wheeled walkers are more common, which have wheels on the front legs and rubber tips on the back legs. The patient/resident pushes the walker about 6 to 8 inches in front of his/her feet. Rubber tips on the back legs usually prevent the walker from moving while the patient/resident is standing. Some walkers may have a braking action when weight is applied to the walker's back legs. Pouches, baskets, and trays are generally attached to the walker and can be used for needed items. This permits more independence and free the hands to grip the walker.

Canes

Canes are walking aids used for weakness on one side of the body. They usually help to provide support and balance. A cane should be held on the strong side of the body (i.e. if the right leg is weak, the cane should be held in the left hand). The size of the cane tip is almost 6 to 10 inches to the side of the foot. The grip should be on the level with the hip. The patient/resident walks as follows:

- **Step I:** The cane is moved ahead 6 to 10 inches.
- **Step II:** The weaker leg that is opposite to the cane is moved forward even with the cane.
- **Step III:** The stronger leg is moved forward and it should be ahead of the weak leg and the cane.

Braces

Braces are walking aids that support weak body parts. They also correct and prevent joint deformities or joint movement. Plastic, metal, or leather is used for braces. A brace is usually applied over the knee, ankle, or back. The skin and bony points under braces should be kept dry and clean. This may prevent skin breakdown.

Nursing assistants should report redness or signs of skin breakdown at once. They should also report complaints of discomfort or pain. The nurse supervisor usually assesses the skin under braces every shift. The care plan suggests when to apply and remove a brace.

Other assistive methods may include service animals (Seeing Eye and Hearing Ear dogs), use of Braille (a system of touch reading and writing for blind persons), modifications to accommodate wheelchair access, and disabled parking.

Relationship between the Patient/Resident's Self-Esteem and Family Involvement in Care

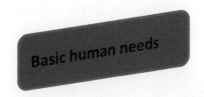

Basic human needs

Nursing Assistants have a professional and legal duty to ensure residents' basic human needs are met. The seven basic needs are further subdivided into subcategories. In each need, the Nursing Assistant has a key role to play. If these needs are not met, Maslow contended that the outcome would be physical illness, mental health issues, and/or psychiatric illness. Maslow warned that if physiological needs are not met, those under a Nursing Assistant's care could become very ill or even die, If a resident's safety needs are not met, posttraumatic stress could occur.

Typically, humans arrive at different stages of the hierarchy along life's path. At different times they might have a deficit in a certain stage. If this happens, that person may abandon the pursuit of a higher stage. He/she regresses to a lower stage to have more fundamental needs met. Not everyone reaches the top of the hierarchy. Things like poverty, injury, financial setbacks or illness may interfere with development in Maslow's hierarchy.

Physiological

Physiological needs are necessary to maintain life. These basic needs are required by all animals—including humans. They are the primary focus of infants.

Every human being has some basic physiological needs including food, oxygen, water, shelter, elimination, sleep, and sex.

It is important that Nursing Assistants recognize the importance of meeting residents' physiological needs. As front-line resident care providers, Nursing Assistants are in a position to note whether residents' basic needs are being met.

Safety and security needs

Safety and security issues gain attention after physiological needs are met. This shift to safety needs includes things like physical and mental health concerns, freedom from war, physical and financial security. Safety and security needs may include clothing, protection from a danger or harm, freedom from illness, injury, harm, fear, stability and order, family, economics

Sense of belongingness

Once physiological, safety, and security needs are met, residents will seek a sense of belonging. The resident will begin to focus on the need to have a feeling of community and being loved. These needs are usually met by friends, family, and romantic partners. In residential long-term care facilities this need to belong is often met by residents, staff, caregivers, and/or outside service providers.

Often residents in a long-term care facility lose contact with friends and family. Other residents, facility staff, and service providers become a community for these residents. As primary caregivers, Nursing Assistants are in a position to nurture resident interaction and encourage involvement.

Esteem

Esteem is feeling good about oneself. It is a sense of self-worth. Esteem is necessary for self-actualization. When a sense of community is met a resident may work toward esteem. Before esteem can be achieved, a resident needs love and a sense of belonging. Self-confidence and acceptance from others are important components of esteem.
The Nursing Assistant has a vital role to play in building resident esteem. Caring is at the heart of the Nursing Assistant–resident relationship. Through verbal and

nonverbal interaction, the Nursing Assistant can develop resident self-esteem and confidence.

Self-actualization

Self-actualization involves the ability to be self-sufficient. It is the ability to achieve one's potential. Self-actualization varies from person to person. Engineers have self-actualized when they can complete a project satisfactorily. When architects complete a drawing that excites their clients, they have achieved self-actualization.

When a resident can complete his/her daily activities unassisted and is happily involved in the activities of the facility, he/she is self-actualized.

Methods of Assisting the Patient/Resident to Meet the Basic Needs

Therapeutic communication

Therapeutic communication makes use of various techniques. These are aimed at preserving and enhancing the resident's physical, mental, and emotional well-being. Nursing Assistants provide patients with empathy, information, support and caring. It is also important that they maintain professional distance and objectivity with residents.

1. Patient/resident-centered and goal oriented

Therapeutic communication involves face-to-face interaction between the residents and their caregivers. The goal is to inform residents and involve them in decision making about their care. Therapeutic communication focuses on maintaining and advancing the physical and emotional well-being of each resident. The nursing team uses therapeutic communication techniques to provide information, engage, and support residents.

2. Verbal or non-verbal communication

While many therapeutic communication techniques involve getting and giving information from residents, Nursing Assistants also use non-verbal techniques.

Documentation Process and the Nurse Assistant's Role in Care Planning

Resident Assessment Instrument (RAI)

The utilization of the components of the RAI provides information about a patient/resident's functional status, weaknesses, strengths, and preferences, as well as offering guidance on further assessments once issues have been identified. The MDS has almost 450 items to addresses clinical and functional aspects of the patient/resident such as physical functioning, sensory, cognition, oral health, nutrition, skin, mobility, elimination, clinical conditions or diseases, etc.

The MDS only indicates if the patient/resident has a problem; however, it does not determine the cause of the problem. Therefore, there are Care Area Assessment resources that are available to help nurses do further assessments specific to the identified problem (e.g. dehydration, delirium). The RAI process drives the care plan that is developed for the resident. The MDS is an excellent teaching tool to use with students in the nursing home setting.

The Minimum Data Set (MDS)

The Omnibus Budget Reconciliation Act of 1987 (OBRA) requires the Minimum Data Set (MDS) for nursing center residents. It provides comprehensive information about the patient/resident. Examples include communication, memory, hearing and vision, physical function, and activities. The nurse uses the observations of the nurse assistant to complete the MDS. The MDS is initiated when the patient/resident is admitted to the center. It is edited and updated before each care conference. A new MDS should be completed once a year and whenever an important change occurs in the patient/resident's health status.

Nursing Diagnosis

The RN uses assessment information and observations to make a nursing diagnosis. A nursing diagnosis demonstrates a health issue that can be managed by nursing measures. It is usually different from a medical diagnosis i.e. the identification of a problem or condition by a physician. Stroke, cancer, heart attack, and diabetes are examples of medical diagnoses. A patient/resident can have multiple nursing diagnoses. These may change as assessment information changes. For example, "Acute pain" can be added after surgery.

Planning

Planning involves setting goals and priorities. Priorities are what is most important for the patient/resident. Goals are aimed at the patient/resident's highest level of well-being and function such as physical, social, emotional, and spiritual. Goals promote normal health and prevent health issues.

The nursing care plan (care plan) is a written guideline about the patient/resident's nursing care. It has the patient/resident's nursing diagnoses and goals. It also has actions or measures for each goal. The care plan is usually used as a communication tool. Nursing staff use it to see what care to provide. The care plan helps to make sure that nursing team members provide the same care. Each healthcare agency has a care plan form. It can be found in the medical record. The care plan may change as the patient/resident's nursing diagnoses change.

464

Helpful Resources

Chambers, R. (2018). Getting organised for supporting self care as a general practice team. *Supporting Self Care in Primary Care*, 43-52. https://doi.org/10.1201/9781315383408-5

Chipu, M., & Downing, C. (2020). Professional nurses' facilitation of self-care in intensive care units: A concept analysis. *International Journal of Nursing Sciences*, *7*(4), 446-452. https://doi.org/10.1016/j.ijnss.2020.08.002

Davis, M. C. (1994). The rehabilitation nurse's role in spiritual care. *Rehabilitation Nursing*, *19*(5), 298-301. https://doi.org/10.1002/j.2048-7940.1994.tb00826.x

Halpern, L. W. (2017). Early ambulation is crucial for improving patient health. *AJN, American Journal of Nursing*, *117*(6), 15. https://doi.org/10.1097/01.naj.0000520240.29643.e2

Hopkins, R. O., Suchyta, M. R., Kamdar, B. B., Darowski, E., Jackson, J. C., & Needham, D. M. (2017). Instrumental activities of daily living after critical illness: A systematic review. *Annals of the American Thoracic Society*, *14*(8), 1332-1343. https://doi.org/10.1513/annalsats.201701-059sr

Jette, A. M. Activities of daily living and instrumental activities of daily living. *Encyclopedia of Health & Aging*. https://doi.org/10.4135/9781412956208.n3

Karper, W. B. (2016). Effects of exercise, patient education, and resource support on women with fibromyalgia: An extended long-term study. *Journal of Women & Aging*, *28*(6), 555-562. https://doi.org/10.1080/08952841.2016.1223954

Mlinac, M. E., & Feng, M. C. (2016). Assessment of activities of daily living, self-care, and independence. *Archives of Clinical Neuropsychology*, *31*(6), 506-516. https://doi.org/10.1093/arclin/acw049

Schoenfeld, B. J., & Grgic, J. (2020). Effects of range of motion on muscle development during resistance training interventions: A systematic review. *SAGE Open Medicine*, *8*, 205031212090155. https://doi.org/10.1177/2050312120901559

Talley, K. M., Wyman, J. F., Savik, K., Kane, R. L., Mueller, C., & Zhao, H. (2015). Restorative care's effect on activities of daily living dependency in long-stay nursing home residents. *The Gerontologist*, *55*(Suppl 1), S88-S98. https://doi.org/10.1093/geront/gnv011

Wu, X., Li, Z., Cao, J., Jiao, J., Wang, Y., Liu, G., Liu, Y., Li, F., Song, B., Jin, J., Liu, Y., Wen, X., Cheng, S., & Wan, X. (2018). The association between major complications of immobility during hospitalization and quality of life among bedridden patients: A 3 month prospective multi-center study. *PLOS ONE*, *13*(10), e0205729. https://doi.org/10.1371/journal.pone.0205729

Yeung, K., Lin, C., Teng, Y., Chen, F., Lou, S., & Chen, C. (2016). Use of and self-perceived need for assistive devices in individuals with disabilities in Taiwan. *PLOS ONE*, *11*(3), e0152707. https://doi.org/10.1371/journal.pone.0152707

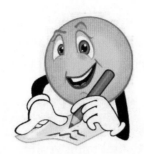

Chapter Fifteen:

Observation and Charting

Outline

I: Word Elements Used in Medical Terms

II: Common Medical Abbreviations

III: Observation and Senses Used to Observe a Patient/Resident

IV: Objective and Subjective Observations

V: Types of Charting Documents and Their Uses

VI: How to accurately complete ADL assessment for MDS?

VII: Procedures used for recording a patient/resident's chart

Words Elements Used in Medical Terms

Parts of words

Most of the medical terms consist of two or three components i.e. prefix, root, and suffix.

Prefix

The prefix is the beginning part of a word that is placed before a root and changes the meaning of the word. Not all medical words have a prefix. Prefixes can never be used alone. A prefix is usually added before the root to make the root more specific. For example, the prefix "olig" (small amount, scant) is placed before the root "uria" (urine) to make the word "oliguria", which means a scant amount of urine.

Root

The foundation of a word is called the word's root. All medical words have at least one root (some may have two), which may be the beginning part of the word. The root is the foundation of the word that contains the basic meaning of the word. It is combined with another root, suffix, or prefix. For example, in the word "cholecystectomy", the root is "cholecyst", which means "gallbladder" and the suffix is "ectomy", which means "removal of." So the word cholecystectomy is used for "removal of the gallbladder."

Suffix

The suffix is the ending part of the word that is placed after a root. Most medical words usually contain a suffix. A suffix changes the meaning of the word. They can never be used alone.

Combining vowel

A combining vowel joins a root to another suffix or root. For example, thermometer (therm heat; meter measuring device)

When translating a medical term, it should begin with the suffix. For example, the word "nephritis" means "inflammation of the kidney". It was formed by combining "nephro" (kidney) and "itis" (inflammation). Medical words are formed by combining multiple word components. It should be remembered that prefixes always come before roots and suffixes always come after roots. A root can be combined with other roots, prefixes, and suffixes. For example:

- The prefix "dys" (difficult) is combined with the root "pnea" (breathing) to forms the word "dyspnea". It means difficulty breathing.
- The root "mast" (breast) is combined with the suffix "ectomy" (removal or excision) to form mastectomy, which means removal of a breast.
- The prefix "endo" (inner) with the root "card" (heart) and the suffix "itis" (inflammation) to form "endocarditis, which means inflammation of the inner part of the heart.

Common Medical Abbreviations

Abbreviations are the short forms of words or phrases. They save space and time when recording observations. Each agency may have a list of accepted abbreviations. The nurse assistant should obtain the list when he/she is hired and should use only those on the list. If not sure about using an abbreviation, he/she should write the term out in full. The nurse assistant notices that the members of the health care team often use abbreviations while communicating with each other. Using appropriate abbreviations can make communication more efficient by saving space and time. Sometimes abbreviations are formed from the beginning letters of each word in a phrase, such as "DON" is used for "director of nursing." Others may be just shortened versions of a word, such as "cath" is used for "catheter." In many cases, abbreviations used in health care do not look to link to the words they stand for at all, such as "NPO", which means "nothing by mouth". It is originated from the Latin phrase "nils per os".

Common abbreviations	Meaning
Abd	Abdomen
Ac	Before a meal
ADLs	Activities of daily living
Adm	Admitted
AM	Morning
Amt	Amount
Amb	Ambulate
Approx	Approximately
ASAP	As soon as possible
Bid	Twice a day
BM	Bowel movement
BP	Blood pressure
BR	Bed rest
Cath	Catheter
CBR	Complete bed rest
Cc	Cubic centimeter
c/o	Complains of
CPR	Cardiopulmonary resuscitation
Disch	Discharge
DR	Dining room
H_2O	Water
HOB	Head of bed
I & O	Intake and output
IV	Intravenous
Liq	Liquid
Meds	Medications
Ml	Milliliter
NPO	Nothing by mouth
N & V	Nausea and vomiting
O	Oral
O_2	Oxygen
oc-bed	Occupied bed
OOB	Out of bed
OT	Occupational therapy
Pc	After meals
PM	Afternoon, evening
PRN	As needed

Q	Every
Qd	Every day
Qh	Every hour
Rehab	Rehabilitation
Resp	Respiration
ROM	Range of motion
SOB	Shortness of breath
ST	Speech therapy
STAT	Immediately
Tid	Three times a day
TPR	Temperature, pulse, respirations
TY	Tympanic
UTI	Urinary tract infection
VS	Vital signs
WA	While awake
w/c	Wheelchair
Wt	Weight

Observation and Senses Used to Observe a Patient/Resident

Observation is using the senses of hearing, sight, taste, touch, and smell to collect information. It is basically an assessment tool that depends on the use of the five senses (hearing, sight, touch, taste, and smell) to discover useful information about the patient/resident. This information links to characteristics of the patient/resident's appearance, functioning, primary relationships, and environment.

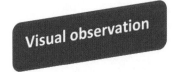

Visual observation

Sight provides lot of useful clues that a nurse assistant must continually process when assessing the patient/resident. A few examples of visual observations to consider are general appearance, mannerisms, body movements, mode of dress, facial expressions, nonverbal communication, interaction with others, skin color and appearance, use of space, and cleanliness. Visual observation can be used to collect subjective data, such as when noting the patient/resident's facial expression and body language. Visual observation can also be used to collect objective data.

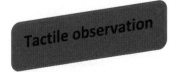

Tactile observation

The sense of touch provides an abundance of valuable information about the patient/resident. For example, palpation or touching of the skin may evaluate factors such as temperature, muscle strength, edema, moisture, rash, or swelling.

470

Hearing allows a nurse assistant to listen actively to the patient/resident and family as they interact with him/her and other members of the healthcare team. Specialized equipment can also be used to listen for information. For example, collection of data through auscultation (listening to the lung, heart, or bowel sounds with a stethoscope) and hearing the sounds of the pulse when measuring blood pressure with a stethoscope and sphygmomanometer.

Olfactory or gustatory observation

The sense of smell identifies multiple different odors that can be specific to a patient/resident's condition or state of health. Some pathogenic infections may have specific, identifiable odors. Olfactory observation includes noting breath and body odors, which might indicate poor hygiene, alcohol intoxication, or metabolic acidosis. The senses of taste and smell may also help to detect harmful chemicals in the air. It should be noted that a patient/resident who lacks a sense of smell is often anorexic (lacks an appetite) because smell stimulates specific taste sensations.

Objective and Subjective Observations

The nurse assistant spends a great deal of time with patients/residents in his/her care. As a result, he/she will often be the first to notice a change in the patient/resident's condition, abilities, or emotional status that should be reported to the licensed nurse. Observations about the patient/resident's condition may take two main forms:

Objective observations

These are related to information that is obtained directly, using one of five senses. For example, the nurse assistant may feel that a patient/resident's skin is dry and hot, or he/she may measure a patient/resident's blood pressure using a blood pressure cuff.

Subjective observations

Subjective observations are related to information that cannot be detected with one of five senses or cannot measure using equipment. For example, a patient/resident may tell that he/she has a headache or that he/she did not sleep well the night before. These are subjective observations because a nurse assistant cannot detect the patient/resident's pain or tiredness with his/her own senses. Instead, he/she must rely on what the patient/resident is telling.

The nurse assistant should report observations that indicate changes in the patient's:
- Mood
- Level of independence
- Behavior Mental awareness
- Vital signs
- Urine or bowel movements
- Skin condition or color
- Appetite
- Sleep habits
- Comfort level

If the nurse assistant is in doubt about whether he/she should report an observation to the nurse, he/she should remember "When in doubt, report" guidelines. It is best to report and share observations with the licensed nurse and let the nurse determine whether an additional follow-up is required. It should be remembered that the members of the health care team who do not have the opportunity to spend as much time with the patient/resident as the nurse assistant do depend heavily on the nurse assistant's observations.

Observations to report at once

- A change in the patient/resident's ability to respond
- A responsive patient/resident no longer responds
- A non-responsive patient/resident starts to respond
- A change in the patient/resident's mobility
- The patient/resident cannot move a body part
- The patient/resident starts to move a body part
- Complaints of sudden pain
- A reddened or sore area on the patient/resident's skin
- Complaints of a sudden changing in the patient/resident's vision
- Complaints of difficulty breathing
- Abnormal respirations
- Complaints or signs of difficulty swallowing
- Vomiting
- Bleeding
- Dizziness
- Vital signs beyond their normal ranges (pulse, temperature, respirations, and blood pressure)

Types of Charting Documents and their Uses

The medical record

The medical record or chart is the legal account of a patient/resident's condition and response to care and treatment. The health team uses this account to share information about the patient/resident. The medical record is a permanent legal document that can be used in court as legal evidence of the patient/resident's problems, care, and treatment. Healthcare agencies have policies about the patient/resident's medical records and who can access them. In some healthcare agencies, nursing assistants record care and observations. Professional healthcare staff involved in the patient/resident's care can review charts. If the nurse assistant has access to charts, he/she has a legal and an ethical duty to keep information confidential. If not involved in the patient/resident's care, the nurse assistant has no right to review the patient/resident's chart. Doing so is against of privacy.

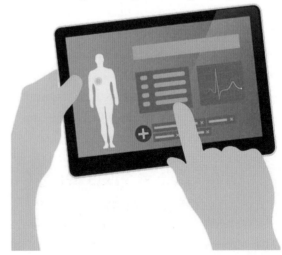

Common components of the medical record include:

Admission details: These are gathered when the patient/resident is admitted to the agency. It includes the patient's identifying information.

Health history: It is completed by the nurse. The nurse asks about past and current illnesses, signs and symptoms, medications, and allergies.

Flow sheets and graphic sheets: These are used to record observations, care measures, and measurements (made daily, every shift, or 3 to 4 times a day). Information may include vital signs (temperature, pulse, respirations, and blood pressure), weight, intake and output, doctor visits, bowel movements, and routine activities.

Progress notes and nurses' notes: They are used to demonstrate observations, the care given, and the patient/resident's response and progress. They are used to record information about treatments, some medications, procedures, and the care given. In long-term healthcare facilities, summaries of care demonstrate the patient/resident's progress toward meeting goals and response to care.

The comprehensive care plan

OBRA requires a comprehensive care plan that is a written guide about the patient/resident's care. The plan has the patient/resident's problems, goals for care, and actions to take. For example, Mr. Wayne is weak from illness and cannot do exercise. The MDS shows that he cannot perform activities of daily living (ADLs). A care plan is established to resolve the problem. The goal is for Mr. Wayne to perform his own ADLs. Actions to help Mr. Wayne reach the goal are:

- Occupational therapy to work with Mr. Wayne on ADL daily
- Physical therapy to work with Mr. Wayne on exercises daily
- Nursing staff to walk Mr. Wayne 25 yards twice daily. The comprehensive care plan also demonstrates the patient/resident's strengths. For example, Mr. Wayne can feed himself. This feeding strength increases his independence. The health team helps Mr. Wayne continue to feed himself that increases his independence.

Nursing care plan

The nursing care plan is a written guide about the patient/resident's nursing care. It has the patient/resident's nursing diagnoses and goals. It also contains measures or actions to meet each goal. The nursing care plan is a communication tool. Nursing staff use this tool to see what care to provide. The nursing care plan helps ensure that nursing team members provide the same care. Each healthcare agency may have a care plan form that is found in the medical record. The plan is carried out and may change as the patient/resident's nursing diagnoses change.

ADL sheet

It is a checklist to assess a patient/resident's functioning level as it relates to Instrumental Activities of Daily Living (IADL) and Activities of Daily Living (ADL). ADL sheet can provide help in determining the level of assistance that a patient/resident's needs. The nurse assistant should use it to document care at each shift for activities of daily living 2. ADL sheet is a record on which most healthcare facilities have the care work chart.

How to Accurately Complete ADL Assessment for MDS?

The Minimum Data Set

The Omnibus Budget Reconciliation Act of 1987 (OBRA) requires the Minimum Data Set (MDS) for nursing center residents. It provides comprehensive information about the patient/resident. Examples include communication, memory, hearing and vision, physical function, and activities. The nurse uses the observations of the nurse assistant to complete the MDS. The MDS is initiated when the patient/resident is admitted to the center. It is edited and updated before each care conference. A new MDS should be completed once a year and whenever an important change occurs in the patient/resident's health status.

Resident Assessment Instrument (RAI)

The utilization of the components of the RAI provides information about a patient/resident's functional status, weaknesses, strengths, and preferences, as well as offering guidance on further assessments once issues have been identified. The MDS has almost 450 items to addresses clinical and functional aspects of the patient/resident such as physical functioning, sensory, cognition, oral health, nutrition, skin, mobility, elimination, clinical conditions or diseases, etc. The MDS only indicates if the patient/resident has a problem; however, it does not determine the cause of the problem. Therefore, there are Care Area Assessment resources that are available to help nurses do further assessments specific to the identified problem (e.g. dehydration, delirium). The RAI process drives the care plan that is developed for the resident. The MDS is an excellent teaching tool to use with students in the nursing home setting.

Assessment Reference Day (ARD)

The Assessment Reference Day (ARD) is the day that signifies the end of the look back period. This ARD can be used to base responses to all MDS coding items.

The major of the ARD is to establish a common temporal reference point for all staff members of the team participating in the patient/resident's assessment. Although team members may work on competing a patient/resident's MDS on different days, establishment of the ARD ensures the commonality of the assessment period.

The ARD is the last day of MDS observation period. This day refers to a specific endpoint in the process of MDS assessment. Almost all MDS items refer to the patient/resident's status over a defined time period, most frequently the 7 day period ending on this date. The ARD sets the defined endpoint of the common observation period, and all MDS items refer back in time from this point. For example, when the ARD is March, the look back period of observation will start from March 2 until March 8.

Activities of Daily Living (ADLs)

It is very important to encourage patients/residents to become as independent as possible. The nurse assistant should assist patients/residents by providing them physical care and encouragement and by helping them with self-care. It is important for all patients/residents to perform as much self-care as possible. When the rehabilitation team has thoroughly assessed the patient/resident and determined what functional capacity is realistic, a comprehensive plan of retraining in ADLs is initiated.

There are two categories of ADL section:

Patient/resident ADL Self-performance

The ADL self-performance determines what the patient/resident can actually do for himself or herself or/and how much physical or verbal assistance is required by staff members during all shifts.

Patient/resident ADL support

These are activities and support provided by staff members and valuable for evaluating patients/residents with early-stage disease.

Self-performance codes

- 0= INDEPENDENT (NO TALK – NO TOUCH): No help or staff helps oversight provided. It was done one or two times during the last 7 days.

- 1= Supervision (TALK – NO TOUCH): Supervision, oversight, cues (verbal), encouragement (with voice), and observation (the patient/resident has been watched thru the open door) provided three or more times during the last seven days OR supervision and physical assistance provided, but only one or two times during the last 7 days.

- 2= LIMITED ASSISTANCE (TALK AND TOUCH): The patient/resident is highly involved in physical activity. He/she received physical help in guided maneuvering of limbs or other non-weight-bearing assistance on three or more occasions OR limited assistance and more weight bearing support provided, but for only one or two times during the last 7 days.

- 3= EXTENSIVE ASSISTANCE (TALK, TOUCH, AND LIFT): The patient/resident performed part of the activity, but weight bearing assistance. (Someone lifted a part of the body) was required.

- 4 = TOTAL DEPENDENCE: The patient/ resident didn't lift a finger to help with any part of the activity. There will be the full staff performance of the activity during the last seven-day period. There is complete non-participation and non-involvement by the patient/resident in almost all aspects of the ADL tasks.

- 8= Activity didn't occur. Over the last 7 days, the ADL activity was not performed by the staff or the patient/resident. The particular activity did not occur at all during the last 7 days.

Staff performance codes

- 0 = NO STAFF PERFORMANCE REQUIRED and there is no set up or physical help from staff.

- 1= SET UP HELP ONLY: Maybe a nurse assistant undid a cover, set the wheelchair at bedside, or placed the walker in front of the patient/resident.

- 2= ONE PERSON physical assistance. It can be considered as: 2 = the resident and the nurse assistant.

- 3 = 2 OR MORE PHYSICALLY ASSISTED. It can be considered as: 3 = the resident, the nurse assistant, and someone else.

- 8 = ADL activity didn't occur DURING THE ENTIRE 7 days.

Procedures Used for Recording a Patient/Resident's Chart

Because the medical record or chart is a legal document, the following principles should be strictly followed when writing in the record:

- The nurse assistant should make sure that he/she has the correct chart or ADL sheet.
- The notes should be written manually on paper first and then should be checked for spelling as well as accuracy.
- All the events should be recorded in proper sequence.
- The nurse assistant should always follow the facility's policies and standards while writing in the medical record.
- The nurse assistant should be concise and should use appropriate abbreviations and terms as per agency's policies.
- **Ballpoint pen with black ink should be used** if the entries are handwritten.
- The **patient/resident's name and any other information as the facility mandates** must be clearly written. The information should be included on every page of the record.
- The nurse should note the **date and time** at the beginning of each entry. The nurse assistant should record his/her signature at the end. For example; K. Park, Nurse Assistant or J. John, NA.
- If an incorrect entry is made, the nurse assistant should **draw a single line through the mistake**. The nurse assistant should write "error," the name of the individual making the change, the reason for correction, and the date next to the entry. The nurse assistant should **not erase** or obliterate any part of the record.

Most facilities usually use a computerized charting system. Confidentiality and privacy are important factors for using computerized charting systems. To fulfil the requirements of confidentiality and privacy, systems must be password protected. Each user should receive a personal password that should be never shared with others. Sharing or using another's password may be grounds for termination. If a practice is using electronic health records (EHR), the system typically restricts access to certain information from those users who do not need or have authorization to view it.

- If a facility is using the digital record-keeping system, the changes must be recorded and traceable in the same manner as handwritten records.
- **Every aspect of a patient/resident's care must be documented**. Legally, it is practically impossible to prove a certain action was taken unless it was recorded and documented in the patient/resident's medical record.

Legal issues of charting

Patient's/resident's record or chart is a legal document that can be used in a court of law. Information in the medical record must be kept confidential. Information regarding the patient/resident's health in the chart must be objective, accurate, and truthful. The Nurse Assistant can access only to the medical records of the patients/residents for whom they are caring.

Helpful Resources

Abbreviations and acronyms. (2014). *Nursing & Health Survival Guide: Medical Abbreviations & Normal Ranges*, 5-26. https://doi.org/10.4324/9781315848150-4

Baddeley, A., & Hull, A. (1979). Prefix and suffix effects: Do they have a common basis? *Journal of Verbal Learning and Verbal Behavior*, *18*(2), 129-140. https://doi.org/10.1016/s0022-5371(79)90082-3

Carins, J. (2016). Visual observation techniques. *Formative Research in Social Marketing*, 107-123. https://doi.org/10.1007/978-981-10-1829-9_7

Deschrijver, E., Wiersema, J. R., & Brass, M. (2015). The interaction between felt touch and tactile consequences of observed actions: An action-based somatosensory congruency paradigm. *Social Cognitive and Affective Neuroscience*, *11*(7), 1162-1172. https://doi.org/10.1093/scan/nsv081

Honavar, S. (2020). Electronic medical records – The good, the bad and the ugly. *Indian Journal of Ophthalmology*, *68*(3), 417. https://doi.org/10.4103/ijo.ijo_278_20

Nurses can facilitate quality improvement in primary care practices with electronic medical records. (2008). *PsycEXTRA Dataset*. https://doi.org/10.1037/e459442008-025

SCHNEIDER, M. E. (2006). Electronic records can improve quality of care. *Internal Medicine News*, *39*(9), 66. https://doi.org/10.1016/s1097-8690(06)73480-1

Snyder, J. S., Gregg, M. K., Weintraub, D. M., & Alain, C. (2012). Attention, awareness, and

the perception of auditory scenes. *Frontiers in Psychology, 3.*

https://doi.org/10.3389/fpsyg.2012.00015

Tsai, J., & Bond, G. (2007). A comparison of electronic records to paper records in mental

health centers. *International Journal for Quality in Health Care, 20*(2), 136-143.

https://doi.org/10.1093/intqhc/mzm064

Wolfe, L., Chisolm, M. S., & Bohsali, F. (2018). Clinically excellent use of the electronic

health record: Review. *JMIR Human Factors, 5*(4), e10426. https://doi.org/10.2196/10426

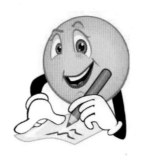

Chapter Sixteen:

Death and Dying

Outline

I: The Five Stages of Grieving

II: Providing End of Life Care

III: Rights of the Dying Patient/Resident

IV: Difference between Signs of Approaching Death and Biological Death

V: Comfort Measures for the Dying Patient/Resident

VI: Hospices and the Nurse Assistant's Role in Providing Hospice Care

VII: Care of the Body After Death

The Five Stages of Grieving

Dr. Elisabeth Kübler-Ross has demonstrated certain phases through which an individual may pass in an attempt to cope with impending death. Formerly referred to as the phases of death and dying, Dr. Elisabeth Kübler-Ross's traditional phases are more commonly linked with the stages of grief and loss. This is because the idea that loss, grief, and death have been identified as separate topics having similar stages of human behavior. Grief is common to all persons; however, not all persons experience grief in the same way. Nursing assistants must be aware that there is no right or correct way to grieve; that is, there is no wrong or right way to experience the pain of loss, grief, or death. Nursing assistants must also be aware that coping with the physical, emotional, and psychological pain of this experience has the potential to be healing and to strengthen those individuals going through this process. Dr. Elisabeth Kübler-Ross's theory suggests that individuals go through five distinct stages of grief after the loss of a loved one i.e. Denial, anger, bargaining, depression, and finally acceptance.

Denial

It is a way of dealing with information that is not easy to accept. Denial lets the individual to put information aside until he/she is emotionally ready to deal with it. In this way, denial helps to protect the individual from overwhelming sadness. An individual who is experiencing denial may insist that members of the health care team are wrong about a diagnosis or may delay following up with recommended tests, care, or treatments. The ideal way to respond to an individual who is experiencing denial is in a honest, yet supportive way. For example, if an individual says to the nurse assistant, "The physician must be wrong. My mother was fine last week, and now they are informing me she might not live another 4 months?" the nurse assistant could respond, "I'm really sorry; this must be very difficult for you." Eventually, the individual will be able to process the information that he/she has been provided and will begin to accept the reality of the condition, but right now he/she cannot. It is important to allow her to process the information at her own pace. It is also important to recognize that throughout the end-of-life period, a person may move back and forth between periods of denial and reality.

Denial is basically the preliminary stage that occurs when the patient/resident does not believe that the diagnosis is right. During this phase, the patient/resident may seek advice from several physicians, expecting that one of them will offer a more acceptable and right prognosis. Because hope is maintained, the patient/resident is susceptible to illegal, unorthodox, or harmful ways of coping with a diagnosis.

Anger

Many patients/residents experience feelings of anger during their end-of-life period. The patient/resident may be angry because he/she feels that the condition is unfair or because he/she feels that maybe there was anything that could have been done to protect the condition. Sometimes

481

the feelings of anger are directed inward, and other times these feelings are directed at others. The patient/resident may even direct his/her anger at a higher being and experience a loss of faith. Patients/residents show anger in different ways. Some patients/residents may become withdrawn and moody, whereas others may criticize others unfairly. If a patient/resident's anger is directed unfairly toward the nurse assistant, it is important for the nurse assistant to remember where that anger may be coming from and to avoid taking it personally.

Bargaining

It is a phase of developing awareness of the situation. An individual bargains or makes deals with God or with herself or himself. The timeframe for this phase may be relatively short. When the time period for bargaining has passed, the patient/resident may make another such bargain, in the expectations of postponing death indefinitely.

Depression

Depression occurs when the patient/resident realizes that he or she is going to die and that nothing can stop him/her from dying. Unlike some forms of psychologically diagnosed depression, this phase and form of depression can be considered a normal and healthy phase. However, it may be beneficial for the patient/resident and family members to receive psychotherapy, including medication.

Acceptance

Acceptance is a stage of peaceful resignation. The patient/resident feels at peace with the future and what the future holds. The patient/resident may experience a sense of calmness and of being able to let go and further move on. Acceptance does not mean that the patient/resident has given up his/her hope. It simply means that the patient/resident has emotionally reached a place that allows him/her to be at peace with the reality of the condition.

Providing End of Life Care

Caregivers having not much previous experience with death and dying, so much worry about their abilities to provide end-of-life care. Preparation of end-of-life care can also make caregivers uncomfortable because it needs them to think about their own mortality. For many individuals, this may be very frightening. To effectively help others through the end-of-life phase, the nurse assistant must first address his/her own feelings about death and dying and the concerns that he/she may have about providing end-of-life care.

The cultural and spiritual or religious beliefs and past experiences of a caregiver with death and dying can influence how he/she feels about death and dying. Providing end-of-life care can be mentally and emotionally difficult, but it can also be extremely rewarding. The nurse assistant will help all the patients/residents in his/her care to meet their social, physical, emotional, and spiritual needs. These needs do not go away during the end-of-life phase; in fact, these needs may increase during this period. By helping the patient/resident to meet these needs and showing compassion and empathy, the nurse assistant can make a significant difference in the end-of-life phase for the patient/resident and his/her family members.

Emotional needs of the dying patient/resident

There are certain emotional needs of the dying patients/residents that may include:

- Contact with their loved ones including friends and family members.
- Proper communication with the patient/resident through listening and touching.
- Expression of emotions including anger, guilt, anxiety, frustration, and depression.
- Reminiscence that can be achieved through recalling life experiences and listening important things.

Providing emotional support

The end-of-life phase is a phase of emotional preparation, for both the patient/resident and those close to the patient/resident. A patient/resident's feelings about death can be influenced by multiple different factors, including:

- The patient/resident's culture.
- The patient/resident's religious or spiritual beliefs.
- The patient/resident's past experiences with death (for example, deaths of friends or family members).
- The patient/resident's sense of having lived a complete and full life.
- The patient/resident's current quality of life (for example, if the patient/resident has had a long struggle with an illness, death may be considered as a release from a state of suffering).

Cultural and spiritual needs

Attitudes and behaviors about death differ among different cultures. In some cultures, dying persons are cared for at home by the family members. Some families prepare the body themselves for burial. Spiritual needs are linked to the human spirit and religious beliefs. Many individuals strengthen their religious beliefs when dying. Religion provides comfort for the dying individual and the family members. Attitudes and behaviors about death are closely linked to the religion. Some people believe that life after death is free of hardships and suffering. They also believe in reunion with friends and family members after death. Many believe misdeeds and sins are punished in the afterlife. Others do not totally believe in the afterlife. To them, death is just an end of life. There are also religious beliefs about the form of body after death. Some people believe the dead body keeps its physical form. Others believe that only the soul or spirit is present in the afterlife. Many religions practice rituals and rites during the dying process and at the time of death. Blessings, prayers, scripture readings, and religious music are the major sources of comfort.

Respecting cultural and religious customs

Many cultures and religions have their own rituals and customs relating to death. Specific rituals and rituals may have to be done before or at the time of death, or as a component of the care that is provided after death. Ahead of time, the nurse assistant should make sure that he/she is aware if something special needs to be done. This information should be recorded in the patient/resident's care plan. If the cultural or religious practices are not properly followed, the family may experience additional unnecessary grief. Not only will the family has to deal with the loss of a loved one, but the family may also feel anger or guilt associated with not performing an important ritual. Some patients/residents may request and receive visits from clergy members throughout the end-of-life phase. The nurse assistant should report a patient/resident's request to see a clergy member to the nurse immediately, so that the necessary arrangements can be made for the visit.

Physical needs

Dying process may take a few minutes, hours, days, or weeks. Body processes become slow. The patient/resident becomes weak. Physical changes occur in levels of consciousness. As the patient/resident weakens, basic needs should be met. Every effort should be made to promote psychological and physical comfort. The patient/resident should be allowed to die in peace and with dignity.

Throughout the end-of-life phase, ensuring the patient/resident's physical and psychological comfort is important. Conditions that a dying patient/resident may experience in the months leading up to death may include pain, digestive problems, and shortness of breath. These situations can be uncomfortable for the patient/resident and distressing to the

family. It is important for nursing assistants to become familiar with these conditions, and recognize them when they occur. Nursing assistants should report them promptly so that steps can be taken to relieve them.

Pain
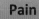

Some dying patients/residents do not have pain. Others may have severe pain. The nurse assistant should always report signs and symptoms of pain at once. The nurse can give pain-relief medications to control or prevent pain. Skin care, back massages, personal and oral hygiene, and proper alignment may promote comfort. The nurse assistant should do frequent position changes and supportive devices. The patient/resident should be turned slowly and gently. The nurse assistant should always follow the care plan to prevent and control pain.

Breathing problems

Difficulty breathing (dyspnea) and shortness of breath are common end-of-life problems. Oxygen administrations and Semi-Fowler's position can be helpful. An open window for fresh air may also help some patients/residents to breathe in fresh air. Noisy breathing (death rattle) is common as death nears. This is due to mucus collecting in the airway. These measures may help for managing breathing problems:
- The side-lying position
- Proper suctioning by the nurse
- Medications to reduce the amount of mucus

Vision blurs and fails gradually. The patients/resident turns toward light. A darkened room may frighten the patient/resident. The eyes may be half-close and half-open. Secretions may collect in the corners of eye. Because of blur vision, the nurse assistant should explain who he/she is and what he/she is doing to the patient/resident or in the room. The room should be lightened properly. However, bright lights and glares should be avoided.

Good eye care is required for these patients/residents. If the eyes remain open, a protective ointment may be applied by the nurse. Then the eyes should be covered with moist pads to prevent injury. Hearing is one of the last senses lost. Many patients/residents can hear until the moment of death. Even unconscious patients/residents may hear. The nurse assistant should always assume that the patient/resident can hear and should speak in a normal voice. He/she should provide reassurance and explanations about care to the patient/resident and should offer words of comfort.

The nurse assistant should avoid topics that could upset the patient/resident and should not talk about him/her. Speech becomes difficult. It may be difficult to understand the patient/resident. Sometimes the patient/resident cannot even speak. The nurse assistant should anticipate the patient/resident's needs and should not ask questions that require long answers. Despite speech problems, the nurse assistant must talk to the patient/resident.

Oral hygiene promotes comfort. The nurse assistant should provide routine mouth care if the patient/resident can eat and drink. He/she should provide frequent oral hygiene as death nears and when taking oral fluids is hard. Oral hygiene is required if mucus collects in the mouth and the patient/resident cannot swallow. A lip balm may help dry the patient/resident's lips. Irritation and crusting of the nostrils can occur. Oxygen cannula, nasal secretions, and naso-gastric tube are common causes.

The nose should be carefully cleaned the nose and a lubricant should be applied as directed by the nurse and the care plan. Body temperature rises and circulation fails as death nears. The skin becomes pale, cool, and mottled (blotchy). Bathing, skin care, and preventing pressure ulcers are necessary.

Gowns and linens should be changed as needed. Although the skin feels cool and clammy, only light bed coverings are required. Blankets may make the patient/resident feel warm and cause restlessness. However, the nurse assistant should observe for signs of cold. Hunching shoulders, shivering, and pulling covers up may indicate that the patient/resident is feeling cold. Drafts should be prevented and more blankets should be provided.

Nutrition

Vomiting, nausea, and loss of appetite are common at the end of life. The physician may order medications for nausea and vomiting. The nurse assistant may need to feed the patient/resident. Small, favorite, and frequent meals may help loss of appetite. Loss of appetite is common as death nears. The patient/resident may choose not to drink or eat. The nurse assistant should not force the patient/resident to eat or drink and should report refusal to eat or drink to the nurse.

Elimination

Fecal and urinary incontinence may occur. Incontinence products or bed protectors should be used as directed. Perineal care should be provided as needed. Urinary retention and constipation are common. Urinary catheters and enemas may be needed. The nurse assistant should always follow the care plan for catheter care.

The patient/resident's room

A comfortable and pleasant room should be provided to the patient/resident. It should be well ventilated and well lit. Unnecessary equipment should be removed. Some equipment is upsetting to look at (drainage containers, suction machines). If possible, these items should be kept out of the patient/resident's sight. Pictures, cards, mementos, flowers, and religious items provide comfort. The patient/resident and family should arrange the room as they wish. This helps meet love, esteem, and belonging needs. The room should reflect the patient/resident's choices.

Emotional and mental needs

Emotional and mental needs are very personal. Some patients/residents are anxious or depressed. Others may have specific concerns or fears. Examples include:

- Severe pain
- How and when death will occur?
- What will happen to family and friends?
- Dying alone

Simple measures may soothe the patient/resident—touch, back massages, holding hands, soft lighting, and music at a low volume.

Providing assistance with repositioning according to the patient/resident's care plan

Many patients/residents lose their ability to reposition themselves as their condition worsens. Assisting with repositioning according to the patient/resident's care plan minimizes the patient/resident's risk for pressure sores and promotes comfort by ensuring proper body alignment. If equipment is available to assist with repositioning, the nurse assistant should be sure to use it properly.

The Rights of the Dying Patient/Resident

- The right to be treated as a living human being until death.
- The right to maintain a feeling and sense of hopefulness, however changing its focus may be.

- The right to be cared for by those caregivers who can maintain a feeling and sense of hopefulness, however changing this may be.
- The right to express emotions and feelings about death in one's own way.
- The right to participate in all relevant decisions concerning one's care.
- The right to be cared for by sensitive, compassionate, and knowledgeable people who will try to understand one's needs.
- The right to expect continuing medical care and nursing attention, even though the objectives may change from "cure" to "comfort" goals.
- The right to have all questions answered fully and honestly.
- The right to seek spirituality and express religious and/or spiritual experiences, whatever these may mean to others
- The right to be free from physical pain.
- The right to express emotions and feelings about pain in one's own way.
- The right of children and family to participate in death.
- The right to understand the process of death in a proper way.
- The right to die in peace and dignity.
- The right to not die alone.
- The right to expect that the sanctity of the human body will be respected after death.
- The right to retain individuality and not to be judged for one's decisions which may be contrary to beliefs of others.

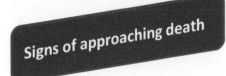

Difference between Signs of Approaching Death and Biological Death

Signs of approaching death

As death nears, these signs may occur fast or gradually:

- Weak, rapid, or irregular pulse
- Decreased blood pressure
- Pale, cool, and moist skin
- Coolness and mottling of the feet and hands
- Incontinence
- Periods of increased, shallow breathing followed by periods of decreased respiration
- A gargling sound with breathing due to mucus in the airway
- Loss of consciousness
- Loss of movement
- Loss of the ability to communicate
- Decrease of peristalsis. Abdominal distention, nausea, vomiting, and fecal incontinence are common.

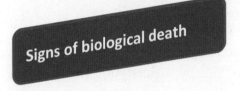

Signs of biological death

The signs of biological death may include no pulse, no respirations, and no blood pressure. The pupils become fixed and dilated. A physician determines that death has occurred and he or she pronounces the person dead.

Identification of signs of biological death

Drying of cornea

These signs include the loss of their original color by the iris, the appearance of the covering of the eye with a whitish film called "herring shine", and the cloudiness of the pupil.

The phenomenon of "cat pupil"

The eyeball is squeezed with the forefinger and thumb, if an individual is dead, then his/her pupil will change shape and turn into a narrow gap called the "cat pupil". In a living individual, this phenomenon is not possible.

Decrease of body temperature

The body temperature gradually drops, almost 1 degree Celsius every hour after death. Therefore, according to these signs, death can only be certified after 2–4 hours and later.

Cadaverous spots

Cadaverous spots of purple color may appear on the underlying parts of the corpse. If it lies on the back, then they can be determined on the head behind the ears, on the back of the hips and shoulders, and on the back and buttocks.

Rigor mortis

Rigor mortis is the post-mortem contraction of skeletal muscles "from top to bottom".

Comfort Measures for the Dying Patient/Resident

Comfort is a basic component of end-of-life care. It involves physical, social, mental and emotional, and spiritual needs.

The major comfort goals are to:

- Relieve or prevent suffering to the extent possible.
- Respect and follow end-of-life wishes. Dying patients/residents may want family and friends present. They may want to talk about their worries, fears, and anxieties. Some patients/residents want to be alone.
- **Listening:** The patients/residents need to talk and share their concerns and worries. The patient/resident should be allowed to express their feelings and emotions in his/her own way.
- **Touch:** Touch shows concern and care when words cannot. Sometimes the patient/resident does not want to talk but needs someone nearby. The nurse assistant should not feel that he/she need to talk. Silence, along with touch, is a meaningful and powerful way to communicate.

Some patients/residents may want to see a spiritual leader. They may also want to take part in religious practices. The nurse assistant should provide privacy during prayer and spiritual moments. The patient/resident has the right to have religious objects nearby such as pictures, medals, writings, and statues etc. These valuables should be handled with care and respect.

All individuals have the right to a comfortable and peaceful death. For many individuals, this means selecting to forego life-sustaining treatments, such as cardiopulmonary resuscitation (CPR) or mechanical ventilation at the end of life, if having these treatments will prolong their suffering. When a patient/resident chooses to forego life-sustaining treatments at the end of life, the patient/resident's primary care provider will write an order called as "do-not-resuscitate (DNR) order". This DNR order means that the health care team should not start mechanical ventilation or CPR if the patient/resident's heart stops or breathing stops.

When a patient/resident has a DNR order, all members of the health care team should be aware of this order, so that the patient/resident's wishes can be honored. A desire to forego life-sustaining treatments at the end of life phase does not mean that the patient/resident wishes to forego all care at the end of life. Instead, many patients/residents choose to receive only supportive (comfort) care (care that will make the patient/resident more comfortable but will not prolong the patient/resident's life, such as administration of pain medications, oxygen therapy, and personal care). In many states, these personal wishes are communicated through a do-not-resuscitate/comfort care (DNR-CC) order. As a component of comfort care, palliative treatments may be offered to relieve

uncomfortable symptoms without actually curing the disease that is causing the symptoms. For example, if a patient/resident has a tumor that is pressing on another organ and causing severe pain, surgery may be performed to minimize the size of the tumor to relieve the severe pain. In this case, the surgery is palliative because it was performed to provide pain relief, not to treat the cancer.

Sometimes comfort care may also involve eliminating routine treatments or procedures that are no longer of benefit to the patient/resident, such as providing a therapeutic diet, routine weight measurements, or routine blood glucose measurement. The major goal of comfort care is to help the patient/resident have the best quality of life up until the time of death.

Hospices and the Nurse Assistant's Role in Providing Hospice Care

A hospice is a health care program or agency for patients/residents who are dying. Such patients/residents no longer respond to treatments aimed at cures. Usually these patients/residents have less than 6 months to live.

Hospice care

The main focus of hospice is on the physical, social, emotional, and spiritual needs of dying patients/residents and their families. Often the patient/resident has less than 6 months to live. Hospice care does not involve treatment or life-saving measures. Pain relief and comfort measures are more stressed in hospice care. The major goal is to improve quality of life.

Follow-up care and support groups for survivors are major components of hospice services. Hospice also involves support for the health team to help deal with a patient/resident's death.

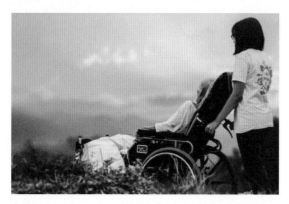

Hospice is a model of care that mainly focuses on providing comfort care to individuals who are dying, and on supporting their families, during the end-of-life phase. The hospice model of care is usually based on several core beliefs such as:

- Dying is a normal and expected component of the life cycle.
- The dying individual should not be separated from family, friends, and other support systems.
- Care for the dying individual and family must address the individual's and family's physical, social, emotional, and spiritual needs.
- Care for the dying individual seeks to relieve pain and other distressing symptoms that an individual may experience during the end-of-life phase.
- Care seeks to help the individual die with dignity, by honoring the individual's preferences for end-of-life care.

Evolution of the hospice nursing

The word hospice is derived from a medieval word meaning "to provide shelter for travelers on difficult and hard journeys." The concept of hospice acknowledges that not all diseases are curable and focuses management of uncomfortable symptoms. The primary and driving force behind the modern hospice movement was Dame Cicely Saunders, who founded St. Christopher's Hospice in 1967 in London. She stated that healthcare workers should perform everything possible not only to help individuals die peacefully, but also to support and help them "to live until they die." In 1974, Florence Wald started the first U.S. hospice in New Haven, Connecticut as a home care program. It was later named the Connecticut Hospice. Other early hospice projects were situated in Boonton New Jersey, and Tucson Arizona. Legislation in the U.S. has greatly influenced the hospice movement. For example, managed care plans, government agencies, and private insurance are now allowed to pay for hospice care. In 1991, Congress passed the Patient Self Determination Act (PSDA) to allow people more freedom regarding end-of-life care.

The hospice concept

Most U.S. hospice programs are community-based and independent or divisions of hospitals, nursing homes or home health agencies. There are some independent hospice corporations. Most hospices admit patients/residents with cancer, as well as other diagnoses; many other admit patients/residents with AIDS (acquired immunodeficiency syndrome). Almost 80-90% of hospices in the U.S. admit terminally ill children. Many hospices require patients/residents to have primary caregivers at home; other programs may consider individual cases. About half of U.S. hospices admit patients/residents who need high-tech therapies, such as tube feedings, intravenous (IV) medications, or supplemental oxygen. Most hospice patients/residents are older than 75, although they can be of any age.

Major goals of a hospice

The hospice care mainly focuses on four major areas of human needs:
- Physical
- Psychological/emotional
- Social/cultural
- Spiritual

The major goals of hospice are:
- Relief of severe and distressing symptoms
- Provision of professional care and a safe environment
- Assurance that the patient/resident and family will not be abandoned

Characteristics of a hospice

For a hospice agency, the following criteria must be fulfilled:
- The hospice should be a centrally administered, autonomous program and staff members and family caregivers mainly provide care, with backup inpatient medical services.

- The goal should be symptom control (intensive palliative care), instead of curative measures. Patients/residents should remain as alert and comfortable as possible.
- The major unit of hospice care should be the patient/resident and his or her family. The term "family" refers to a patient/resident's significant others, whether related by blood or not.
- Team members of a hospice agency should practice interdisciplinary care, under a qualified physician's guidelines and consultation should be available at all times, day or night. Specially trained volunteers should also be available to provide their services.
- Proper support should always be available for hospice staff and for the patient/resident's caregivers.
- Hospice services must be extended to the family during the bereavement period for at least one year.
- Hospice services must be centered on a patient/resident's needs, not on financial resources.

Providing care in hospice nursing

- The nurse assistants should emphasize on the positive things and should focus on what can be done, not on problems.
- They should provide practical solutions to control the patient/resident's symptoms.
- They should not try to predict the exact time of death and should not get involved in family disputes.

- They should allow the patient/resident and family to express spiritual feelings in the way they desire.
- They should respect the patient/resident's cultural customs and beliefs and should maintain his/her sense of humor.
- They should allow the patient/resident to be alone or stay with the patient/resident, depending on what he or she desires.
- They should recognize that acting out behaviors by the family and the hospice patient/resident is a normal part of grieving.
- They should be honest and should explain what is happening.
- They should allow the patient/resident and family to maintain hope, at whatever level.
- They should provide care within scope of practice as recommended by the multidisciplinary team.

Care of the Body after Death

Care of the body after death is called as post-mortem care. The nurse assistant may be asked to assist the nurse. Post-mortem care starts when the patient/resident is pronounced dead. Post-mortem care is performed to maintain a proper appearance of the body. Skin damage and discoloration are prevented. Personal items and valuables should be gathered for the family. The right to privacy and the right to be treated with respect and dignity apply after death. Within 3 to 4 hours after death, rigor mortis occurs. Rigor mortis is the rigidity or stiffness (rigor) of skeletal muscles that occurs after death (mortis). The body should be positioned in normal alignment before rigor mortis occurs. The family may want to see the dead body. The body should appear in a natural and comfortable position.

Depending on the employer's policy, the nurse assistant may be responsible for assisting with postmortem care. Postmortem care involves positioning, cleaning, and identifying the body. After death, the bowels and bladder may empty, so the skin needs to be cleaned and the linens and clothing should be changed. The body can be wrapped in a cloth covering known as a shroud. Certain rituals may need to be followed according to the patient/resident's cultural or religious beliefs. The nurse assistant should make sure that he/she is aware of these rituals and that the necessary arrangements have been done to permit the rituals to be carried out according to the family's wishes. When the nurse assistant is providing postmortem care, he/she should ensure privacy and should handle the patient/resident's body with respect and care.

In some healthcare agencies, the dead body is prepared only for viewing by the family. The funeral director completes post-mortem care and sometimes an autopsy is also performed. An autopsy is the examination of the dead body after death. It is performed to determine the cause of death. The coroner or medical examiner may order an autopsy. The family can also request to know the cause of death.

Encouraging comfort and safety

Standard Precautions and the Bloodborne Pathogen Standard should be followed in post-mortem care. The nurse assistant may have contact with body fluids, blood, secretions, and excretions.

Providing postmortem care

The nurse assistant should provide assistance for providing post-mortem care in following ways:

1. Hands should be washed properly.
2. The nurse assist should gather all supplies:
   - Gloves
   - Bed protector
   - Bath blanket
   - Clean gown
   - Wash cloth
   - Towel
   - Wash basin
   - Soap
   - Identification tags (one or two, depending on whether a shroud is used)
   - Envelope or plastic bag for small personal items and an inventory sheet
   - Shroud (if used)
   - Clean linens (if needed)
3. The nurse assistant should knock, greet the patient/resident and should ensure his/her privacy.
4. The procedure should be explained thoroughly to the patient/resident.
5. Equipment should be adjusted for proper body mechanics and safety: the bed should be raised to a comfortable working height. It should be ensured that the wheels on the bed are locked.
6. The over-bed table should be covered with the paper towels. The nurse assistant should arrange his/her supplies and should fill the wash basin with warm water. The wash basin should be placed on the over-bed table.
7. The nurse assistant should put on the gloves and should lower the head of the bed. The body should be placed in the supine position.
8. The person's eyes should be closed.
9. With approval from the nurse, the nurse assistant should remove any medical equipment.
10. Jewelery should be removed and placed in the envelope or plastic bag designated for the patient/resident's belongings. The nurse assistant should record each item on the inventory sheet as he/she removes it.

11. If the patient/resident wears dentures and they were not in the patient/resident's mouth at the time of death, the nurse assistant should replace the dentures in the patient/resident's mouth and close the patient/resident's mouth.

12. The bath blanket should be placed over the body, and the patient/resident's clothing should be removed. The body should be washed and dried, and then dressed in the clean gown.

13. An identification tag should be put around the patient/resident's ankle.

14. The linens should be replaced, if necessary. The bed protector should be placed under the patient/resident's buttocks. The top sheet should be drawn over the patient/resident's legs and torso to make a cuff. The patient/resident's face should not be covered.

15. If the family would like to see the body, the nurse assistant should clean up his/her work area and should dim the lights before inviting the family back in. Proper privacy should be provided and the nurse assistant should leave the room.

16. After the family leaves, the nurse assistant should return to the room and complete the postmortem care procedure.

17. If a shroud is to be used:

- The nurse assistant should unfold the shroud on the bed and the patient/resident's body should be placed on it.
- The top of the shroud should be folded down over the patient/resident's head.
- The bottom of the shroud should be folded up over the patient/resident's feet.
- The sides of the shroud should be folded over the patient/resident's body and the ends should be taped together.
- An identification tag should be attached to the shroud.

18. Hands should be properly washed, and observations should be reported and recorded at the end of the procedure.

Helpful Resources

Carlson, M. D., Morrison, R. S., Holford, T. R., & Bradley, E. H. (2007). Hospice care: What

services do patients and their families receive? *Health Services Research*, *42*(4), 1672-1690.

https://doi.org/10.1111/j.1475-6773.2006.00685.x

Condic, M. L. (2016). Determination of death: A scientific perspective on biological

integration. *Journal of Medicine and Philosophy*, *41*(3), 257-278.

https://doi.org/10.1093/jmp/jhw004

Corr, C. A. (2018). Elisabeth Kübler-Ross and the "Five stages" model in a sampling of

recent American textbooks. *OMEGA - Journal of Death and Dying*, *82*(2), 294-322.

https://doi.org/10.1177/0030222818809766

Goncalves, S. A. (2020). Death and dying and postmortem care: Essential addition to senior

skills day. *Journal of Nursing Education*, *59*(1), 60-60. https://doi.org/10.3928/01484834-

20191223-17

Goodman, A. E. (2011). Do not resuscitate (DNR) orders. *Essence of Anesthesia Practice*,

130. https://doi.org/10.1016/b978-1-4377-1720-4.00116-3

Lai, X. B., Wong, F. K., & Ching, S. S. (2018). The experience of caring for patients at the

end-of-life stage in non-palliative care settings: A qualitative study. *BMC Palliative Care*,

17(1). https://doi.org/10.1186/s12904-018-0372-7

Lewis, S. L. (2012). Palliative care in the neonatal intensive care setting. *Journal of Hospice & Palliative Nursing*, *14*(2), 149-157. https://doi.org/10.1097/njh.0b013e31823f0c71

Meyer, M. J., & Weidner, N. J. (2013). Do-not-Resuscitate orders in the OR. *Oxford Medicine Online*. https://doi.org/10.1093/med/9780199764495.003.0006

Oechsle, K. (2019). Current advances in palliative & hospice care: Problems and needs of relatives and family caregivers during palliative and hospice care—An overview of current literature. *Medical Sciences*, *7*(3), 43. https://doi.org/10.3390/medsci7030043

Pastan, L., & L. Beaman, S. (2018). The five stages of grief. *Grief and the Healing Arts*, 2-17. https://doi.org/10.4324/9781315231594-2

Patient rights at the end of life. (2020). *Professional Case Management*, *25*(2), E7-E8. https://doi.org/10.1097/ncm.0000000000000428

Peace, S., & Katz, J. (2003). End of life in care homes. *End of Life in Care Homes: A Palliative Care Approach*, 195-200. https://doi.org/10.1093/acprof:oso/9780198510710.003.0012

Stroebe, M., Schut, H., & Boerner, K. (2017). Cautioning health-care professionals. *OMEGA - Journal of Death and Dying*, *74*(4), 455-473. https://doi.org/10.1177/0030222817691870

Williams, R. S. (2016). Managing bodies, managing persons: Postmortem care and the role of the nurse. *The New Bioethics*, *22*(2), 133-147. https://doi.org/10.1080/20502877.2016.1194660

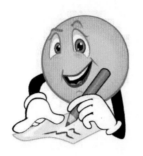

Chapter Seventeen:

Patient/Resident Abuse

Outline

I: Elder Abuse and Types of Elder Abuse

II: Issues Related to Elder Abuse

III: The Nurse Assistant Role in Recognizing and Preventing Elder Abuse

IV: The Nurse Assistant Role in Reporting Abuse and Neglect

What is an abuse?

Abuse is the wilful infliction of harm, injury, unreasonable confinement, intimidation, or punishment on another that results in physical harm, pain, or mental anguish. An individual can commit abuse by actively doing something to another individual (for example, by verbally tormenting, hitting the individual, or threatening the individual). Failing to provide proper care for someone who is dependent on others for that care is also a kind of abuse. Abuse can take multiple different forms.

Abuse can occur to anyone, and anyone can be an abuser. Individuals who depend on others for routine care, such as children and the elderly, are at the greatest risk for being abused. Caregivers can be at great risk for committing abuse when the stress of providing proper care becomes overwhelming. Even professionals like nurse assistants may experience on-the-job stress that can lead to abuse. Abuse is never an acceptable behavior, and behaving like an abusive manner can lead to the end of the one's career in health care.

Abuse is a crime that can occur at home or in a health care agency. All patients/residents must be protected from abuse. This includes patients/residents in a coma. The abuser is usually a caregiver or family member or caregiver. The abuser can be a neighbor, friend, landlord, or other person. Both women and men are abusers. Both women and men can be abused. All patients and residents, regardless of gender and age, are vulnerable. Older people and children are at risk for abuse.

Elder Abuse and Types of Elder Abuse

Older adults, especially those who have multiple different health problems and depend on others for care, are particularly vulnerable to being abused. This is known as elder abuse, and it can occur in different forms. An older adult who is being abused is often hesitant to report abuse, especially when he or she relies on the abuser for care. When caring for older patients/residents, the nurse assistant should be alert to changes in the patient/resident's behavior or appearance that might indicate that abuse is occurring.

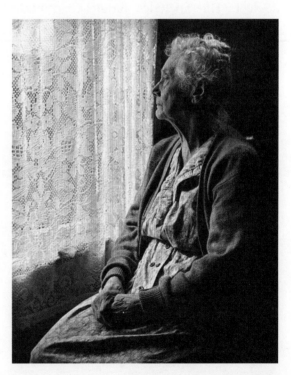

Elder abuse can occur in following forms:

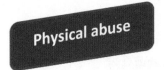

Physical abuse involves inflicting, or threatening to inflict, injury or physical pain. Slapping, hitting, grabbing, pinching, kicking, hair-pulling, or beating are examples of physical abuse. It also includes corporal punishment (punishment inflicted directly on the body) such as lashing, beatings, and whippings. Depriving the older adults of a basic need is also physical abuse.

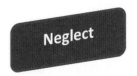

Failure to provide an older adult with the services or goods to avoid physical harm, mental illness, or mental anguish is called neglect. This includes failure to provide clinical care or treatment, clothing, food, shelter, hygiene, or other needs.

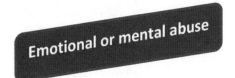

This involves inflicting mental pain, distress, or anguish through nonverbal or verbal acts. Harassment, ridicule, humiliation, and threats of punishment are examples. It may also include being deprived of basic needs such as food, care, clothing, a home, or a place to sleep.

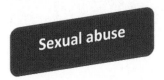

The older adult can be harassed about sex or is attacked sexually. The victim may be forced to perform sexual acts out of fear of physical harm or punishment.

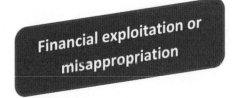

Exploitation means to use unjustly. Misappropriation means to unfairly, dishonestly, or wrongly take for one's own use. The older adult's resources (property, money, assets) can be mis-used by another person. Or the resources can be used for the other individual's profit or benefit. The victim's money can be stolen or used by another individual. It is also mis-using an individual's property. For example, children sell their father's house without his consent.

Federal and state laws recommend and require the reporting of elder abuse. If the nurse assistant suspects an elder abuse, he/she should discuss the matter and his/her observations with the nurse. The nurse assistant should provide as many details as possible. The nurse contacts members of health team as required. The nurse may also contact community agencies that investigate elder abuse. They act at once if the situation is life-threatening. Sometimes the courts or police are involved.

Type of abuse	Possible signs	Examples
Physical abuse: Deliberately harming another person	• Bruises, cuts, or other signs of injury • Burns that occur in unusual places or have unusual patterns	• Pulling the hair • Biting • Burning • Shaking • Choking • Using restraints inappropriately
Emotional abuse: Degrading or threatening another person	• Person may be fearful or withdrawn especially in the presence of the individual who is abusing	• Teasing a person in cruel way • Humiliating a person • Refusing to speaking to the person • Ignoring the person • Using restraints inappropriately
Sexual abuse: Forcing the person for sexual activities	• Scratches, bruises, or cuts around the breasts, buttocks, or genitals • Unexplained rectal or vaginal bleeding • Person may be fearful or withdrawn especially in the presence of the individual who is abusing	• Inappropriately touching a person's buttocks, breasts, or genitals • Forcing a person to involve in sexual activities • Making sexually suggestive comments • Sexually exploiting the person
Neglect: Failing to meet a dependent person's basic needs	• Signs of poor personal hygiene • Weight loss • Dehydration • Pressure sores	• Failing to provide water, food, clothing, or shelter • Failing to assist the person with personal hygiene
Financial exploitation: Misusing another person's asset or money	• Person reports that assets or money are missing • Unpaid bills	• Stealing a person's money • Using a person's cheque or credit card • Withdrawing money from the person's bank account

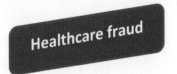

There are multiple different types of healthcare frauds, committed by healthcare providers or hospital staff. These may include billing twice for the same service, overcharging, falsifying Medicaid or Medicare claims, and charging for service that was not provided.

Issues Related to Elder Abuse

Older adults, especially those who have multiple different health problems and depend on others for care, are particularly vulnerable to being abused. This is known as elder abuse, and it can occur in different forms. An older adult who is being abused is often hesitant to report abuse, especially when he or she relies on the abuser for care. When caring for older patients/residents, the nurse assistant should be alert to changes in the patient/resident's behavior or appearance that might indicate that abuse is occurring.

Federal and state laws recommend and require the reporting of elder abuse. If the nurse assistant suspects an elder abuse, he/she should discuss the matter and his/her observations with the nurse. The nurse assistant should provide as many details as possible. The nurse contacts members of health team as required. The nurse may also contact community agencies that investigate elder abuse. They act at once if the situation is life-threatening. Sometimes the courts or police are involved.

As discussed earlier, elder abuse may occur in multiple different forms like physical abuse, verbal abuse, involuntary seclusion, financial abuse, psychological abuse (mental/emotional abuse), sexual abuse, neglect, abandonment, and healthcare fraud.

Difference between negligence and abuse

Negligence

Negligence is failure to perform what a careful and reasonable individual would be expected to perform in a given situation. Examples of negligence may include:

- A nurse assistant is usually trained in how to use the mechanical lift. While using the lift to move a patient/resident from the bed to a chair, the nurse assistant forgets or fails to lock the brakes on the lift, resulting in injury to the patient/resident.
- A nurse assistant is supporting a patient/resident to get out of bed. The patient/resident repeatedly informs the nurse assistant that he/she is feeling dizzy, but the nurse assistant encourages him/her to stand up anyway, because he/she does not have enough time to wait for the patient/resident's dizziness to pass. The patient/resident stands up and then experiences a fall.
- A nurse assistant is asked to perform a task that he/she has not been trained to perform it. Instead of refusing to do the task, the nurse assistant tries to perform the task and causes injury to the patient/resident.

Abuse

Abuse is the willful infliction of harm, injury, unreasonable confinement, intimidation, or punishment on another that results in physical harm, pain, or mental anguish. An individual can commit abuse by actively doing something to another individual (for example, by verbally tormenting, hitting the individual, or threatening the individual). Failing to provide proper care for someone who is dependent on others for that care is also a kind of abuse. Abuse can take multiple different forms.

Signs of elder abuse

- Living conditions are unclean, unsafe, or insufficient.
- The individual is not clean. His/her clothes are dirty.
- There are signs of poor fluid intake and poor nutrition.
- Assistive devices are missing or broken.
- Medical needs are not properly met.
- Conditions behind the injuries are strange or look impossible.
- New and old injuries including bruises, welts, pressure marks, fractures, scars, punctures etc.
- Complaints of itching or pain in the genital area.
- Bruising or bleeding around the buttocks, breasts, or in the genital area.
- Burns on the hands, feet, buttocks, or other parts of the body. Cigars and cigarettes cause small circle-like burns.
- Pressure sores or contractures.
- The individual seems very quiet or withdrawn.
- Unexplained withdrawal from routine activities.
- The individual seems anxious, fearful, or agitated.
- Sudden changes in alertness.
- Depression.
- Sudden changes in financial conditions.

- The individual does not seem to want to talk or answer questions.
- The individual is restrained or locked in a certain area for long periods.
- The individual cannot reach toilet facilities, water, food, and other needed items.
- Tense or strained relationships with a caregiver.
- Frequent arguments with a caregiver.
- The individual seems anxious to please the caregiver.
- Medications are not taking properly. Medications are not bought or too little or too much of the medications are taken.
- Emergency visits may be frequent.
- The individual may change doctors often.

OBRA Requirements

State rules, the Omnibus Budget Reconciliation Act of 1987 (OBRA), and accrediting agencies do not allow agencies to employ individuals who were convicted of neglect, abuse, or mistreatment. Before hiring, the agency should comprehensively check the applicant's work history. All references should be checked properly. Efforts must be carried to find out about any criminal records. The agency should also check the nursing assistant registry for determination of neglect, abuse, or mistreatment. It should also be checked for mis-using or stealing an individual's property. OBRA needs these actions if abuse is suspected within the center:

- The matter should be reported at once to:
  - The administrator

- Other representatives as required by federal and state laws
- All claims of abuse should be thoroughly investigated.
- The center should prevent further possibilities for abuse while the investigation is in progress.
- Investigation results must be reported to the center administrator within 4-5 days of the incident. They should also be reported to other representatives as required by federal and state laws.
- Corrective actions should be taken if the claim is found to be correct.

The Nurse Assistant's Role in Recognizing and Preventing Elder Abuse

The Nurse Assistant's role in recognizing elder abuse

Elder abuse can be recognized as:
- The individual is not clean. His/her clothes are dirty.
- There are signs of poor fluid intake and poor nutrition.
- New and old injuries including bruises, welts, pressure marks, fractures, scars, punctures etc.
- Complaints of itching or pain in the genital area.
- Bruising or bleeding around the buttocks, breasts, or in the genital area.
- Burns on the hands, feet, buttocks, or other parts of the body. Cigars and cigarettes cause small circle-like burns.
- Pressure sores or contractures.

- Tense or strained relationships with a caregiver.
- Frequent arguments with a caregiver.
- The individual may change doctors often.

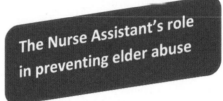

The Nurse Assistant's role in preventing elder abuse

Elder abuse can occur for a variety of different reasons, and there are no definitive factors that demonstrate all elder mistreatment. If a nurse assistant can identify risk factors, he/she will be more likely to spot and prevent abuse. Nursing assistants should be constantly working to prevent instances of abuse before they happen. Abuse is however sometimes hard to prevent, as the victim may not easily acknowledge or report the incidence of abuse. In order to prevent abuse, nursing assistant need to:

Recognize: The nurse assistant must be able to recognize the signs and symptoms of abuse and should believe that he/she can report allegations to management without suffering negative consequences.

Educate: Nursing assistants must receive proper education specific to caring for their residents that will improve knowledge, competence, and self-esteem. The education will prepare the nurse assistant to respond appropriately and immediately to difficult situations, effectively resolve different types of conflicts, and increase their empathy. By providing them proper education, burnout and stress in turn may decrease. Education should also be provided along with awareness to the individuals being cared for, as an educated person is less likely to be a victim.

Work with staff to decrease stress/burnout: Ensuring sufficient staffing in all areas of care is one of the greatest ways to decrease staff stress and burnout.

Assist with staffing ratios: Providing professional staffing and adequate supervision are key components to preventing abuse.

Patient/resident safety and abuse prevention techniques

Patient/resident safety and abuse prevention techniques may include:

- The facilities should be equipped with effective monitoring systems.
- Nursing assistants should follow institutional policies and procedures related to patient care.
- Healthcare facilities should arrange trainings on elder abuse and neglect for employees at regular basis.
- There should be proper awareness, clear guidance, and appropriate education on durable power of attorney and how it should be used.
- The facility should promote regular visits of friends, family members, social workers, and volunteers.
- There should be appropriate coordination of services and resources among different community agencies, organizations, and support groups.

How to rectify situations that could possibly lead to abuse?

1. The facility should provide appropriate services to relieve the burden of caregiving, such as respite care, education, housekeeping and meal preparation, support groups, and day care.
2. There should be proper estate planning that may include:

Living Wills: A living will is about measures that maintain or support life when death is likely. Ventilators, tube feedings, and resuscitation are examples. A living will may instruct physicians:

- Not to begin measures that prolong dying
- To remove certain measures that prolong dying
-

Durable Power of Attorney for Health Care: This advance directive provides the power to take health care decisions to another individual. That individual is often called a health care proxy. Generally this is a family member, lawyer, or friend. When an individual cannot take health care decisions, the health care proxy can do so. This advance directive does not cover financial or property matters.

"Do Not Resuscitate" Orders: "No code" or "Do not resuscitate" (DNR) orders mean that the individual will not be resuscitated. The individual is permitted to die with dignity and peace. The provider writes the DNR order after consulting with the individual and family. The provider and family take the decision if the individual is not mentally able to do so.

3. There should no signing of documents without first consulting an attorney or family member.
4. The nurse assistant should not provide personal information (e.g. credit card, social security number).
5. The nurse assistant should tear up shred credit card receipts, bank statements, or financial records before disposing of them.

Mandated reporter

A mandated reporter is an individual who is legally required to report any risk or suspicion of child abuse or neglect to the relevant authorities. These laws are made to protect children from being abused and to finish any possible abuse or neglect at the earliest possible stage.

The role of the mandated reporter

Making a comprehensive report of suspected child abuse is difficult. There are always suspicions about how the parents will react. The ideal way to reduce the difficulty of reporting is to be fully prepared for the experience and to understand the reporting process and requirements that should be triggered by making a comprehensive report.

Self-care techniques for caregivers

Here are some useful tips for handling the major challenges for caregivers:
- Caregivers may need to ensure their availability around the clock to fix meals, take care of laundry and cleaning, provide nursing care, drive to physician's appointments, and pay bills. All these tasks may increase their stress.
- Caregivers should make sure that they have proper time to rest. They should also take appropriate care of their needs.
- The Caregiver should ask a family member or friend to help out for a few hours, or on weekends, so that he/she can take some time for himself/herself.
- Caregivers should observe for signs of stress, such as loss of appetite or difficulty with sleep, impatience, lack of concentration, or memory problems. They should pay attention to changes in their mood, a loss of interest in routine activities, or an inability to accomplish usual tasks.
- They should eat a well-balanced diet and drink plenty of water every day.
- They should exercise by taking short walks daily or at least 2-4 times a week.
- They should listen to guided relaxation recordings or relaxing music.
- They should schedule short rest periods between their activities and should make it a priority to get a good night's sleep.
- They should be realistic and should not overload their daily to-do list.
- They should find a few hours several times a week for activities that they find enjoyable and meaningful.
- They should keep the lines of communication open among their loved one, family, friends, and the health care team.
- Caregivers should share their feelings with family members or other

caregivers. They may also join a support group.

The Nurse Assistant's Role in Reporting Abuse and Neglect

Anyone who knows of an elderly patient/resident being neglected or abused is obligated to notify the proper authorities. Reporting procedures may vary from state to state. In a long-term care facility, the nurse assistant who suspects abuse of a resident by either a professional caregiver or a family member should first report it to his or her supervisor. Nursing assistants should be well aware with any statements or laws that their state has in place to protect the elderly and residents of long-term care facilities. Nursing assistant should ask their supervisor for copies of relevant legal documents. Every state has a department or an office that deals with elderly abuse and neglect. There can be different names for these offices (e.g., human services, health and welfare, adult protective services, and department of aging). Nursing assistants should write down the name and number of their state agency and know where they can access it at all times.

Reporting resources

Adult Protective Services (APS)

Adult Protective Services (APS) programs promote the independence, safety, and quality-of-life for vulnerable adults who are being (or are in danger of being) abused, neglected, or financially exploited by others. Adult Protective Services (APS) is a social services program governed by state and local governments serving older adults and adults with disabilities who require support because of abuse, neglect, or financial exploitation. In all states, APS is charged with responding and receiving to reports of adult maltreatment. It is working closely with a wide variety of allied professionals and clients to maximize the safety and independence of clients. Most APS programs serve both younger and older vulnerable adults.

Long-Term Care Ombudsmen

Long-term care Ombudsmen are advocates for patients/residents of nursing homes, assisted living facilities, and board and care homes. Ombudsmen provide significant information about how to find a facility and what to do to receive quality care. They are professionally trained to resolve problems.

States' Long-Term Care (LTC) Ombudsman programs generally work to resolve issues related to the health, welfare, safety, and rights of individuals who live in LTC facilities, such as nursing homes, assisted living facilities, board and care homes, and other residential care communities. Ombudsman programs encourage policies regarding consumer protections to improve long-term supports and services at the local, facility, state, and national levels.

Eldercare Locator

The Eldercare Locator is the primary step to finding useful resources for older adults in any U.S. community. It is a free national service regulated by the Administration on

Aging to provide an instant connection to beneficial resources that enable older adults living independently in their communities. It also offers appropriate support for caregivers. The Eldercare Locator is governed by The National Association of Area Agencies on Aging to find useful resources for older adults in any U.S. community.

National Center on Elder Abuse (NCEA)

National Center on Elder Abuse (NCEA) provides the latest and updated information regarding research, news, best practices, training, and resources on elder abuse, neglect, and financial exploitation to professionals and general public. It disseminates relevant information to professionals and public, and provides technical training and support to states and to community-based organizations.

The NCEA was established by the U.S. Administration on Aging in 1988 as a national elder abuse resource center. After amendments made to Title II of the Older American Act in 1992, the NCEA was granted a permanent home at Administration on Aging.

Helpful Resources

Browne, A. (2011). Advance directives and living wills. *The Picture of Health*, 385-391. https://doi.org/10.1093/acprof:osobl/9780199735365.003.0065

Cook, I., Kirkup, A. L., Langham, L. J., Malik, M. A., Marlow, G., & Sammy, I. (2017). End of life care and do not resuscitate orders: How much does age influence decision making? A systematic review and meta-analysis. *Gerontology and Geriatric Medicine, 3,* 233372141771342. https://doi.org/10.1177/2333721417713422

Elder abuse in long-term care facilities. (2016). *Elder Abuse and Nursing.* https://doi.org/10.1891/9780826131539.0004

Friedman, L. S., Avila, S., Liu, E., Dixon, K., Patch, O., Partida, R., Zielke, H., Giloth, B., Friedman, D., Moorman, L., & Meltzer, W. (2017). Using clinical signs of neglect to identify elder neglect cases. *Journal of Elder Abuse & Neglect, 29*(4), 270-287. https://doi.org/10.1080/08946566.2017.1352551

Glendenning, F. (1999). Elder abuse and neglect in residential settings: The need for inclusiveness in elder abuse research. *Journal of Elder Abuse & Neglect, 10*(1-2), 1-11. https://doi.org/10.1300/j084v10n01_01

Goergen, T. (2001). Stress, conflict, elder abuse and neglect in German nursing homes: A pilot study among professional caregivers. *Journal of Elder Abuse & Neglect, 13*(1), 1-26. https://doi.org/10.1300/j084v13n01_01

Harris, D. K., & Benson, M. L. (2000). Theft in nursing homes: An overlooked form of elder abuse. *Journal of Elder Abuse & Neglect*, *11*(3), 73-90. https://doi.org/10.1300/j084v11n03_05

Kuwahara, R. T. (2001). More on living wills, death, and dying. *Western Journal of Medicine*, *175*(1), 18-18. https://doi.org/10.1136/ewjm.175.1.18

Myhre, J., Saga, S., Malmedal, W., Ostaszkiewicz, J., & Nakrem, S. (2020). Elder abuse and neglect: An overlooked patient safety issue. A focus group study of nursing home leaders' perceptions of elder abuse and neglect. *BMC Health Services Research*, *20*(1). https://doi.org/10.1186/s12913-020-5047-4

Phelan, A. (2015). Protecting care home residents from mistreatment and abuse: On the need for policy. *Risk Management and Healthcare Policy*, 215. https://doi.org/10.2147/rmhp.s70191

Pillemer, K., Burnes, D., Riffin, C., & Lachs, M. S. (2016). Elder abuse: Global situation, risk factors, and prevention strategies. *The Gerontologist*, *56*(Suppl 2), S194-S205. https://doi.org/10.1093/geront/gnw004

Post, L., Page, C., Conner, T., Prokhorov, A., Yu Fang, & Biroscak, B. J. (2010). Elder abuse in long-term care: Types, patterns, and risk factors. *Research on Aging*, *32*(3), 323-348. https://doi.org/10.1177/0164027509357705

Wang, X. M., Brisbin, S., Loo, T., & Straus, S. (2015). Elder abuse: An approach to identification, assessment and intervention. *Canadian Medical Association Journal, 187*(8), 575-581. https://doi.org/10.1503/cmaj.141329